Infantile Anterior Segment Disorders

Ilse Broekaert · Francesco Buonfiglio ·
Adrian Gericke · Ken K. Nischal ·
Sarah Zwingelberg

Infantile Anterior Segment Disorders

Springer

Ilse Broekaert
Department of Paediatrics
Faculty of Medicine and University
Hospital Cologne
University of Cologne
Cologne, Germany

Adrian Gericke
Department of Ophthalmology
University Hospital Mainz
Mainz, Rheinland-Pfalz, Germany

Sarah Zwingelberg
Department of Ophthalmology
University Hospital of Cologne
Köln, Nordrhein-Westfalen, Germany

Francesco Buonfiglio
Department of Ophthalmology
Johannes Gutenberg University Mainz
Mainz, Rheinland-Pfalz, Germany

Ken K. Nischal
Division of Pediatric Ophthalmology
Children's Hospital of Pittsburgh
Pittsburgh, PA, USA

ISBN 978-3-031-68557-6 ISBN 978-3-031-68558-3 (eBook)
https://doi.org/10.1007/978-3-031-68558-3

This Springer imprint is published by the registered company Springer Nature Switzerland AG
The registered company address is: Gewerbestrasse 11, 6330 Cham, Switzerland

What You Will Find in This Book

- Introduction to target-oriented anamnesis history, clinical exam and diagnostics in infantile anterior segment disorders
- A succinct, comprehensive description of the most important clinical scenarios in infantile anterior segment disorders and their differential diagnoses with illustrations.
- Up-to-date and scientifically reviewed therapy options for the specific infantile anterior segment disorders.

Prologue

The present work is intended to give a condensed overview of the clinical features, diagnostic tools, molecular genetics and the current treatment options of infantile anterior segment disorders.

For this purpose, a literature search was performed on "Pubmed". In addition, this book presents own clinical multicenter data of the University Hospital of Cologne of the Department of Ophthalmology and the Department of Pediatric Diseases, the Department of Ophthalmology of the Children's Hospital of Pittsburgh and the University Hospital of Mainz of the Department of Ophthalmology in order to give you an optimal, scientifically up-to-date and clinically relevant insight into the exciting subject of infantile anterior segment disorders.

Contents

Chapter 1
Anatomy, Physiology and Embryology

Ilse Broekaert

Abstract The anterior segment of the eye consists of the cornea, the iris, the lens and the aqueous humor. It is a complex sensory organ allowing to process visual stimuli from our surroundings. The development of the eye involves a series of cascading cellular events, orchestrated by molecular signals that activate and deactivate genetic programs. There are an increasing number of genetic mutations causing disorders of the anterior segment of the eye. For ophthalmologists, establishing a strong understanding of ocular embryology is critical to recognize and manage congenital eye disorders, comprehending the mechanisms of ocular diseases, and ultimately contributing to the development of innovative treatments.

Keywords Anatomy · Physiology · Embryology · Anterior segment of the eye · Genetic mutation

1.1 Anatomy and Physiology of the Anterior Segment of the Eye

The anterior segment of the eye consists of the cornea, the iris, the lens and the aqueous humor, which provides nutrients to the avascular cornea and lens (Fig. 1.1).

Light is directed into the eye by passing through the transparent dome-shaped front section known as the **cornea** (Fig. 1.2). Positioned behind the cornea is the aqueous humor, a fluid-filled space within the eye that is consistently produced. In order to maintain a steady eye pressure, the aqueous humor is drained from the eye via the drainage angle. Moving beyond the anterior chamber, we encounter the iris, housing muscles responsible for the constriction (sphincter pupillae) and dilation (dilator pupillae) of the pupil.

Its dynamic function regulates the amount of light entering the posterior part of the eye. Directly posterior to the pupil lies the lens, which adjusts its shape to focus light toward the back of the eye. The lens is suspended from the eye wall by delicate fibers called zonules. The lens is surrounded by the lens capsule.

I. Broekaert et al., *Infantile Anterior Segment Disorders*,
https://doi.org/10.1007/978-3-031-68558-3_1

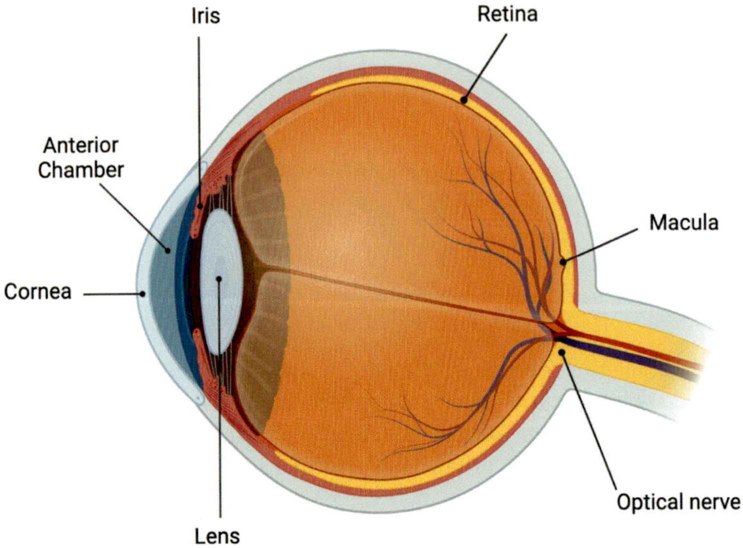

Fig. 1.1 Schematic lateral view of the eye. Created by Sarah Zwingelberg with Biorender.com

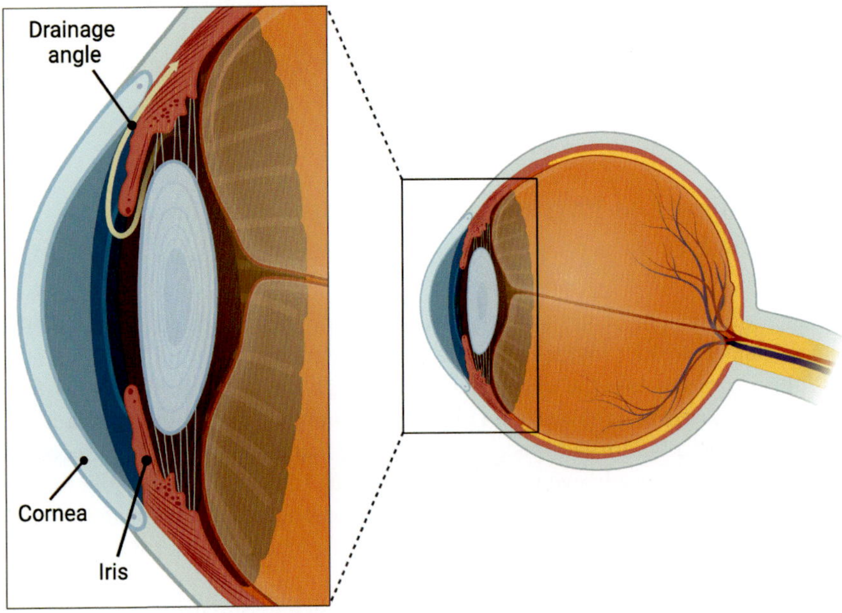

Fig. 1.2 Schematic lateral view of the anterior segment of the eye. Created by Sarah Zwingelberg with Biorender.com

By helping to focus light as it enters the eye, the cornea and the lens both play important roles in ensuring clear vision. The cornea contributes 70% of the eye's focusing power, while the lens provides the remaining 30%.

1.2 Embryology of the Anterior Segment of the Eye

The development of the eye is complex involving a series of cascading cellular events, orchestrated by a series of molecular signals that activate and deactivate genetic programs. For ophthalmologists, establishing a strong understanding of ocular embryology is critical to recognize and manage congenital eye disorders, comprehending the mechanisms of ocular diseases, and ultimately contributing to the development of innovative treatments.

In the early stages of embryonic development, the eye undergoes gastrulation, wherein the blastula transforms into a gastrula—a three-layered structure comprising the endoderm, mesoderm, and ectoderm layers. By the third week of development, these three layers organize into a flat disc-like structure known as the trilaminar disc.

Soon after gastrulation, the embryo undergoes neurulation (Fig. 1.3). During neurulation, a sheet of cells referred to as the neural plate folds on itself to form the neural tube.

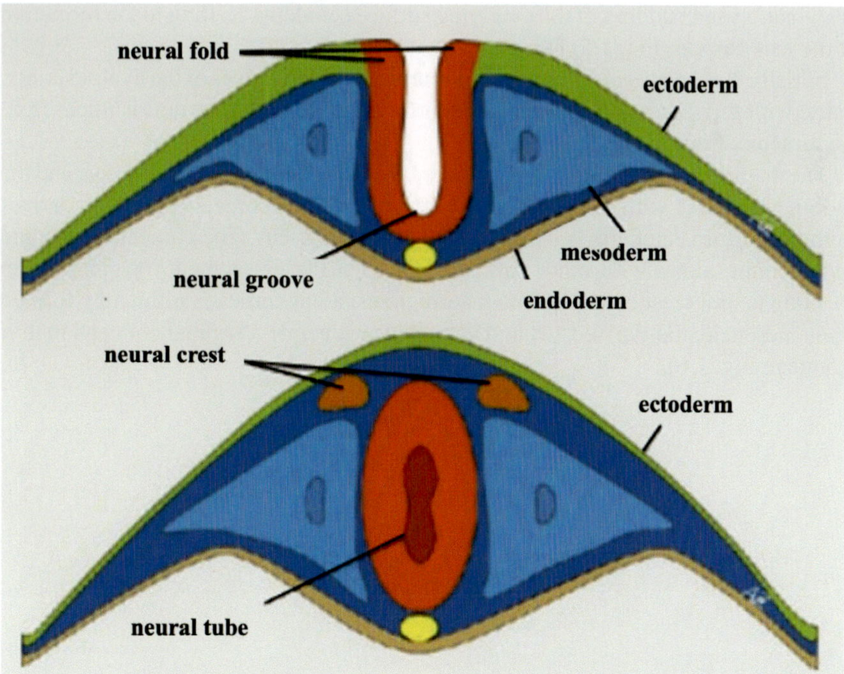

Fig. 1.3 Schematic view of the neurulation process with formation of the neural tube

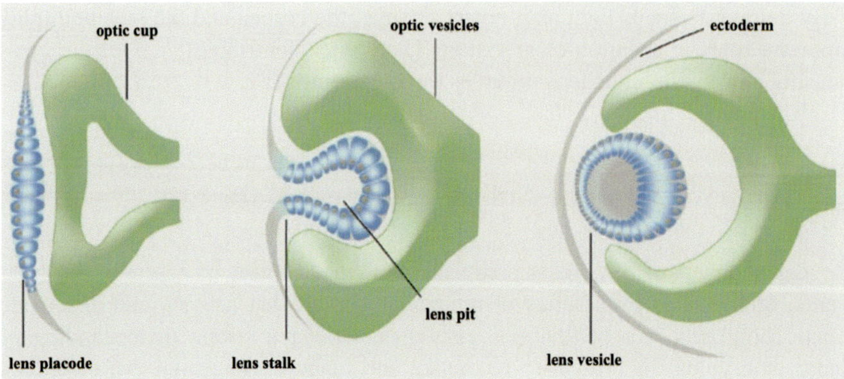

Fig. 1.4 Schematic view of the evagination of the optic vesicle and the formation of the optic stalk

At day 23 of gestation, the optic pits appear on the neural tube, which develop into the optic vesicles on day 25 (Fig. 1.4). As the optic vesicles extend outward toward the surface ectoderm, the proximal portion of the vesicle constricts to form the optic stalk, which forms the future optic nerve.

The distal portion invaginates to form the optic cup forming the future retina, iris, and ciliary body (Fig. 1.5).

The formation of the **lens** commences with the optic vesicle inducing inward invagination and budding of the overlying surface ectoderm, leading to the formation of the lens vesicle (Fig. 1.5) [1].

Initially, the developing lens acquires nutrition via derivatives of the hyaloid artery. Later, with the regression of the hyaloid artery, the lens receives nourishment from the **aqueous humor**.

The mature **cornea** is composed of three layers: the epithelium, the stroma, and the endothelium, each with distinct embryologic origins. The corneal epithelium derives from the surface ectoderm proximal to the developing lens. The corneal stroma and endothelium, along with other structures of the anterior segment, originate from invading neural crest cells [2]. The mature, transparent cornea is ultimately formed when mesenchymal-derived stromal keratocytes generate a stromal collagen matrix (compare Fig. 1.6).

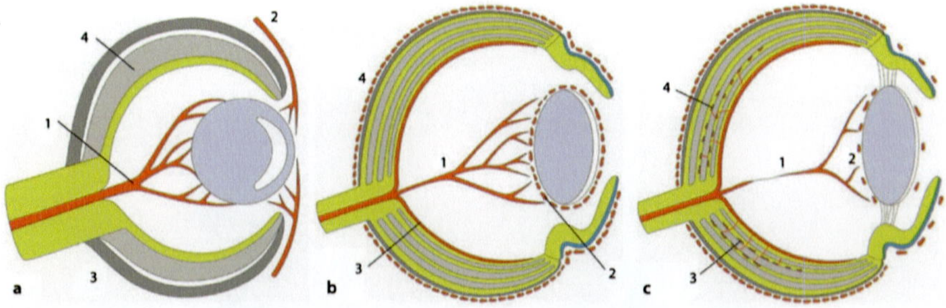

Fig. 1.5 Schematic view of the formation of the optic cup, lens vesicle and the vascular development of the eye through the interaction of the optic vesicle and the overlying surface ectoderm. During the 6th week, the interior of the eye is predominantly supplied by the hyaloid artery (1), which extends into the eye through the optic cup fissure towards the embryonic lens primordium. Vessels from the long posterior ciliary arteries (2) extend from the anterior rim of the optic cup to the iris primordium and the anterior surface of the lens, forming the anterior pupillary membrane, where their capillaries communicate with those from the hyaloid artery. 3 Outer optic cup layer. 4 Inner optic cup layer. b By the 20th week, a dense capillary network, the tunica vasculosa lentis (2), has formed around the lens. Concurrently, as the retina enlarges, a vascular network develops on the inner retina, giving rise to the inner vascular plexus (3) by the 20th week. Similarly, to supply the retinal pigment epithelium and outer retina, a dense capillary network, the choriocapillaris (4), has developed immediately beneath the retinal pigment epithelium. c By the 34th week, a significant portion of the capillaries of the tunica vasculosa lentis (2) have regressed. There are also clear signs of regression of the hyaloid artery (1), which begins in the area of the vitreous body and progresses towards the lens and the optic disc during further development. At the posterior pole, the intermediate (3) and deep (4) intraretinal vascular plexuses have already formed. This process of retinal vascularization continues centrifugally toward the ora serrata and is typically completed only after birth

The **iris** and the ciliary body are product of the anterior rim of the optic cup (compare Fig. 1.6). Additionally, neural crest cells contribute to the production of the iris stroma, and the presence of melanocytes determines the color of the iris.

The inner and outer layers of the anterior rim, induced by surrounding mesenchymal development, give rise to the posterior and anterior portions of the iris epithelium, respectively [3]. The intrinsic muscles of the iris, namely the sphincter pupillae and dilator pupillae, originate from the surrounding neuroectoderm. In contrast, the ciliary muscle, responsible for changing the shape of the mature lens, is derived from invading neural crest cells [4].

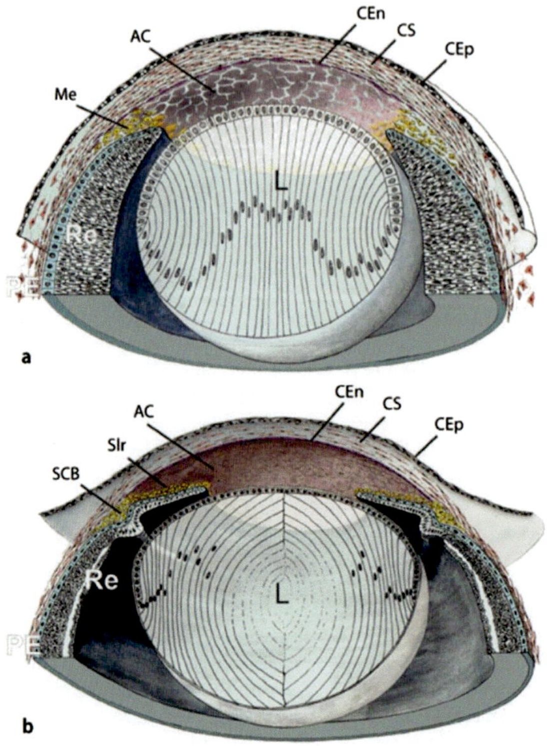

Fig. 1.6 Schematic representation of the development of the anterior segment of the mammalian eye. a The cells of the corneal primordium, adjacent to the lens, progressively flatten, form apicolateral cell contacts, and eventually differentiate into the corneal endothelium (CEn). At the end of this process, the principal layers of the cornea have formed, with the corneal epithelium (CEp) arising from the superficial ectoderm and the keratocytes of the corneal stroma from the mesenchymal cells between the corneal epithelium and endothelium. Immediately after the differentiation of the corneal endothelium, the lens (L) separates from the corneal primordium, creating a fluid-filled space, the primitive anterior chamber (AC), between the two structures. Concurrently, there is further migration of neural crest cells, now reaching the angle between the corneal primordium and the anterior rim of the optic cup. b The anterior rim of the optic cup elongates to form the iris and ciliary body. Cells in the chamber angle continue migrating anteriorly to form the stroma of the iris (SIr) and ciliary body (SCB)

1.3 Genes Associated with Ocular Embryology

Several genes play crucial roles in the embryonic development of the eye (Table 1.1).

Table 1.1 Notable genes implicated in ocular embryology

Gene	Genetic function	Reference
PAX6	"Master" gene in the development of the eye; mutations are associated with coloboma, microphthalmia, and Peter's anomaly	[5]
SSH	Responsible for the division of the eye field into two globes; mutations are associated with cyclopia	
PAX2	Essential for optic stalk formation and the closure of the retinal fissures	[6]
Rx	Essential for optic vesicle evagination and PAX6 expression, may also play a role in retinal differentiation and proliferation [4]	
BMP4	Induces the surface ectoderm that overlies the optic vesicle to form a lens placode	
Nrl	Important regulator of rod photoreceptor development	

References

1. Fuhrmann S. Eye morphogenesis and patterning of the optic vesicle. Curr Top Dev Biol. 2010;93:61–84.
2. Creuzet S, Vincent C, Couly G. Neural crest derivatives in ocular and periocular structures. Int J Dev Biol. 2005;49(2–3):161–71.
3. Davis-Silberman N, Ashery-Padan R. Iris development in vertebrates; genetic and molecular considerations. Brain Res. 2008;1192:17–28.
4. Zhao S, Chen Q, Hung FC, Overbeek PA. BMP signaling is required for development of the ciliary body. Development. 2002;129(19):4435–42.
5. Zagozewski JL, Zhang Q, Eisenstat DD. Genetic regulation of vertebrate eye development. Clin Genet. 2014;86(5):453–60.
6. Torres M, Gomez-Pardo E, Gruss P. Pax2 contributes to inner ear patterning and optic nerve trajectory. Development. 1996;122(11):3381–91.

Chapter 2
Childhood Glaucoma

Francesco Buonfiglio and Adrian Gericke

Abstract Childhood glaucoma stands as a prominent cause of of blindness among children, contributing to more than 18% of irreversible visual impairment in infants globally. This condition holds a heightened level of significance compared to adult glaucoma due to its potential to inflict severe damage on the developing visual systems, leading to impactful changes such as corneal enlargement, amblyopia, and myopia. Despite being acknowledged as a rare ailment, the aftermath of childhood glaucoma raises considerable societal concerns on a global scale, affecting both the quality of life for patients and imposing substantial costs on healthcare systems. Given the profound implications for public health and affected individuals, an up-to-date and comprehensive exploration of childhood glaucoma becomes imperative within the scientific community. Within this framework, this chapter aims to present a detailed overview of the current understanding of clinics, diagnostics, genetics, and pathophysiology associated with childhood glaucoma. Furthermore, we provide a concise summary of the prevailing conservative and surgical treatment options essential for managing this incapacitating disorder.

Keywords Blindness · Childhood glaucoma · Diagnosis · Pathophysiology · Therapy

2.1 Introduction

The term "glaucoma" encompasses a range of ocular diseases characterized by progressive optic nerve atrophy and early detectable visual field loss, often associated with elevated intraocular pressure (IOP) [1, 2]. Globally, it stands as the second leading cause of irreversible visual impairment [3, 4]. Childhood glaucoma, also referred to as pediatric glaucoma, is a distinct subtype occurring exclusively in childhood, defined by national criteria (<18 years of age in the US or $\leq$ 16 years of age in Europe, UK, UNICEF). It is invariably secondary to elevated IOP, encompassing a heterogeneous spectrum of congenital and acquired disorders [5]. The damage to ocular structures depends on the duration and severity of uncontrolled elevated IOP.

I. Broekaert et al., *Infantile Anterior Segment Disorders*,
https://doi.org/10.1007/978-3-031-68558-3_2

Left untreated, this condition leads to injuries culminating in structural and functional impairment of the optic nerve, progressively causing irreversible vision loss [5].

The incidence rates and prevalence of childhood glaucoma vary widely by country [6–10]. For example, in a US county, the estimated incidence of childhood glaucoma is around 2.29 per 100,000 individuals under the age of 20 (or 1:43,575), with traumatic and surgical etiologies being the most common subtypes. In the UK, an epidemiological investigation found an annual incidence of congenital primary form at around 1:18,500 live births [11, 12]. Overall, in America, Australia, and Europe, childhood glaucoma has been reported to occur at rates ranging from 1:10,000 to 38,000 live births, categorizing it as a rare disease [6, 11, 13–16]. However, higher prevalence rates are observed in specific populations, such as in Saudi Arabians (1:3000), Indians (1:3300), and Slovakian gypsies (1:1250) [13, 17–19].

Despite being recognized as rare, childhood glaucoma is a major cause of blindness in children, contributing to over 18% of irreversible visual loss in infants globally [20–25]. Consequently, the economic burden is substantial and significantly relevant for global public health systems.

A cost-of-illness study in the US by Liu et al. revealed an average annual cost of care for childhood glaucoma of $21,441.61 per affected individual, corresponding to a 1100% increase over adult glaucoma costs and an 800% increase in pediatric patient healthcare costs. The study highlighted that the annual costs are generally higher in the first year, averaging $46,293.62 per patient [26].

These findings underscore that, apart from visual field loss occurring in adult glaucoma, childhood glaucoma can lead to more severe injuries on the developing visual systems, resulting in significant changes such as buphthalmia, corneal aberrant enlargement, amblyopia, and myopia [5, 6]. However, due to its rarity and initial subtle clinical manifestations, childhood glaucoma is often misdiagnosed or diagnosed late, leading to delayed treatment initiation [12, 27, 28].

Therefore, a profound understanding of the clinics and diagnostics of childhood glaucoma is crucial to enhance the chances of prompt management, vital for preventing progression to blindness and limiting the devastating consequences in children, thereby averting high costs for healthcare systems worldwide. This chapter aims to provide an up-to-date and comprehensive overview of the diagnostics, clinics, genetics, and pathophysiology of childhood glaucoma. Additionally, we present major existing conservative and surgical approaches to treat this disabling condition.

2.2 General Aspects in Childhood Glaucoma

2.2.1 Definition of Childhood Glaucoma and Childhood Glaucoma Suspect

During the 9th World Glaucoma Association meeting in Vancouver, Canada, in 2013, a significant milestone was achieved by international experts and leading researchers in the field. They introduced the Childhood Glaucoma Research Network (CGRN) classification system, a groundbreaking international consensus guide specifically dedicated to childhood glaucoma [5]. This classification system focused on clinics and utilized standardized outcome criteria with the aim of providing tangible benefits to both clinical practice and research related to this group of diseases [5, 6]. The CGRN definition of childhood glaucoma underscores the clinical importance of five key criteria: intraocular pressure (IOP) levels, optic disc configuration, perimetric findings, the presence of myopia, and corneal changes. These criteria and their corresponding signs are succinctly summarized in Table 2.1. Notably, the diagnosis of childhood glaucoma necessitates the presence of at least two or more of these signs, ensuring a comprehensive and robust assessment [5, 6, 29].

Notably, the CGRN classification system extends its applicability to the assessment of individuals considered as glaucoma suspects, where the diagnosis of childhood glaucoma is hypothesized but not definitively demonstrated.

Table 2.2 furnishes a comprehensive overview of the criteria for identifying glaucoma suspects, along with their corresponding signs. Establishing the diagnosis of a childhood glaucoma suspect entails the presence of at least one or more of these signs, ensuring a nuanced evaluation [5].

Table 2.1 Definition of childhood glaucoma according to the criteria of the childhood glaucoma research network (CGRN) classification system [5]

Clinical criteria	IOP	Optic disc	Perimetry	Myopia	Corneal findings
Signs or Findings	> 21 mmHg	• Progressive increase in cup-disc ratio • Cup disc asymmetry of > 0.2 when the optic discs are of similar size • focal rim narrowing	Detectable visual field defects, consistent with glaucoma, in absence of other possible etiopathogenetic drivers	Presence of myopic shift or progressive myopia combined with enhanced ocular dimensions, out of keeping with normal growth	• Presence of corneal edema • corneal diameter: • ≥ 11 mm in neonates • > 12 mm in child < 1y • > 13 mm any age • Presence of Haab striae

Table 2.2 Definition of childhood glaucoma suspect according to the criteria of the CGRN classification system [5]

Clinical criteria	IOP	Optic disc	Perimetry	Corneal findings
Signs or findings	> 21 mmHg on two separate occasions	Suspicious optic disc configuration, possibly suggesting glaucoma	Suspicious visual field defects, possibly suggesting glaucoma	In a context of normal IOP: • Increased corneal diameter • Increased axial length

The significance of establishing a standardized definition for childhood glaucoma becomes evident in its potential to facilitate prompt intervention upon confirmed diagnosis or, in the case of glaucoma suspects, enable continuous monitoring for a timely diagnosis and treatment. The definitions put forth by the CGRN aim to address challenges related to misdiagnosis or delayed diagnosis, which frequently pose substantial hurdles in clinical practice.

Within the realms of research and clinical trials focusing on childhood glaucoma, the CGRN classification system's definitions have proven invaluable, offering global researchers a framework for evaluating diagnoses of childhood glaucoma or glaucoma suspects [29]. Numerous studies have embraced these definitions and outcomes, utilizing the CGRN classification system to reevaluate diagnoses or suspects in trials and epidemiological investigations [30–35].

Noteworthy is a recent systematic review by Sarohia and colleagues, which scrutinized outcome measures employed in randomized controlled trials for childhood glaucoma. The review revealed a heterogeneous array of measurements, with IOP being the most frequently studied primary outcome [36]. Based on these findings, the authors advocate for a new consensus in childhood glaucoma studies, as, apart from IOP, the remaining outcomes are inconsistently utilized [36].

2.2.2 Classification and General Epidemiology of Childhood Glaucoma

The CGRN classification system has systematically categorized childhood glaucoma into two overarching subgroups [5]:

1. Primary Forms: Intricately linked to specific genetic backgrounds and not associated with other pathological conditions, this category includes:
    (a) Primary Congenital Glaucoma (PCG)
    (b) Open Angle Juvenile Glaucoma (JOAG)
2. Secondary Forms: Associated with related conditions and further subdivided into:
    (a) Glaucoma associated with non-acquired ocular anomalies
    (b) Glaucoma associated with non-acquired systemic anomalies
    (c) Glaucoma associated with acquired conditions
    (d) Glaucoma following cataract surgery

For a detailed overview of each subcategory, as outlined in the CGRN guidelines, refer to Table 2.3, which succinctly summarizes the main characteristics [5].

Table 2.3 Overview on the different categories and subcategories of childhood glaucoma according to the CGRN classification system [5]

	Categories	General aspects and Subcategories according to the CGRN
Primary forms	Primary congenital glaucoma	• Isolated angle anomalies (± mild congenital iris anomalies); • Meets glaucoma definition, usually with ocular enlargement; • Subcategories based on age of onset 1. Neonatal or newborn onset (0–1 month); 2. Infantile onset (> 1–24 months); 3. Late onset or late-recognized (> 2 years); – Cases with normal IOP and optic discs but typical signs of PCG which do not show signs of progression may be indicated as spontaneously arrested PCG
	Juvenile open angle glaucoma	• Meets glaucoma definition with no ocular enlargement; • No congenital ocular anomalies or syndromes; • Open angle (normal appearance);
Secondary forms	Associated with non-acquired ocular anomalies	• Includes conditions of predominantly ocular anomalies present at birth which may or may not be associated with systemic signs; • Common following associations are reported: – Axenfeld Rieger anomaly – Peters anomaly – Aniridia – Microphthalmos and microcornea – Ectopia Lentis
	Associated with non-acquired systemic diseases	• Conditions predominantly of systemic disease present at birth which may be associated with ocular signs • Common following associations are reported: – Phacomatoses, such as the Sturge-Weber Syndrome – Connective tissue disorders – Metabolic disorders – Chromosomal disorders, such as the Trisomy 21

(continued)

Table 2.3 (continued)

	Categories	General aspects and Subcategories according to the CGRN
	Associated with acquired conditions	• Condition not inherited or present at birth; • Common following associations are reported: – Uveitis – Trauma – Steroid-induced – Retinopathy of prematurity
	Following cataract surgery	• Meets glaucoma definition after cataract surgery is performed and is subdivided into three categories based upon cataract type: 1. Congenital idiopathic cataract 2. Congenital cataract associated with ocular anomalies/systemic disease 3. Acquired cataracts (no previous glaucoma)

Significantly, the CGRN classification system offers notable advantages owing to its relative simplicity, global applicability, and the presence of definite and unequivocal criteria [29].

From an epidemiological perspective, the various forms of childhood glaucoma exhibit substantial variability across different geographic locations. A retrospective Canadian study, encompassing 306 children with glaucoma, revealed that congenital causes were the most prevalent (approximately 38% of all cases), followed by aphakic glaucoma, accounting for around 20% of cases [16]. A comprehensive Chinese study involving 1055 patients with childhood glaucoma similarly identified congenital glaucoma as the predominant form, with cases presenting at a younger age (<2 years), while acquired forms manifested in older individuals (10–15 years of age) [37]. In contrast, a study at a tertiary referral center in the United States highlighted traumatic childhood glaucoma as the most common, followed by the congenital form [38]. A study in Germany demonstrated a higher occurrence of acquired forms (61%) compared to congenital forms (39%) [25].

In Brazil, Lopes and colleagues found a slightly higher rate of congenital forms than acquired forms (44% vs. 42%) [39]. Meanwhile, in Egypt, congenital forms were the most prevalent, followed by acquired subtypes [40].

A large international prospective multicenter study conducted by the CGRN Study Group, encompassing 441 children and 691 eyes, concluded that the most common diagnoses for children with newly diagnosed glaucoma, in order of frequency, were PCG, glaucoma after congenital idiopathic cataract surgery, and glaucoma associated with trauma [41].

Collectively, these diverse epidemiological findings underscore the complex heterogeneity of childhood glaucoma, involving variations in disease genetics and pathophysiology. Additionally, they highlight distinct incidence and/or prevalence rates of primary and secondary forms across different ages of onset. Notably, congenital presentations warrant prompt diagnosis and treatment before the age of 2, while acquired forms are typically diagnosed and managed later, between 10 and 15 years of age.

2.2.3 *Medical History and Diagnostic Considerations*

Childhood glaucoma is often characterized by a classic symptomatic triad, including.

epiphora without discharge, blepharospasm, and photophobia, primarily attributed to corneal changes [6]. Anamnesis should consider the age of onset and gestational history, with a particular emphasis on familial, syndromic, and ocular history, given the genetic associations with certain conditions [5, 6].

Early diagnosis and prompt initiation of treatment are crucial to minimize visual impairment in childhood glaucoma [5, 6]. Examination under anesthesia (EUA) or sedation may be necessary for diagnosis or surgical intervention. In cases of uncertain diagnosis or progression, appropriately timed follow-up or repeated examination under anesthesia or sedation is advisable [5, 6]. Childhood glaucoma is defined by elevated IOP and characteristic optic disc cupping. IOP measurement and gonioscopy are vital diagnostic tools. Chronic elevation in IOP can lead to pathological changes in susceptible structures like the cornea, resulting in diameter enlargement and increased axial length, leading to progressive myopia [5, 6]. Evaluation should include the investigation of Haab striae on the cornea, as it serves as an important diagnostic criterion [5].

Optic disc appearance is also crucial, as elevated IOP can cause cupping and focal rim narrowing in the optic nerve, confirmed by perimetry showing corresponding visual field deficiencies [5].

A recent Brazilian retrospective study revealed different referral reasons for children to a tertiary glaucoma clinic based on age groups [42]. In the neonatal period, corneal opacity, buphthalmia, tearing, and photophobia were common referral reasons. However, beyond the neonatal period, additional signs such as cup-to-disc ratio, IOP, and myopic shift were reported as reasons for referral [42].

2.2.3.1 Anterior Eye Segment Examinations

Intraocular pressure (IOP): Accurate measurement of IOP is crucial in the anterior eye examinations for the diagnosing childhood glaucoma. However, various factors, such as the type of tonometer, eye movements, and corneal alterations (e.g., edema and opacities), can significantly influence the measurement, potentially leading to errors in IOP assessment [5, 6]. Hence, a diagnosis of childhood glaucoma should not rely solely on IOP measurement [5]. The Goldmann applanation tonometry is widely used for IOP measurement, whereas the Perkins tonometer (Haag-Streit UK), a hand-held version of Goldmann applanation, is recommended during EUA [5]. Another commonly employed tonometer is the Tonopen™ (Reichert, Inc., NYA) [5, 6]. A notable advancement in IOP measurement for children is represented by rebound tonometry, such as the iCare™ (iCare Finland), which significantly improves IOP assessment [6]. This method allows IOP measurement without topical anesthesia, providing a reasonably accurate estimation compared to the Goldman method and reducing the need for EUA [43, 44]. Ideally, IOP assessment should be conducted in a dimly lit room with the child comfortable, not crying or squeezing, to minimize the risk of falsely elevated values [6]. Measurement can be taken in the vertical or supine position, and are generally well tolerated [45, 46]. Importantly, differences in IOP values obtained by the iCare rebound tonometer and Goldman tonometer tend to rise with increasing central corneal thickness (CCT) [47, 48]. A recent study on rebound tonometry in glaucoma and ocular hypertension patients highlighted the influence of age, CCT, and time of day on measurements, emphasizing the importance of considering these factors in IOP evaluation [49].

Central corneal thickness (CCT): The measurement of the CCT by pachymetry is a fundamental diagnostic tool in childhood glaucoma. Thinner corneas may lead to an underestimation of IOP, while thicker corneas may cause an overestimation compared to the actual value [5]. Of note, CCT varies significantly based on age and race.

A multicenter investigation by the Pediatric Eye Disease Investigator Group revealed that in normal infants, median CCT tends to increase with age from 1 to 11 years [50]. In addition, racial differences were observed, with White and Hispanic infants having thicker corneas than African American infants [50]. CCT values also differ in various forms of childhood glaucoma. For example, PCG cases displayed a mean CCT of around $543.3 \pm 66.9\ \mu m$, while secondary forms such as Sturge-Weber syndrome, aphakic glaucoma, and aniridia exhibited higher CCT values [51]. Eyes with aphakia and aniridia were found to have the thickest CCT values, while anterior segment dysgenesis and uveitis had the thinnest [52]. Infants with JOAG had thinner central corneas than normal subjects [53]. In aphakic eyes after congenital cataract surgery, thicker corneas were observed compared to eyes with congenital cataracts, suggesting a postoperative increase in CCT [54].

Importantly, elevated IOP in aphakic patients should be primarily considered in connection with optic disc appearance, corneal diameters, axial lengths, and refraction, rather than relying solely on CCT [5, 55].

Taken together, caution should be exercised when interpreting CCT values in children with glaucoma. Standard formulas for IOP-to-CCT correction may not be applicable due to the wide range of CCT values observed in infants. Instead, CCT values should be considered in the overall context of the examination, rather than relying solely on them for typical IOP adjustments [5, 52].

Corneal diameter measurement: Precise measurement of corneal diameter in infants, particularly those under the age of 3, is critical as corneal enlargement is indicative of elevated IOP [5, 6]. Physiologically, the average corneal diameter at birth ranges from 10 to 10.5 mm horizontally, showing a tendency to increase by 0.5–1.0 mm in the first year of life, ultimately reaching an adult value of 11.7 mm by the age of 7 years [6]. A corneal diameter exceeding 11 mm in neonates, or surpassing 12 mm in a child under 1 year of age, or in any age group exceeding 13 mm, may signify IOP-induced corneal damage [5, 6].

In cases of abnormal corneal diameter enlargement, it is essential to consider primary megalocornea during the differential diagnosis for childhood glaucoma. Primary megalocornea is a rare, congenital, bilateral, and typically X-linked recessive condition characterized by abnormal enlargement of the anterior eye segment, even in the absence of elevated IOP [56]. Megalocornea presents with features such as aberrant corneal enlargement (13–18 mm), reduced corneal thickness, normal endothelial cell density, and the absence of Haab striae [5]. In addition, megalocornea can be associated with other etiologies such as connective tissue disorders like Marfan syndrome or recessive LTBP2 mutations linked to a secondary form of childhood glaucoma [5].

Axial length (AL) and refraction: Axial elongation is a characteristic feature of childhood glaucoma and requires thorough investigation. Increased AL leads to secondary high axial myopia and scleral thinning [57]. AL assessment can be conducted during EUA or in a clinical setting, requiring serial measurements at 3–4 month intervals, considering the impact of growth in infants [5, 6]. Estimates by Sampaolesi indicate that, at the age of one month, the 5th and 95th percentiles of normal AL are 17.2 and 20.25 mm, respectively [58]. Recent literature emphasizes a substantial increase in AL growth during the first 10 months of life, with minimal growth after 36 months [59]. Asymmetric AL assessments compared to normal or megalocornea eyes may indicate a potential diagnosis of glaucoma [60]. An incremental increase in AL on serial measurements and asymmetry between eyes may suggest inadequate IOP control during follow-up [5], while improvements due to glaucoma treatment are reflected in reduced AL values and stabilization of the AL growth curve, aligning with the normal axial growth curve [61, 62].

Cycloplegic refraction can be performed in the clinic, or retinoscopy can be conducted during EUA [5]. Effective control of childhood glaucoma can result in myopia stabilization [5, 63]. Notably, a significant reduction in hyperopia and the presence of myopia both serve as evidence of glaucoma in children [63]. Loss of hyperopia can also suggest glaucoma in aphakic patients [63]. In addition, astigmatism at oblique axes or irregular astigmatism may occur, especially in the presence of Haab striae [5].

Gonioscopy: The development of the chamber angle progresses from birth to 2 years of age, with the gonioscopic appearance stabilizing, and the chamber angle recess becoming evident around 4 or 5 years of age [64]. In newborn eyes, the iris insertion into the angle is flat, resulting in the absence of a peripheral angle recess. Conversely, eyes with PCG exhibit a higher-than-normal iris insertion [5]. In aphakic children, the angle may be closed and present smooth peripheral anterior synechiae [5].

Gonioscopy serves the purpose of distinguishing primary from secondary glaucomas [5, 65]. Changes observed in the angle during gonioscopy may suggest Axenfeld Rieger anomaly rather than PCG, and such cases may respond less favorably to angle surgery. [5]. Additionally, extensive peripheral anterior synechiae identified through gonioscopy in uveitic glaucomas can preclude angle surgery [5].

While the described characteristics of the chamber angle are generally well detectable during gonioscopy, this diagnostic tool is recommended to be performed at least once when possible. However, visualizing the angle structures can be challenging, necessitating special techniques to enhance detectability of angle structures [65]. Novel modalities can also be employed for better visualization and gonio-photographic evidence of various angle disorders [65].

Anterior segment optical coherence tomography (OCT) and ultrasound biomicroscopy (UBM): In cases involving corneal edemas or opacities, such as those associated with Peters anomaly, anterior segment OCT and UBM prove to be invaluable, providing a clear view of intraocular structures [5]. Anterior segment OCT allows for qualitative and quantitative assessment of anterior segment structures relevant to the pathogenesis and the anatomical changes in glaucoma. It aids in follow-up, facilitating the assessment of approaches and success follow-up evaluations, facilitating the assessment of treatment approaches and success [66, 67].

Gupta et al. demonstrated that that anterior segment spectral domain (SD)-OCT can identify angle dysgenesis, characterized by abnormal tissue with a detectable hyperreflective membrane or the absence of Schlemm's canal (SC), providing in vivo evaluation of eyes with childhood glaucoma [68]. UBM scans enable visualization of a thin, stretched-out ciliary body and abnormal tissue at the iridocorneal angle, particularly in patients with PCG [69].

UBM imaging contributes additional information on anterior chamber angle dysgenesis and helps characterize the form of glaucoma, aiding in the selection of the most appropriate surgical option [70]. A clinical limitation of UBM is its requirement for the patient to be in a supine position with the use of a water bath in contact with the eye, making it suitable for assessment during EUA [5].

2.2.3.2 Posterior Eye Segment Examinations

Fundus evaluation: The optic disc configuration holds significant importance for diagnosing and tracking the progression of childhood glaucoma. In particular, documentation of the optic nerve head (ONH) is crucial for capturing initial changes in glaucomatous damage, facilitating early diagnosis and management in children [71]. Key parameters such as optic nerve size, cup-disc ratio, focal areas of rim loss, and nerve fiber layer defects should be detected, preferably with mydriasis [5]. Comparative documentation, allowing for a side-by-side analysis of the optic disc's appearance at baseline and during follow-up, is critical for evaluating both diagnosis and treatment response [5, 71].

Retinal imaging: Advancements in design and technology have led to high-resolution imaging of the pediatric retina, with the development of wide- and ultra-wide field photographs over the last decades [72]. For example, the RetCam fundus image, designed for wide-field photography, has been instrumental in glaucoma management, providing images of the optic disc and anterior chamber angle [73].

The MII (Make in India) RetCam, a smartphone-based fundus imaging system, has shown promise in low-resource areas for monitoring retinopathy of prematurity and may have potential applications in monitoring and detecting glaucoma in children [74–77].

Periocular photographs, including corneal opacity, corneal enlargement, and globe enlargement, have also proven valuable for deep learning devices, serving as promising tools for diagnosing missed childhood glaucoma cases [78]. However, despite these advancements, fundoscopy remains a fundamental diagnostic step in childhood glaucoma, enabling the detection of positive treatment responses, such as cupping reversal, commonly observed in successfully treated childhood glaucoma [5, 79].

OCT imaging: The SD-OCT facilitates assessment of the retinal fiber nerve layer (RNFL) at the optic disc, making it a crucial diagnostic tool in childhood glaucoma [80]. Macular OCT aids in evaluating the RNFL and visualizing macular configuration, particularly valuable in cases of altered ONH morphology due to high myopia or axial elongation [81, 82]. A combination of OCT imaging of both the ONH and macula is recommended for screening and diagnosing childhood glaucoma [77].

A normative database of RNFL thickness in children proves valuable in assessing disease severity or treatment response [77]. In a focused investigation, the mean retinal nerve fiber layer (RNFL) thickness was found to be approximately 93–94 μm. Additionally, the study reported a decrease in RNFL thickness of 1.9 μm for every 1 diopter increase in myopic shift and a decrease of 1.9 μm for every millimeter increase in AL [83]. As the RNFL thickness tends to diminish with myopic shift or axial length elongation, attempts have been made to establish a normative RNFL thickness with refractive errors. For example, Goh and colleagues determined a mean spherical equivalent refraction of approximately -3.20 ± 3.51 D, and a mean AL of approximatively 24.39 ± 1.72 mm, resulting in an estimated mean average RNFL thickness of 99.00 ± 11.45 μm [84].

Given the low compliance of children during routine OCT imaging, alternative methods, including handheld OCT and overhead-mounted OCT, have been developed to perform this essential examination in infants with glaucoma [85–88].

Perimetry: Conducting perimetric evaluations in children poses unique challenges, underscoring the importance of employing the shortest possible test duration [5]. Additionally, it is advisable to perform repeated assessments to confirm deficits [5]. Unlike the classic sequential progression observed in adults, visual field loss in children with glaucoma follows a distinctive pattern [89]. Studies dedicated to PCG have emphasized that arcuate scotomas are the most common defects, with cases detected at age ≤ 1 month and having a baseline IOP > 30 mm Hg tending to exhibit more substantial visual field damages [90]. In this context, the 'OPTIC' (Optimal Perimetric Testing In Children) study recommends static perimetry for children under

10 years of age, while a combined static/kinetic technique may be more appropriate for older children [91].

However, it is noteworthy that the OPTIC study did not reach a consensus on defining progressive visual field loss or on the utility of perimetry over an individual's lifetime, underscoring the imperative need for further research [92].

Table 2.4 summarizes the main anamnestic criteria, examinations, findings and diagnostic tools in childhood glaucoma.

Table 2.4 Overview on the diagnostics in childhood glaucoma

Diagnostics	Signs, findings, diagnostic tools
History and anamnesis	• Symptomatic triad: 1. Epiphora without discharge 2. Blepharospasm 3. Photophobia • Age of onset: – Congenital forms detectable in neonates – Secondary forms detectable in older children • Gestational history • Family history • Syndromic history • Ocular history
Anterior eye segment examinations	*Intraocular Pressure*: via the Goldmann Applanation Tonometry, Perkins Tonometer, Tonopen™, iCare™, iCare Pro
	Central Corneal Thickness: congenital forms present thinner corneas, while secondary forms ticker corneas. *Note*: it is not recommended to adjust the IOP estimation according to the value of the central corneal thickness
	Corneal Diameter: > 11 mm in neonates, or > 12 mm in a child < 1 year of age, or > 13 mm in any age group indicative for raised IOP-induced corneal damage
	Axial Length: values at the age of one month correspond to the 5th percentile and 95th percentile of around 17.2 and 20.25 mm, respectively. An axial elongation is typically found in childhood glaucoma
	Cycloplegic Refraction: a progressive myopia is indicative of axial elongation or it is suggestive of negative response to the therapy, while a loss of hyperopia can also be indicative of glaucoma in aphakic patients
	Gonioscopy: – iris insertion in PCG is typically higher than normal – in aphakic children, the angle can be closed, presenting anterior synechiae – in uveitic glaucomas, may be detected peripheral anterior synechiae
	Anterior Segment OCT: an angle dysgenesis in the form of abnormal tissue with detectable hyperreflective membrane or an absence of the Schlemm's canal can be identified in childhood glaucoma
	Ultrasound Biomicroscopy: visualization of a thin, stretched-out ciliary body and abnormal tissue at the iridocorneal angle, in most of patients with PCG

(continued)

Table 2.4 (continued)

Diagnostics	Signs, findings, diagnostic tools
Posterior eye segment examinations	*Fundus Evaluation*: via mydriasis – Optic nerve size – Cup-disc ratio – Focal areas of rim loss – Nerve fiber layer defects Helps to detect typical pathological findings in childhood glaucoma: – Progressive increase in cup-disc ratio – Cup disc asymmetry of > 0.2 – Focal rim narrowing
	Retinal Imaging: RetCam Fundus Image helps obtaining wide-field photographs
	OCT imaging: – SD-OCT allows the RNFL assessment of the optic disc – Macular OCT particularly valuable in case of altered morphology of the ONH due to high myopia or axial elongation
	Perimetry: a static perimetry in children < 10 years of age, and a combined static/kinetic technique in older children are suggested. *Note*: However, currently there is no agreement about defining progressive visual field loss

2.2.4 *Differential Diagnosis in Childhood Glaucoma*

According to the CGRN, several conditions should be taken into consideration in the context of the differential diagnosis in case of PCG (Table 2.5).

Two significant conditions deserving attention, particularly linked to corneal pathologies, are highlighted by the CGRN group: X-linked megalocornea and the congenital hereditary endothelial dystrophy (CHED) [5].

2.2.4.1 X-linked Megalocornea

X-linked megalocornea is an inherited eye disease characterized by congenital bilateral enlargement of the anterior eye segment, presenting a horizontal corneal diameter of ≥ 13 mm, notably in the absence of elevated IOP [5]. Additionally, characteristics described in the literature include reduced corneal thickness, a deep anterior chamber, corneal arcus, mosaic stromal corneal degeneration, atrophy of the iris stroma, miosis secondary to decreased function of the dilator muscle, iridodonesis and tremulousness, as well as subluxation or dislocation of the lens [93–96].

This genetic basis of this disorder involves mutant variants in the Chordin-like 1 gene (*CHRDL1*) [56].

The CHRDL1-encoded protein plays a crucial role in embryonic bone formation, retinal angiogenesis, neuronal differentiation, and the development of the anterior eye segment [97, 98]. A total of 21 disease-causing *CHRDL1* variants have been

Table 2.5 Overview on the differential diagnosis in childhood glaucoma according to the CGRN classification system [5]

Categories	Conditions to be considered in the differential diagnosis with PCG
Secondary glaucoma forms	Glaucoma associated with non-acquired ocular anomalies or with non-acquired systemic disease or syndrome
Alternative causes of corneal anomalies	– Corneal / ocular enlargement 1. X linked megalocornea 2. Congenital high myopia 3. Connective tissue disorders (*e.g.*, Marfan syndrome, osteogenesis imperfecta) 4. LTBP2 mutations
	– Corneal haziness 1. Obstetric trauma 2. Corneal dystrophies (*e.g.*, PPMD, CHED) 3. Metabolic disorders (*e.g.*, mucopolysaccharidoses, mucolipidoses, cystinosis) 4. Infection (*e.g.*, congenital rubella without IOP increase or other signs of glaucoma) 5. Peters anomaly / sclerocornea (without IOP increase or other signs of glaucoma)
Alternative causes of epiphora	1. Nasolacrimal duct obstruction 2. Conjunctivitis 3. Corneal abrasion/keratitis
Alternative causes of optic nerve defects	Congenital optic nerve cupping 1. Physiologic cupping of large optic nerves 2. Optic nerve hypoplasia with periventricular leukomalacia 3. Optic nerve coloboma 4. Optic nerve pit 5. Other optic nerve abnormality

identified, resulting in loss of function [99, 100]. A recent study by Dudakova et al. reported seven novel *CHRDL1* mutant variants, revealing that some heterozygous female carriers may exhibit mild corneal thinning, evolving into a keratoconus pattern in some individuals [101].

2.2.4.2 Congenital Hereditary Endothelial Dystrophy

The congenital hereditary endothelial dystrophy (CHED) is characterized by bilateral corneal opacification and results from an autosomal dominant (CHED1) or recessive (CHED2) mutation affecting the corneal endothelium [5].

The autosomal recessive form is the most common and severe [102]. Pathophysiologically, corneal opacification in CHED results from stromal edema and thickening of the Descemet's membrane due to endothelial dysfunction [103].

The CHED mutation has been identified in the *SLC4A11* gene, located on chromosome 20p13 [104]. This gene encodes a transmembrane protein, a bicarbonate transporter that counteracts the osmotic gradient, pumping fluid from the stroma into the aqueous humor (AH) [104–106]. Mutant variants of *SLC4A11* reported in CHED induce synthesis of a truncated protein incapable of reaching the cellular membrane and performing its function [107]. Consequently, stromal edema, disruption of collagen fibrils, and thickening of the Descemet's membrane occur, ultimately leading to corneal opacification. In the following chapter of congenital corneal opacities this topic will discuss be this topic in more detail.

2.2.5 *Childhood Glaucoma Flowchart*

The CGRN has developed a classification system flowchart (Fig. 2.1), useful in the clinical practice, with the purpose to facilitate and accelerate the differential diagnosis, the diagnosis and the classification in the different subcategories of childhood glaucoma [5, 29, 108].

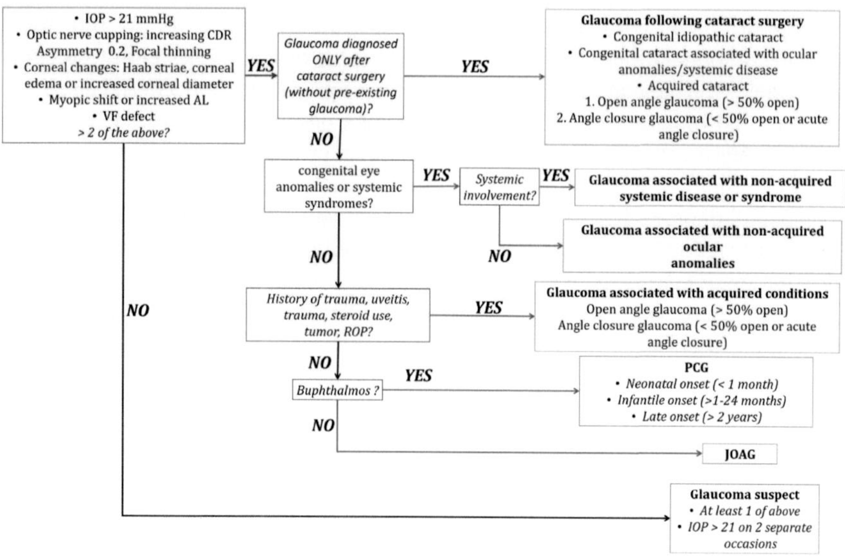

Fig. 2.1 *Childhood glaucoma flowchart according to the CGRN classification system* [5]. CDR: cup-to-disc ratio; JOAG: juvenile open-angle glaucoma; IOP: intraocular pressure; PCG: primary congenital glaucoma; ROP: retinopathy of prematurity; VF: visual field

2.3 Forms of Childhood Glaucoma

2.3.1 Primary Forms

According to a retrospective study of the CGRN conducted in 2016, PCG and JOAG account for 32% and 7.4% of all cases of childhood glaucoma, respectively, thereby representing the most prevalent group of glaucomatous disorders in infants [30].

2.3.1.1 Primary Congenital Glaucoma

Definition, epidemiology and prognosis: PCG is a rare form of glaucoma, accounting for 1–5% of all cases [109]. It manifests bilaterally in around 70% of cases, and usually the severity of involvement is asymmetrical [110–112]. Remarkably, even though rare compared to adult forms, PCG is the most common type of childhood glaucoma and a major cause of blindness in children [112–114], reaching rates of prevalence of around 32% in infants affected by glaucoma [30]. As described in Sect. 2.2, the prevalence rates of PCG are anyway very variable in dependence of geographical sites and ethnic origins [112]. In particular, western countries such as the UK and the US, present an incidence rate amounting to approximatively 1 per 10–20,000 live births [15, 115–118]. In contrast, the incidence of PCG appears higher in the Middle East, including Saudi Arabia, where consanguineous marriages are more prevalent, with an estimated incidence rate of 1 per 2500 live births [17, 118, 119]. In populations with a higher incidence, the onset of PCG tends to occur in earlier ages, with a mean age of presentation ranging by 3–4 months in Asians, Saudi Arabians, and Indians while the onset is generally described later, by 11 months of age, in Western countries [13, 118, 120]. The gender appears also to have a role in the epidemiology of PCG, showing males a slight predominance in both Western and Asian populations, and accounting for approximatively 65% of cases [13, 118, 120].

From a prognostic perspective, PCG is recognized as a sight-threatening condition, able to progress to irreversible visual loss also after many years of IOP stability [121].

An initial angle surgery is therefore usually performed within the first year of life, while critical ages for further glaucoma surgery are by 2–5 years [33]. The prompt surgical therapy in children afflicted by PGC is crucial, as these patients can achieve an acceptable visual acuity especially in cases of timely intervention and close follow-up [113].

Genetics: PCG is an autosomal recessive disorder that presents a large heterogeneity in disease-related loci and very variable levels of penetrance among diverse populations [122]. Even though the precise etiology of PCG remains to be explained, several mutant pathogenic variants of diverse genes have been discovered and examined, in view of their contribution to the etiopathogenesis of PCG. Above all, the *CYP1B1* gene located in the locus GLC3A on the chromosomal region 2p21–22, appears to be implicated in the anterior segment development and has a central role in the development of PCG [123–125]. In the current literature, the *CYP1B1* emerges as the most studied gene associated with PCG, presenting over 150 known pathogenic variants that, in the last decades, have been detected in affected individuals [122]. The *CYP1B1* encodes a homonymous protein, the cytochrome P450, family 1, subfamily B and polypeptide 1, which has the function of catalyzing the NADPH-dependent mono-oxygenation of xenobiotics and endogenous molecules [126, 127].

The *CYP1B1* gene is expressed in various tissues of the human body and of the eye, like for example the cornea, the ciliary body as well as the iris and the retina, and importantly, it may contribute in the development of the trabecular meshwork (TM) [123, 128]. In this regard, a noteworthy investigation conducted by Zao and associates on mice lacking the *CYP1B1* gene (*CYP1B1*$^{-/-}$), revealed as a consequence of the loss of function of *CYP1B1*, increased oxidative stress as well as a decreased synthesis of the protein periostin, which collectively lead to structural changings and ultimately to a dramatic dysfunction of the TM [129].

However, many other loci have been investigated in PGC, like among others the GLC3B (1p36.2–36.1), GLC3C (14q24.3), and GLC3D (14q24.2–24.3) [118, 122, 130].

Of note, in the GLC3D locus is sited the gene *LTBP2*, encoding the latent transforming growth factor (TGF)-β binding protein 2 protein, expressed in the anterior eye segment and ciliary body, and fundamental for the organization and formation extracellular matrix, possibly for its effect on TGF-β signaling and the ECM of TM [122]. In this regard, Suri et al. demonstrated in an in vitro investigation on human TM cell cultures, that *LTBP2* knockdown via siRNA, and events of oxidative stress may be responsible of apoptosis in TM through the TGFβ and the bone morphogenetic protein (BMP) signaling pathway [131].

A prior study by Inoue and coworkers showed that *LTBP2* mutants may present an abnormal domain structure, that obstruct the secretion of this protein, finally blocking the formation of microfibril bundles in ciliary zonulas [132]. Collectively, these studies have demonstrated that mutant variants of *LTBP2* represent possible causes of congenital structural abnormalities that culminate in the onset of PCG.

In addition, other genes like *MYOC* (lq24.3–q25.2), *COL1A1* (17q21.33), *FOXC1* (*F*orkhead B*ox C1*, 6p25.3), appear to possibly contribute to PCG, as their encoded proteins possess regulatory functions in the development of the anterior eye segment, and in particular of the trabecular meshwork [133]. *MYOC* encodes for the protein myocilin, expressed in TM, sclera, ciliary body and retina, which in mutant variations elicit structural changings of TM and ciliary body, blocking the flow of aqueous humor and ultimately causing an elevation of IOP [134].

FOXC1 is a member of the winged helix/forkhead family of transcription factors that mediate the craniofacial, cardiovascular and ocular development [135, 136]. It has been detected in the periocular mesenchyme cells, being critical to originate ocular structures such as the iris, cornea, and TM, and thereby pivotal in regulating the flow of the aqueous humor [122, 137, 138]. An investigation by Smith and associates on mice lacking *FOXC1* in homozygosis (*FOXC1*$^{-/-}$) and in heterozygosis (*FOXC1*$^{+/-}$) has reported anterior eye segment anomalies similar to those in humans with anterior segment dysgenesis and congenital glaucoma, like for example small or absence of SC, aberrantly developed TM and iris hypoplasia [139]. Of note, individuals affected by PCG with pathogenic *FOXC1* variants have been reported to present systemic symptomatic, associated with the Axenfeld-Rieger syndrome, like for example hearing loss, heart murmur and developmental delay [122, 140].

COL1A1 (collagen type 1 alpha 1 chain) encodes the pro-α1 chains of type I collagen, a central component of the ECM in the TM, SC and lamina cribrosa [122, 141]. Moreover, mutant variants of *COL1A1* may contribute to an impaired development of CCT, possibly in connection to PCG [142, 143].

Current literature also underscores the role of the angiopoietin 1 (*ANGTP1*) gene, sited in the chromosomal region 8q23.1 and the TEK receptor tyrosine kinase (*TEK,* tunica interna endothelial cell kinase, also known as *TIE2*) gene, located on the chromosomal region 9p21.2, as involved in the pathogenesis of PCG [122].

*ANGTP1*is a glycoprotein able to activate receptors by inducing tyrosine phosphorylation, and serving in blood vessel maturation, being required for the development of SC [144, 145]. *TEK* is a receptor tyrosine kinase, expressed in endothelial cells, and that when dysfunctional induces vascular malformations [146]. In human ocular tissues, the expression level of the TEK receptor is remarkably high in the SC endothelium [147–149]. The ANGPT/TEK pathway has been assessed to be involved in the development of SC and importantly, in the regulation of aqueous humor outflow [147, 150, 151]. Taken together, the ANGPT/TEK pathway appears to preserve the stability of SC and TM functions, while its loss of function drives to a degeneration of TM and SC, further developing into irregular canal formation, ultimately leading to IOP elevation and glaucoma [152–154]. Importantly, the current identified genes just explain the etiology in 5–50% of cases [7]. More recent studies underlined the role of other genes like for example *CPAMD8* (C3 And PZP Like Alpha-2-Macroglobulin Domain Containing 8), *PLOD2* (procollagen-lysine 2- oxoglutarate 5-dioxygenase 2), *GPATCH* (G-Patch Domain Containing 1), and *PRSS56* (Putative Serine Protease 56) in association with PCG, being however the pathogenetic events that derive from their mutations still to be deciphered [7, 155–158].

Of note, the pathogenetic variant mutations of *CYP1B1,* apart from being associated with a higher degree of postoperative haze, earlier onset disease, more severe manifestations and progression, were also described to present a significant penetrance (>90%), collectively suggesting the clinical relevance of genetic screening in predicting the disease prognosis [7, 159–163].

Pathogenesis: Considering the evidences on the genetics of PCG reported in the existing literature, a maldevelopment of the TM, along with a vascular malformation of the SC, structural changings in the ciliary body and anomalies in the ciliary zonulas, are identified to be central pathogenetic drivers of this disorder [151, 154, 164]. Collectively, an arrested maturation of the tissues deriving from the cranial neural crest cells can be recognized as pivotal pathophysiological element [6].Thick trabecular sheets tend to compact, blocking the posterior positioning of the iris which occurs during the development of the anterior eye segment, finally eliciting a more anteriorly location of the iris, that results in the typical appearance of the high insertion, characteristic of "premature" angle [112, 165].

Typical pathophysiological characteristics are also the overlap of ciliary body and TM with the iris and the reduction or complete absence of the SC [166]. As a recent study by Abdeen and coworkers demonstrated, the iris appears thinner in PCG, with a reduced thickness near the iris root, in the middle and also near the pupillary border [167]. In summary, these pathological alterations of the structures responsible of an impaired AH drainage in the anterior eye segment, elicit a chronic and aberrant elevation of IOP. Furthermore, as a consequence of the chronic elevated IOP, corneal damages occur, through edema, increased corneal diameter, Haab's striae or an enlarged axial length [168].

Figure 2.2a provides an illustration of the physiological structure of the anterior eye segment involved in the AH drainage route, while Fig. 2.2b offers a representation of the pathophysiological changings in PCG, highlighting corresponding involvement of the etiologic genetic drivers.

Clinics: PCG is normally detectable in neonates or infants, generally under the age of 6 months [112]. Apart from being classified, according to the CGRN guidelines, into neonatal PCG (<1 month), infantile PCG (>1 month to 24 months), or late-onset PCG (>24 months) [5], Gupta and coworkers recently categorized PCG, emphasizing specific parameters to be considered with the goal to assess the severity of the disease, being each parameter worth 1 point, and resulting a case "severe" in case of total score ≥ 4 [169, 170]:

- **non-severe PCG**:
  - infantile age of onset
  - corneal diameter < 13 mm
  - axial length < 24 mm
  - clear cornea or anyway identification of the corneal structures despite hazes
  - improvement of the corneal haze after IOP lowering
  - surgeries required after IOP control ≤ 2
- **severe PCG**:
  - neonatal age of onset
  - corneal diameter $\geq$ 13 mm
  - axial length $\geq$ 24 mm
  - no identification of the corneal structures due to massive hazes
  - persisting of corneal haze despite IOP lowering
  - surgeries required after IOP control > 2

Along with the classical symptomatic triad represented by epiphora without discharge, photophobia and blepharospasm, frequent sings are corneal opacification, edema, increased corneal diameter, together with an overall enlargement of the eyeball, the so termed Buphthalmos [112, 118, 122]. During gonioscopy, in cases of sufficient corneal transparency, the anterior insertion of the iris is observable, as well as the Barkan's "pseudo-membrane", thin structures covering the anterior chamber angle, called pseudo-membrane because never found in histological analysis [118, 171, 172]. In addition, a thin and hypopigmented iris stroma can be visible as well as hyperemic iris vessels, with vascular tortuosity running in the peripheral iris [112]. The AH outflow block and the consequent accumulation of AH in the anterior

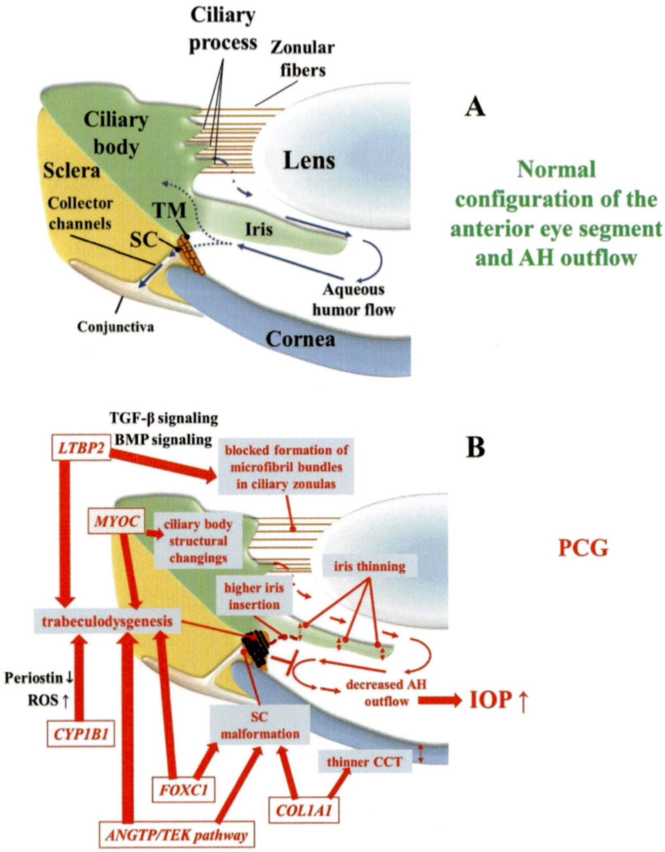

Fig. 2.2 Physiology of the anterior eye segment (**a**) and illustration of the main structural and pathophysiological changings in PCG with corresponding involved genetic mutant variants (**b**). AH: aqueous humor; ANGTP: angiopoietin; BMP: bone morphogenetic protein; CCT: central corneal thickness; COL1A1: collagen type 1 alpha 1 chain; CYP1B1: cytochrome P450, family 1, subfamily B and polypeptide 1; FOXC1: Forkhead Box C1; IOP: intraocular pressure; LTBP2: latent transforming growth factor (TGF)-β binding protein 2; MYOC: myocilin; PCG: primary congenital glaucoma; ROS: radical oxygen species; SC: Schlemm's canal; TEK: tunica interna endothelial cell kinase; TGF-β: transforming growth factor beta; TM: trabecular meshwork

chamber drives to IOP elevation and to a disruption in corneal endothelial integrity [173]. In addition, horizontal lines marking a Descemet membrane rupture, the so called Haab's striae, are generally present and can even persist after IOP reduction through treatment [174]. However, the IOP elevation apart from being responsible of such corneal damages, causes a further extension of the sclera, and importantly a mechanic compression, and thereby injuries, on the ONH.

A typical sing of elevated IOP in these circumstances is the so termed 'Bull's eye' classic clinical feature of PCG, representing elevated IOP-induced growth of the eyeball [122, 175].

2.3.1.2 Juvenile Open Angle Glaucoma

Definition, epidemiology and prognosis: JOAG is a relatively rare form of childhood glaucoma, and its first manifestations generally appear between 4–35 years of age and manifests usually bilaterally [5, 6]. JOAG presents differences with the corresponding adult form (primary open angle glaucoma) for its age of onset, apart from typically showing a significant higher level of IOP elevation, which usually reach values over 40 mmHg [176]. JOAG accounts for 0.2% of all glaucoma cases, with an increasing trend in prevalence through age, showing a predominance in males [177], and being potentially responsible for 3–4% of primary open angle glaucoma [178].

The prognosis in patients afflicted by JOAG is usually positive in cases of early diagnosis and prompt therapy initiation. However, as often occurs in childhood glaucomas, due to the asymptomatic course of the disease, the diagnosis is delayed until advanced stages establish. Reported causes of poor visual acuities are principally the progression of glaucoma, and therefore, the delay of detection of onset, or also surgery and amblyopia [179]. In a long-term follow-up study, with observation periods ranging from 2–14 years, on children affected by JOAG and treated via surgical intervention, the prognosis tends to be satisfactory but the effectiveness of the therapy decreases with the elongation of the follow-up period [180].

Genetics: JOAG presents a large genotypic and phenotypic heterogeneity [6, 181]. It is typically recognized as an autosomal dominant disorder characterized by variable penetrance and expressivity [29, 182, 183]. However, some studies also described an autosomal recessive pattern, with an association with an African ancestry [184]. According to the current literature, *MYOC* mutations are the most common genetic causes [181], with recorded relative high prevalence (around 34%) in the JOAG population compared with the *CYP1B1* mutations (accounting for 2%) [185]. The likelihood of developing glaucoma increases to approximately 50%–87% when carrying a MYOC mutant variant, with this risk escalating in tandem with advancing age of onset [6, 178, 186].

Pathogenesis: Given that MYOC mutations stand out as the most widely acknowledged etiological factors in JOAG, it is unsurprising to observe trabeculodysgenesis characterized by an immature and thickened TM. This condition leads to a compromised development of the anterior chamber angle (goniodysgenesis), ultimately resulting in an elevated IOP due to the accumulation of AH in the anterior chamber [187, 188]. Interestingly, as the age of onset increases, the developmental aberrations of the angle chamber appear to be less evident [189].

An interesting investigation on patients with JOAG revealed that approx. 25% of cases shows unilateral optic neuropathy at presentation, probably in connection with a later age of onset, which may correspond to less severe developmental anomalies of the TM and, thereby, tend to involve only one eye [190].

Figure 2.3 schematically summarizes the etiopathogenesis in JOAG and the main differences with PCG.

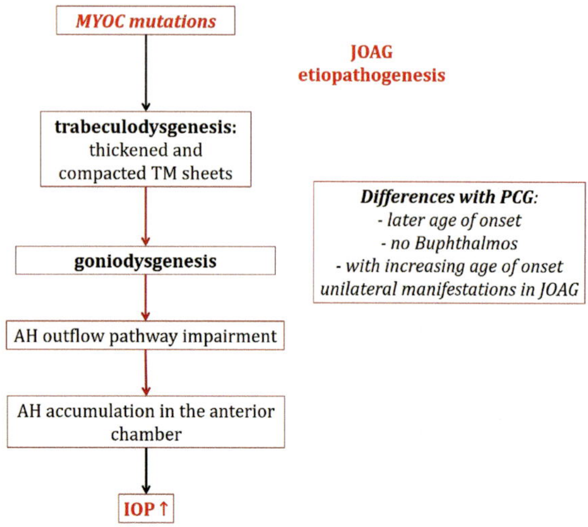

Fig. 2.3 *Scheme on the etiopathogenesis in JOAG and principal clinical differences with PCG.* AH: aqueous humor; IOP: intraocular pressure; JOAG: juvenile open angle glaucoma; MYOC: myocilin; PCG: primary congenital glaucoma; TM: trabecular meshwork

Clinics: In clinical terms, juvenile-onset open-angle glaucoma (JOAG) distinguishes itself from primary congenital glaucoma (PCG) by its later onset. Crucially, JOAG exhibits a notably distinct and less pronounced genetic influence compared to PCG. The absence of buphthalmos is a noteworthy observation in JOAG, marking a relevant aspect for the purpose of differential diagnosis [5, 6, 29].

Gonioscopy enables the observation of an anterior iris insertion or a featureless angle [181]. A recent study by Selvan and colleagues employed cluster analysis to categorize JOAG into four distinct groups, emphasizing the diverse iris characteristics discernible through gonioscopy [181]. Additionally, more than 40% of JOAG-affected eyes may exhibit hyper-reflective membranes covering the trabecular meshwork TM and/or an absent Schlemm's canal SC as visualized through anterior-segment OCT [181].

Pachymetry emerges as a crucial diagnostic tool in JOAG, as corneas in this disorder, similar to PCG, tend to exhibit thinning [191]. Fundus evaluations play a significant role in diagnostics, with JOAG patients typically displaying larger optic discs compared to individuals affected by primary open-angle glaucoma [192].

2.3.2 *Secondary Forms*

2.3.2.1 Glaucoma Associated with Non-acquired Ocular Anomalies

As per the CGRN, these conditions primarily manifest as ocular anomalies present at birth, either with or without systemic signs [5]. The 2016 CGRN study indicates that glaucoma associated with non-acquired ocular anomalies constitutes 8.2% of all cases of childhood glaucoma [30].

Examples of glaucoma linked to non-acquired ocular anomalies include congenital aniridia, Axenfeld–Rieger syndrome, Peters anomaly, congenital ectropion uveae, microphthalmia, oculodermal melanocytosis (also known as nevus of Ota), persistent fetal vasculature, posterior polymorphous dystrophy, and ectopia lentis [29]. Among these, congenital aniridia, Axenfeld–Rieger syndrome, Peters anomaly, and congenital ectropion uveae are the most extensively studied conditions. In the following sections, we delve into the genetics, pathophysiology, and specific clinical aspects of these disorders.

Glaucoma Associated with Congenital Aniridia

Definition, epidemiology and prognosis: Congenital aniridia is a developmental pan-ocular disorder characterized by variable hypoplasia of the iris, and accompanied by foveal hypoplasia, glaucoma, cataract, optic nerve hypoplasia, limbal stem cell deficiency, dry eye disease and meibomian gland dysfunction, nystagmus, and of note, a devastating keratopathy establishing through corneal vascularization and opacification [193–196]. Of note, congenital aniridia can be reported as partial or total absence of iris, but during gonioscopy an iris stump can almost always be observed [197, 198]. The prevalence of congenital aniridia ranges between 1:40,000 and 1:100,000 [199–202]. Currently, no specific environmental factors during pregnancy which could eventually enhance the risk of aniridia are known, and no racial or sex predominance has been reported in the existing literature [194, 199, 203]. According to the current literature, foveal hypoplasia is being recognized as a more common feature than complete iris hypoplasia in congenital aniridia, and as the major visual prognosis determinant, revolutionizing the classical clinical concept in this disorder [204, 205].

However, the risk of developing glaucoma in congenital aniridia amounts to approx. 70%, and generally an aniridic glaucoma emerges in childhood or later in adolescence [206–209].

Moreover, apart from the eye, congenital aniridia is linked with dysfunction in other organs, such as the brain, the pancreas and the auditory system [210–212].

The foveal and the iris hypoplasia, together with the aniridia-associated keratopathy are the most common pathophysiological changings in congenital aniridia, occurring in 80–100% of the cases [195]. Remarkably, corneal ulceration and scarring may escalate and induce severe visual impairment, finally leading to blindness [195, 203]. Due to these dramatic aberrant ocular alterations, the visual prognosis in congenital aniridia tends to be poor, despite the existing surgical treatment options [195, 213].

Genetics: Congenital aniridia is a rare disorder inherited via an autosomal dominant pattern, presenting generally high penetrance and variable expressivity [6, 203]. Importantly, aniridia can be either isolated or syndromic, presenting as a part of the WAGR (Wilms' tumor-aniridia-genital anomalies-retardation), WAGRO (WAGR and obesity) or Gillespie syndromes (non-progressive cerebellar ataxia, intellectual disability, iris hypoplasia) [204].

In around 85–90% of cases, congenital aniridia is due to a mutation in the *PAX6* (Paired-Box-Protein PAX6, also termed Aniridia-Typ-II-Protein AN2 or Oculorhombin) gene (11p13), that encodes a protein serving as a DNA-binding transcription factor and acting on a large number of target genes [203, 214]. This transcription factor has a key-role in the formation and development of the central nervous system, and of the eye [203, 215]. Crucially, *PAX6* results largely dosage sensitive, being a haploinsufficiency, a loss of one functional copy of the gene, related with disease and malformation [216].

In this regard, Davis et al. demonstrated that a *PAX6* haploinsufficiency induces an impaired growth and differentiation of iris and ciliary body, ultimately leading to a dramatic dysgenesis of these tissues [217]. Studies have also shown that a downregulation of *PAX6*, specifically induced in the lens and cornea, causes TM defects [218, 219]. In heterozygote $PAX6^{lacZ/+}$ deficient mice, Baulmann and associates determined a lack in the differentiation of TM cells as well as an absence of the SC [220]. A more recent in vivo and ex vivo investigation by Cole and coworkers on a *small-eye* mouse model ($PAX6^{Sey}$), highlighted the consequence of a *PAX6* deficiency, reporting raised IOP and diminished visual acuity in an age-dependent manner in $PAX6^{Sey}$ mice, and further describing also a local retinal damage and a layer disorganization, displaying activated microglia and astrocytes, suggesting a possible neuroinflammatory response to the *PAX6* deficit [221].

Apart from the *PAX6* gene, mutations in other genes have been linked with congenital total or partial aniridia, like for example in *FOXC1*, *PITX2* (paired-like homeodomain transcription factor 2, also termed pituitary homeobox 2), *TRIM44* (tripartite motif-containing 44), *CYP1B1*, and *FOXD3* (Forkhead Box D3) [198, 222–225].

Pathogenesis: Anomalies in the SC are postulated to represent principle pathogenetic triggers for the early-onset of the aniridic glaucoma, while progressive changes in the iridocorneal angle are presumed to be a leading cause of glaucoma with later onset [203, 226]. In aniridic glaucomas, both open or closed-angle forms can be observed, being however the open-angle variant more common [6]. On the other hand, closed-angle forms may develop when the iris gradually migrates over the TM, progressively establishing a process of angle closure [198].

Figure 2.4 offers a schematic overview on the main structural anomalies in the anterior eye segment during congenital aniridia, as a result of the mutation in *PAX6*, leading to aniridic glaucoma.

Clinics: Slit lamp examination and above all, the gonioscopy represent crucial diagnostic tool in aniridic glaucomas. The angle in individuals affected by aniridia shows a typical iris stump [197]. The TM and ciliary processes are generally observable posterior to the stump, while irregular strands originating from the iris stroma became thicker and moved forward, causing obscuration of the TM, and finally escalating in an angle obstruction and an AH blockage, in a context of progressive angle-closure [198, 227].

The employment of the UBM allows the detection of an iris hypoplasia, along with a hypoplasia of the ciliary body [228]. In addition, congenital aniridia is often associated with abnormalities of the lens and cataract formation, apart from other abnormalities like for example congenital aphakia, or variable degrees of subluxation [227].

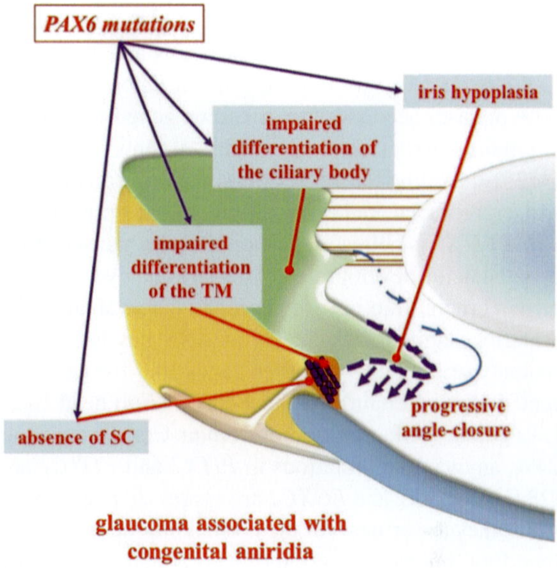

Fig. 2.4 *Scheme on the etiopathogenesis in aniridic glaucoma.* PAX6: Paired-Box-Protein PAX6; TM: trabecular meshwork; SC: Schlemm's canal

Glaucoma Associated with Axenfeld–Rieger Syndrome

Definition, epidemiology and prognosis: The Axenfeld–Rieger Syndrome (ARS) encompasses an heterogenous spectrum of genetic anomalies, defined by neurological, ocular and systemic developmental aberrancies [229]. Its overall prevalence amounts to approximatively 1:50,000–1:100,000 live births, with no racial or gender predilection in the different ethnic groups [230].

Historically, the German ophthalmologist Theodor Axenfeld was the first to describe, in 1920, an individual with an anterior displacement of the Schwalbe's line, the so termed posterior embryotoxon, in combination with corectopia, a displacement of the pupil [231]. Later, in 1935, the Austrian ophthalmologist Herwigh Rieger reported two cases with "mesodermal dysgenesis" and showing iris hypoplasia, pseudopolycoria, and posterior embryotoxon [232]. Originally, the ARS consisted of four separate conditions, such as the Axenfeld anomaly, the Rieger anomaly, the Axenfeld syndrome, and the Rieger syndrome, however, as these entities substantially tend to overlap for their common phenotypic and genotypic characteristics, currently the ARS is indicated as a unified combination of such conditions [230, 233].

As a consequence of genetic anomalies, in ARS aberrant migration of neural crest cells during embryogenesis occurs, leading to a maldevelopment of the anterior chamber structures, involving the ciliary body, the cornea, and the iris stroma, collectively causing secondary glaucoma through an iridogoniodysgenesis [234, 235].

In fact, this maldevelopment is the primary cause of glaucoma in ARS, that fundamentally represents the principle source of morbidity and is usually diagnosed during infancy or childhood, in over half of cases [236–238]. Of note, from a prognostic perspective, even though the vision loss in ARS is commonly due to the progression of glaucoma, also other disorder-related factors impact on the patient outcomes, like for example refractive error, strabismus and amblyopia [235, 237, 239].

Genetics: ARS is inherited in an autosomal dominant manner, being anyway 60% of cases secondary to unknown genetic mutations, while around 40% of cases are mainly associated with mutant variants in the genes *FOXC1* (6p25) and *PITX2* (4q25), encoding for transcription factors critical in modulating the ocular, neurological, craniofacial, and cardiovascular development [135, 237, 240–243]. Specifically, while *PITX2* is believed to be pivotal as a transcription regulator during embryogenesis and in the development of the anterior eye segment structures, *FOXC1* appears to have a crucial role in cardiac, renal, cerebral and also ocular morphogenesis [229]. Anterior segment dysgenesis in ARS has been also reported in association with mutant variants also in other genes like for example *CYP1B1*, *COL4A1*(collagen type 4 alpha 1 chain), *PAX6*, *FOXE3* (*F*orkhead B*ox E3*), *CPAMD8* (C3 And PZP Like Alpha-2-Macroglobulin Domain Containing 8), and *PXDN* (peroxidasin) [244–247], anyway the mutations in *PITX2* and *FOXC1* are the most common described [237]. As *PITX2* and *FOXC1* are expressed in the neural crest cells during embryogenesis, they are critical for the normal migration and differentiation of these cells, and therefore, for the formation of the corneal stroma and endothelium, iris stroma and muscles, ciliary body stroma, TM and AH outflow tracts, and sclera [248–253]. An interesting investigation by Chen and Gage on heterozygous *PITX2* mice (*PITX2*$^{+/-}$), examined the murine model clinically and histologically to describe ocular characteristics of ARS and glaucoma [254]. The authors assessed a postnatal expression of *PITX2* in the corneal endothelium and stroma, iris stroma, TM and SC.

A decreased CCT, along with iris defects, and iridocorneal adhesions were observable in *PITX2*$^{+/-}$ eyes, together with raised IOP and ONH cupping, while a neurodegeneration and significant reductions in ganglion cell density were also detectable [254].

A recent study by Senthil and coworkers, compared the anterior segment anomalies in individuals affected by *PITX2* mutations with those afflicted by *FOXC1* mutations, concluding that corneal alterations were more common in *FOXC1* mutant variants than those with *PITX2* variants, whereas iris abnormalities such as hypoplasia and pseudopolycoria, a condition where multiple pupils are observable in one eye, were on the other hand more frequent in individuals with *PITX2* variants than those with *FOXC1* variants [255]. Another recent investigation by Zhou et al. also compared *PITX2* with *FOXC1* variants in ARS, and examined phenotypically and genotypically eight families [256]. The authors assessed a significantly lower frequency of systemic abnormalities in *FOXC1* than in *PITX2* (58.77% in the *FOXC1* group vs. 89.16% in the *PITX2* group), while no significant differences in ocular abnormalities was observed. Moreover, iris abnormalities and glaucoma were the most frequent clinical manifestations in both groups, and, interestingly, a significant difference in glaucoma (44.06% in the *PITX2* group vs. 54.55% in the *FOXC1* group) could be displayed [256]. However, iris defects in form of peripheral anterior synechiae and posterior embryotoxon were also equally observable in both affected family members. Additionally, a higher frequency of corectopia (35.81% vs. 18.57%) and pseudopolycoria (18.60% vs. 2.95%), was recorded in *PITX2* than in *FOXC1* [256].

Pathogenesis: In the context of ARS, mutations in *PITX2* and *FOXC1* are associated with early-onset glaucoma, and raised IOP is typically due to iridogoniodysgenesis and iris strands that bridge the angle structures [233, 234, 238, 257]. The retention and contraction of primordial embryonic endothelium, and consequent iridocorneal adhesions or the formation of the classic posterior embryotoxon, appear to be the main responsible of the pathophysiological events in ARS [236].

More precisely, a retraction of contiguous tissue between aberrant iris and posterior cornea, tend to move the iris toward the cornea, finally forming iridocorneal adhesions which typically form at a level higher than the Schwalbe's Line [236], whereas, isolated contraction of the aberrant iris tissue, and its condensation, causes an anterior displacement of Schwalbe's line, with the generation of a thickened ridge, the posterior embryotoxon [236]. Figure 2.5 presents photographs of the anterior eye segments of a patient with ARS.

Figure 2.6 illustrates the main events in the etiopathogenesis in ARS that drive to secondary glaucoma, corectopia and pseudopolycoria.

Clinics: Glaucoma in ARS is usually bilateral, but it may asymmetrically involve one eye more severely than the other [230, 239]. Iris defects in ARS vary from very subtle to profound, and, basing on the location of the pupil, corectopia and pseudopolycoria lead to abnormal intolerance to light, a significant photophobia, apart from causing cosmetic concerns to the patients [230].

Through slit lamp examination, a band-shaped keratopathy may be observed, together with corectopia, pseudopolycoria, or eventually partial aniridia [236]. The gonioscopic examination is also here fundamental, as it allows the detection of high iris processes obscure the TM and insert on the posterior embryotoxon or in the iridocorneal angle, fundamental features to document for the diagnosis [236].

In addition to increased IOP and optic nerve cupping, patients affected by ARS < 5–7 years of age may show classic signs usually associated with PCG, like for

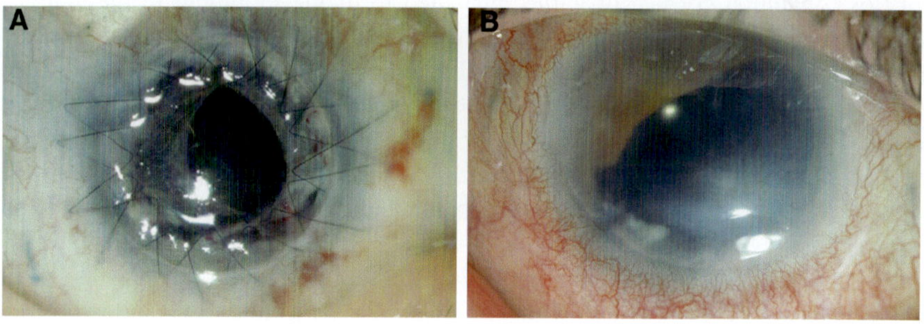

Fig. 2.5 *Eyes of a patient with Axenfeld-Rieger Syndrome.* **a** The right eye already underwent multiple surgeries because of elevated intraocular pressure, lens opacification and dislocation, and because of corneal decompensation. At the 10 o' clock position, at the edge of the freshly reconstructed pupil, the tip of an Ahmed valve tube is visible, which is placed behind the sclera-fixated intraocular lens due to a very flat anterior chamber. **b** At the left eye, corectopia and iris atrophy are visible. The patient suffers from recurrent IOP elevation resulting in redness of the eye and a cloudy cornea. Courtesy of Department of Ophthalmology, University Medical Center Mainz

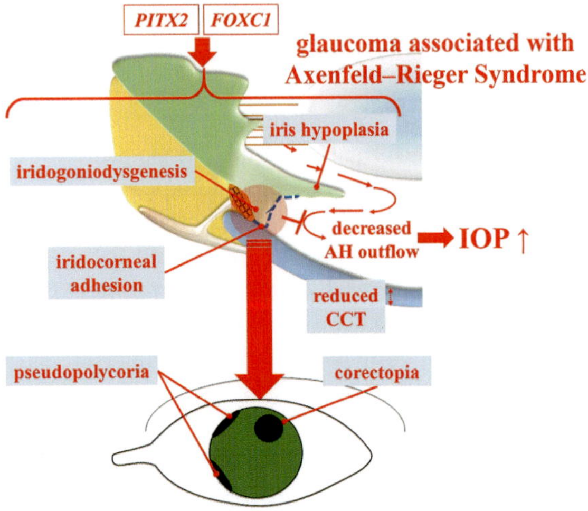

Fig. 2.6 *Scheme on the etiopathogenesis in ARS.* AH: aqueous humor; CCT: central corneal thickness; FOXC1: *F*orkhead B*ox C1*; IOP: intraocular pressure; PITX2: paired-like homeodomain transcription factor 2, also termed pituitary homeobox 2

example buphthalmos, Haab striae, increased corneal diameter and corneal edema [6, 237]. Particular attention is also recommended for strabismus measurements, cycloplegic refraction, and certainly the optic nerve appearance, evaluable through fundus examination and OCT imaging [237].

Glaucoma Associated with Peters Anomaly

Definition, epidemiology and prognosis: Peters anomaly (PA) is an infrequent and typically bilateral disorder characterized by central congenital corneal opacity resulting from anterior segment dysgenesis [258]. Specifically, it falls into the category of congenital corneal opacities attributed to maldevelopment in the anterior segment, also known as kerato-irido-lenticular dysgenesis [259]. PA is identified by a central corneal opacity, with anomalies in the posterior stroma of the cornea involving Descemet's membrane and the corneal endothelium within the opacified region [260–262].

PA is identified by a central corneal opacity, with anomalies in the posterior stroma of the cornea involving Descemet's membrane and the corneal endothelium within the opacified region [263].

PA has an incidence of around 1.2–1.5:100,000 live births, and is bilateral in approx. 80% of cases, with no reported predilection for gender or race [260, 261, 264, 265].

Up to 60% of patients manifest systemic aberrancies or developmental delays like for example craniofacial abnormalities, microcephaly, hypopituitarism, dwarfism, cardiac malformations [266–268]. However, PA is often considered as an isolated ocular disease [269–271], and ocular abnormalities can comprise among others glaucoma, corectopia, keratolenticular touch, anterior polar cataract, aniridia, aphakia, iris hypoplasia, iris coloboma, chorioretinal coloboma, staphyloma, retinal dysplasia, all of those massively impacting on the visual development in children [264, 266–268, 272]. The risk of secondary glaucoma is observed in 50–70% of cases, and up to 50% of patients can present concomitant vision-threatening disorders [260, 273]. Of note, apart from glaucoma, the prognosis in PA is strongly influenced by the central corneal opacification, which is commonly documented and often represents an indication for corneal transplantation in infants [267, 274–276]. In this regard, despite of the progresses in the surgery concerning corneal grafting in children, the treatment presents a higher graft failure rate and worse visual prognosis in children than in adults [273].

Genetics: PA is usually sporadic, being anyway documented also an autosomal dominant and recessive inheritance pattern in consanguineous cases [277]. Mutant genetic variants linked with the occurrence of PA have been found in diverse regulatory genes responsible of a normal development of the anatomic structures in the anterior eye segment, like for example *PAX6*, *PITX2*, *PITX3*, *COL4A1*, *FOXC1*, and *COL6A3* (collagen type 6 alpha 3 chain), being *PAX6* and *FOXC1* the most frequent reported gene mutations [258, 260, 278–281]. As previously described, these genes, in particular *PAX6*, *PITX2* and *FOXC1*, are critical for the normal migration of the neural crest cells during embryogenesis [258].

Their mutations can induce devastating pathogenetic events that in PA culminate in a kerato-irido-lenticular dysgenesis, basis for the establishment of the disorder.

Remarkably, the most common condition related with PA is the so termed Peters Plus syndrome (PPS), an aberrancy linked with diverse systemic conditions such as among others facial dysmorphism, short stature, brachydactyly, central nervous system defects, congenital heart defects, genitourinary abnormalities [282].

However, the classic PPS is defined by the triad of PA, brachydactyly, and short stature [283] and it is inherited in an autosomal recessive manner, linked with biallelic pathogenic variants in the gene *B3GALTL*, that encodes for a putative glycosyltransferase, which when mutant induces glycosylation defects, basis for this congenital malformation syndrome [284, 285].

Pathogenesis: An aberrant migration and an impaired differentiation of neural crest cells in the anterior segment leads to a defective separation of the lens from the surface ectoderm and to an anomalous reattachment of the lens or/and iris to the cornea, fundamental pathophysiological processes in PA [259, 260, 273, 286, 287]. According to an anatomic step-ladder illustration of the pathophysiological changings in PA [260, 288], a simplest form of PA is represented by posterior corneal defect, showing a central damage of the cornea, known as internal corneal ulcer of Von Hippel, observable in the slit lamp examination as a central corneal leukoma. In a more severe variant, iris strands are present, reaching the posterior corneal wall in correspondence of the Von Hippel ulcer, hereby giving rise to an irido-corneal adhesion. Finally, in case of corneo-lenticular touch, the lens adheres with the central posterior corneal wall.

In this context, parallelly to the central corneal opacification, the irido-corneal adhesion and/or the corneo-lenticular contact, prevent the normal AH outflow, generating IOP elevation and therefore secondary glaucoma. Figure 2.7 offers an overview on the glaucomatous etiopathogenesis in PA.

Clinics: Clinically, two relevant classification have been postulated to help physicians in categorizing PA.

The first categorization was introduced by Townsend and colleagues in 1974, and subdivided the disorder into three main groups: (1) cornea with central leukoma only; (2) cornea with central leukoma and corneo-lenticular touch; (3) cornea with central leukoma associated with Rieger mesodermal dysgenesis [289]. A more recent classification system distinguishes two types of PA:

- **Type I:** an irido-corneal adhesion with central corneal opacity is detectable, usually unilateral. This variant is defined as "mild" and rarely associated with systemic abnormalities [290, 291].

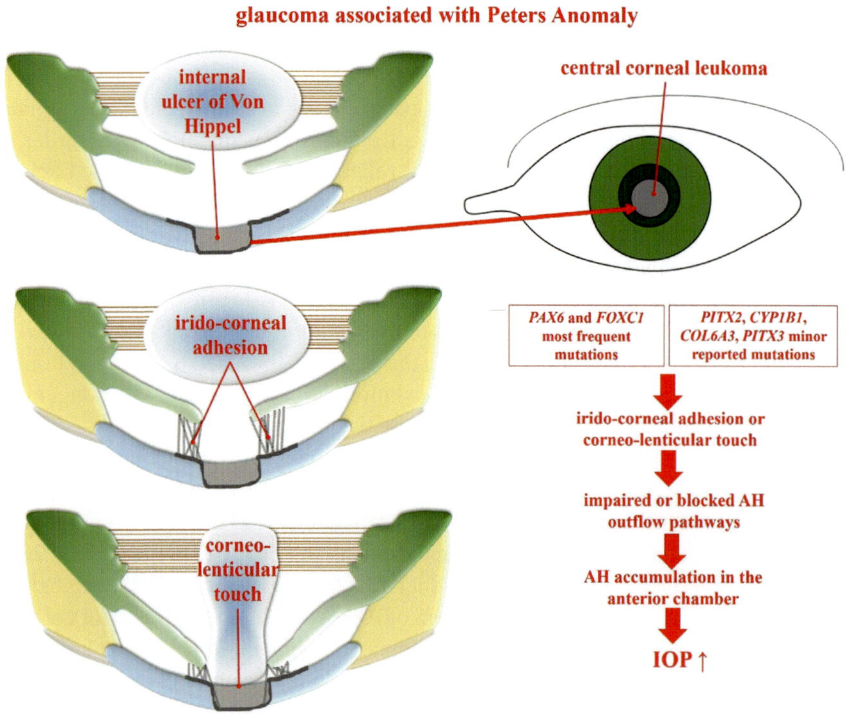

Fig. 2.7 *Scheme on the glaucomatous etiopathogenesis in PA.* AH: aqueous humor; COL6A3: collagen type 6 alpha 3 chain; CYP1B1: cytochrome P450, family 1, subfamily B and polypeptide 1; FOXC1: *F*orkhead B*ox C1*; IOP: intraocular pressure; PAX6: Paired box protein Pax-6, also known as aniridia type II protein (AN2) or oculorhombin; PITX: paired-like homeodomain transcription factor, also termed pituitary homeobox

- **Type II:** a corneo-lenticular touch with the lens directly adherent to the corneal opacity or corneal opacity with cataract is observable. This form is generally bilateral and is identified as "severe", being further associated with systemic anomalies [266, 286].

In relation to the secondary glaucoma associated with PA, of particular importance for the clinical evaluation is once again the gonioscopy, which for example helps detecting iris strands reaching the mid-peripheral cornea in correspondence of the leukoma [288]. In addition, the UBM as well as the anterior segment OCT, become vital for the low visibility of the anterior eye segment structure as a result of the massive central corneal opacity [273]. These diagnostic tools are fundamental for the confirmation of the diagnosis as well as for the preoperative assessment of the structures of the anterior chamber [292, 293].

Glaucoma Associated with Congenital Ectropion Uveae

Generalities: Congenital ectropion uveae (CEU), also known as congenital iris ectropion syndrome, is a rare, non-progressive form of anterior segment dysgenesis, caused by failed regression of primordial endothelium, resulting in hyperplasia of iris pigment epithelium on the anterior surface of the iris [294–297]. Wicherkiewicz in 1891 and Spiro in 1896 were the firsts to describe CEU [298, 299], while the first authors to report CEU in association with glaucoma were Ritch and coworkers in 1984 [296]. CEU is typically unilateral, however it has been described also as bilateral disorder [300, 301].

It has been reported to be associated with some malformation and syndromic disorders such as coloboma, ptosis, neurofibromatosis type 1, Prader-Willi Syndrome, ARS, and facial hemihypertrophy [295, 302–306]. Of note, glaucoma represents a relative frequent complication of CEU, and can manifest at any age from infancy to early adulthood [295–297, 301, 307].

Genetics and Pathogenesis: Little is known on the etiologic drivers and genetic mutations in CEU, leading to the glaucomatous etiopathogenesis. Cases of neonatal-onset of CEU has been described to be caused by distinct *CYP1B1* pathologic variant [308], whereas other cases have been reported to be associated with a *PAX6* mutation [309]. However, from a pathophysiological perspective, the presence of iris pigment epithelium on the iris anterior surface elicits the generation of pathogenetic features such as the anterior insertion of the iris, the dysgenesis of the drainage angle, and finally an impaired AH outflow pathway and IOP elevation, in a context of secondary glaucoma [297, 310]. The anterior insertion of the iris and the consequent TM dysgenesis appears to be the main pathogenetic drivers in CEU [297].

Even though CEU is defined as a non-progressive disorder, some studies have highlighted the connection between CEU and an appearance of progressive open-angle glaucoma derived from the angle dysgenesis [296, 297, 310–313].

Figure 2.8 provides a schematic representation of the glaucomatous etiopathogenesis in CEU.

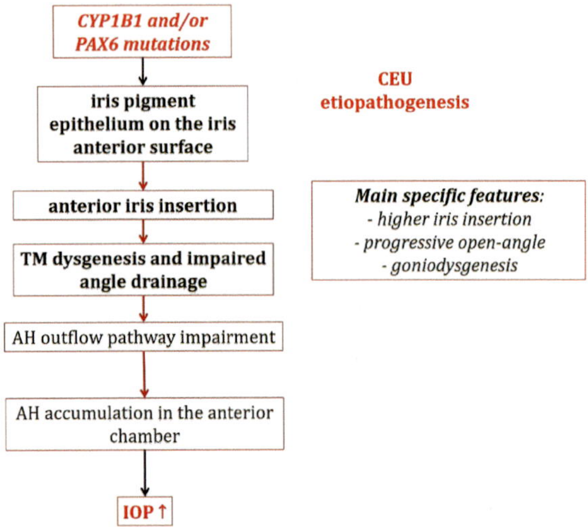

Fig. 2.8 *Scheme on the glaucomatous etiopathogenesis in CEU.* AH: aqueous humor; CYP1B1: cytochrome P450, family 1, subfamily B and polypeptide 1; IOP: intraocular pressure; PAX6: Paired box protein Pax-6, also known as aniridia type II protein (AN2) or oculorhombin; TM: trabecular meshwork

Clinics: The slit lamp examination allows to observe smooth, cryptless iris surface as well as an iris stromal atrophy or hypoplasia [297]. Gonioscopy permits to document an anterior iris insertion, prominent iris processes, pigmentation at the angle, and poorly developed TM. Fundus evaluation normally show healthy optic discs or eventually varying stages of optic nerve injury due to glaucoma [294].

2.3.2.2 Glaucoma Associated with Non-acquired Systemic Diseases

As per the CGRN, these conditions primarily manifest as systemic diseases or syndromes present at birth, either with or without accompanying ocular signs [5]. The 2016 CGRN study reveals that glaucoma associated with non-acquired systemic diseases constitutes 11.5% of all cases of childhood glaucoma [30]. Examples of glaucoma linked to non-acquired systemic diseases or syndromes include [29]:

- **Chromosomal disorders**
  - Trisomy 21
- **Connective tissue disorders**
  - Marfan syndrome
  - Weill–Marchesani syndrome
  - Stickler syndrome
- **Metabolic disorders**
  - Homocystinuria
  - Lowe syndrome
  - Mucopolysaccharidoses

- **Phacomatoses**
  - Neurofibromatosis
  - Sturge–Weber syndrome
- **Rubinstein–Taybi**
- **Congenital rubella**

Well-studied conditions are, even though very rare, the Rubinstein–Taybi syndrome and the Sturge–Weber syndrome. In the next sections, we report on the genetics, pathophysiology and specific clinics of these disorders.

Glaucoma Associated with Sturge–Weber Syndrome

Generalities: Sturge-Weber syndrome (SWS), also termed encephalo-trigeminal angiomatosis, is a rare congenital neurocutaneous disorder, defined by the presence of three major clinical features: a facial port-wine birthmark due to cutaneous capillary malformations in the distributions of the trigeminal nerve, secondary glaucoma, and leptomeningeal angiomatosis [314–316]. This syndrome was first described by Sturge in 1879, and then by Weber in 1922 [317, 318]. Of note, Roach proposed a classification system for SWS, evidencing three specific phenotypes [319]:

- **Type 1**: classical form including facial angioma, leptomeningeal angiomas, and possible glaucoma;
- **Type 2**: with facial angioma and possible glaucoma;
- **Type 3**: leptomeningeal angiomas in the absence of facial angioma.

SWS occurs with an incidence of around 1:20.000–1:50.000, without reported gender predilection [320, 321].

This disorder is probably caused by a failed or absent regression of a primitive cephalic plexus, that leads to the establishment of capillary malformations in a context of underdevelopment of the brain superficial venous drainage and venous hypertension, and parallelly, to the formation of compensatory deep dilated venous vessels [314, 322–324]. As a result, a condition of venous stasis occurs, that in the eye originates prominent epibulbar vessels, diffuse choroidal hemangiomas and secondary glaucoma [324]. Ocular manifestations are described in around 50% of patients with SWS [295]. Glaucoma is recognized as the most common ocular complication, occurring in ca. 30–70% of patients, and as a chronic condition can escalate causing devastating damage of the optic nerve, finally leading to irreversible vision loss, therefore it needs considerable attention in patients with SWS [315, 326–328]. Prognostically, the management of SWS is significantly challenging [6].

Particular complex to perform are surgical interventions to treat glaucoma, due to possible hemorrhages deriving from dilated aberrant episcleral and choroidal vessels [329].

Genetics: SWS presents no familial predisposition and is described as a sporadic disorder, as such not being associated with any specific inheritance pattern [324]. According to the current literature, in SWS occurs a postzygotic, somatic mutation, during early embryogenesis, that namely does not involve the germline, in particular being identified in a gain-of-function variant of the gene *GNAQ* (guanine nucleotide-binding protein G(q) subunit alpha), encoding for the subunit $G_{\alpha q}$ of a G protein [330]. Approximatively 80% of individuals affected by SWS shows the R183Q *GNAQ* pathogenic variant [330–332]. Shirly and associates were the firsts to report this somatic activating mutation, that downstream triggers different signaling pathways, like the PI3K/Akt/mTOR axis, the PLC/PKC/ERK pathway, and the non-canonical Hippo cascade through Rho/Rac, collectively resulting in cell proliferation and inhibition of apoptosis [333]. Additionally, a recent study by Thorpe et al. also identified an alternative mutation in the gene *GNA11* encoding for the subunit $G_{\alpha 11}$ [334].

Pathogenesis: The pathogenesis of glaucoma associated with SWS is complex and, to date, not precisely explained. Anyway, there exist four principle theories [324, 335]:

1. an enhanced episcleral venous pressure deriving from arteriovenous shunts into the episcleral hemangioma [336, 337];
2. aberrant hemodynamic events of the episclera on the anterior eye segment as a result of premature aging of the TM and SC, as described in SWS later-onset glaucoma [338];
3. fluid hypersecretion from the ciliary body or from the choroidal hemangioma [339];
4. mechanical mechanisms and obstructions induced by congenital malformation of the anterior chamber angle guiding to augmented resistance to the AH outflow [340].

However, recently, an interesting study by Wu et al. has shed light on the role of the R183Q *GNAQ* mutation, leading to the pathogenesis of the secondary glaucoma in SWS [341].

Remarkably, the authors identified on the tissue of patients affected by glaucoma and SWS, the mutation in the abnormal scleral tissue presenting dysplastic blood vessels, in 100% of individuals afflicted by glaucoma secondary to SWS. They detected an aberrant activation of the MAPK signaling pathway via ERK and JNK, in endothelial cells of scleral and episcleral blood vessels, suggesting that through the abnormal vascular scleral tissue, may occur a dramatic impairment of the AH outflow pathway may occur, leading to glaucoma in SWS [341]. Figure 2.9 offers a schematic overview on the etiopathogenesis in SWS, and further on the pathogenetic events triggered by the *GNAQ* mutation, driving to secondary glaucoma in SWS.

Clinics: Typically, glaucoma secondary to Sturge-Weber Syndrome (SWS) is characterized by a bimodal presentation: early onset glaucoma in 60% of cases and late onset glaucoma in 40% of patients [325]. Importantly, in SWS, the eye on the side exhibiting the port-wine stain is usually the one affected by secondary glaucoma [327]. Furthermore, in instances of isolated involvement of the port-wine

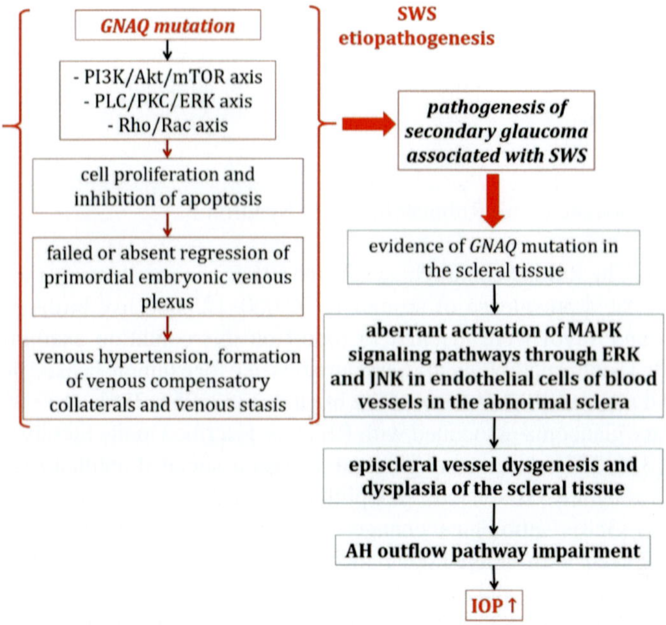

Fig. 2.9 *Scheme on SWS and on its glaucomatous etiopathogenesis.* AH: aqueous humor; Akt: Ak strain transforming (also known as protein kinase B); ERK: extracellular-signal-regulated kinase; *GNAQ*: guanine nucleotide-binding protein G(q) subunit alpha; IOP: intraocular pressure; JNK: c-Jun N-terminal kinase; MAPK: mitogen activated protein kinase; mTOR: mammalian target of rapamycin; PI3K: Phosphoinositide 3-kinase; PKC: protein kinase C; PLC: phospholipase C; TM: trabecular meshwork

birthmark on a unilateral upper eyelid, glaucoma has been reported with a frequency of approximately 21%. This frequency notably increases to 72% in cases of bilateral involvement [321, 342–344].

Open-angle glaucoma is the most common variant described in association with SWS, even though isolated cases of angle-closure have been also reported [325]. A swelling of the ciliary body, along with an anterior rotation of the ciliary processes, and a swelling of the lens have been suggested to represent possible pathogenic events leading to angle closure [345]. An angle neovascularization caused by retinal pathologies and cases of ectopia lentis have been also linked with angle-closure glaucoma in SWS [346, 347].

Anterior eye segment imaging or gonioscopy can help describe the structural anomalies in glaucoma associated with SWS. In particular, flat and anterior iris insertion was reported, along with prominent vascular loops at the iris root, and the presence of blood in SC [325, 337, 338, 348]. Enlarged corneal diameters and myopia are typically detectable in early-onset glaucoma, while in the late-onset variant, no eye enlargement has been described [349, 350]. The slit lamp examination can show dilated conjunctival and episcleral blood vessels [324]. Moreover, apart from IOP measurement and gonioscopy, through a constant monitoring of individuals afflicted by SWS, the fundus evaluation of these subjects is also critical, as choroidal hemangiomas may be present in 71% of cases [315]. Other relevant ocular complications of SWS are iris heterochromia, retinal detachment, strabismus, and homozygous hemianopia [315].

Glaucoma Associated with Rubinstein–Taybi Syndrome

Generalities: The Rubinstein–Taybi syndrome (RSTS) is an extremely rare disorder, with an estimated prevalence of around 1:100,000–125,000 live births [351–353]. Rubinstein and Taybi were the first to report on this condition examining seven patients with specific pathological characteristics like for example beaked nose, broad thumbs, and angulation deformity of the big toes [352, 354, 355].

Secondary glaucoma associated with RSTS is described in the literature firstly in the 1970s [356, 357]. Apart from glaucoma, other associated ophthalmologic signs comprise nystagmus, strabismus, enophthalmos, iris atrophy, high myopia, and optic atrophy [358]. Pathological changes of the anterior and posterior eye segments commonly linked with congenital glaucoma in RSTS are among others corneal edema, enlarged cornea and optic disc cupping [358, 359]. Although described as a rare complication of RSTS [359], congenital glaucoma has been also reported as a relative frequent ocular abnormality in RSTS, along with colobomas and lacrimal duct problems [360]. This is possibly due to the highly overlapping of signs and symptoms in RSTS, resulting in extremely challenging differential diagnosis with other conditions that simulates glaucoma [361]. In fact, RSTS is particularly subject to misdiagnosis, as a result of the substantial lack of specific clinical presentations during the neonatal period [353]. However, the current literature emphasizes the relevance of measuring IOP in RSTS, as glaucoma can lead in these patients to irreversible visual loss [353, 358].

Etiopathogenesis and Clinics: RSTS has been demonstrated to be caused by mutations in the *CREBBP* gene (16p13.3), encoding for the cAMP responsive element binding protein and/or the *EP300* gene (22q13.2), which encoded for the E1A-binding protein 300 [353, 362, 363]. *CREBBP* and *EP300* are homologous genes, possessing key-roles as global transcriptional coactivators [364]. However, in around 35–45% of cases with the clinical phenotype of RSTS, no mutation is observable [358].

Of note, patients without documentable mutation do not present clinical differences compared to patients with recognizable mutation [365]. In fact, although RSTS syndrome is an autosomal dominant inheritance pattern, many patients present new mutations, hereby being documented as sporadic cases [366].

Little is known about the pathogenetic mechanisms that lead to secondary glaucoma in RSTS. However, pre-operative examinations of patients undergoing surgery, displayed via gonioscopic evaluations, a deep anterior chamber, along with a dysgenesis of the irido-corneal angle, abundant basal iris processes, and a flat iris insertion into the TM [359]. Figure 2.10 offers a schematic overview of the etiopathogenesis in glaucoma associated with RSTS.

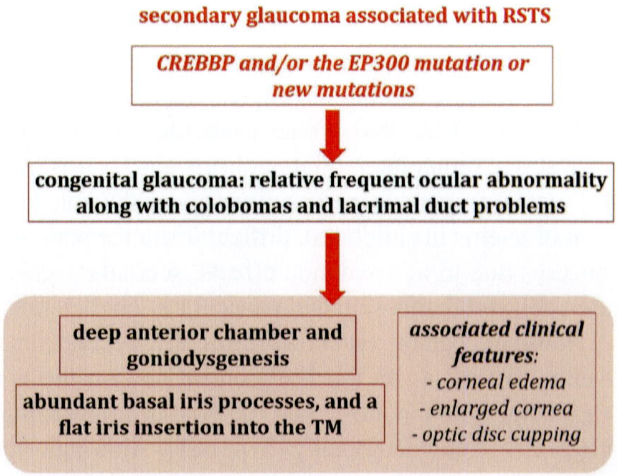

Fig. 2.10 *Scheme on the etiopathogenesis of glaucoma associated with RSTS*. CREBBP: cAMP responsive element binding protein; EP300: E1A-binding protein 300; RSTS: Rubinstein-Taybi syndrome; TM: trabecular meshwork

2.3.2.3 Glaucoma Associated with Acquired Conditions

According to the 2016 CGRN study, glaucoma associated with acquired conditions constitutes 23% of all cases of childhood glaucoma. Consequently, it stands as the second most prevalent cause of glaucoma in children, following the primary forms [30].

The principle acquired conditions and environmental triggers inducing secondary glaucomas in children comprise uveitis, trauma, retinopathy of prematurity (ROP) and corticosteroid therapy.

Uveitic Glaucoma

Epidemiology and prognosis: Children account for approximately 5–10% of the population affected by uveitis, with a reported annual incidence of around 4.3–6:100,000 [367–369]. Remarkably, in pediatric uveitis, visual impairment is more frequent and severe than in adulthood, leading to blindness in 30–45% of cases [370, 371]. Secondary uveitic glaucoma in children, represents the second most frequent complication after cataracts, and among the most common reasons driving to severe visual impairment [372, 373]. According to the current literature, the prevalence of childhood uveitic glaucoma in the pediatric population afflicted by uveitis, is circa 5–25% [374–376].

In the context of the childhood glaucoma, uveitis is the underlying cause in about 6–9% of cases, therefore representing one of the most frequent etiologic drivers of glaucoma in childhood [377, 378]. Importantly, children affected by uveitis present an innate predisposition to develop glaucoma compared to adults, further showing the eventuality of manifesting specific severe complications as the disease progresses, such as for example amblyopia [376, 379]. Notably, the occurrence of uveitic glaucomas fundamentally depends on the underlying disorder, on its severity and on its duration [380]. In this regard, it is noteworthy reporting that approximatively the half of all pediatric uveitis (ranging between 41 and 47%), is due to juvenile idiopathic arthritis (JIA), which thereby represents the most prevalent disorder in children with uveitis [367, 372, 381]. Other systemic disorders leading to pediatric uveitis are sarcoidosis, tubulointerstitial nephritis and uveitis, and Blau syndrome [382].

From a prognostic perspective, given the substantially asymptomatic development of uveitis in childhood, difficulties in the pediatric ocular examination, therapy concerns due to age and side effects, secondary glaucomas are underdiagnosed or often delayed diagnosed, and particularly challenging to treat [383, 384].

However, patient outcomes critically depend on the type and duration of the uveitis, as well as on the IOP control and on the management of the devastating intraocular inflammation, with the goal of minimizing the risk of amblyopia and of progressive optic neuropathy [376, 385]. Although steroid as well as corticosteroid-sparing treatments have served to progress in the control of the inflammation [386], improvements of visual prognosis in childhood uveitic glaucomas are difficult to achieve, considering the concerns linked with the underlying uveitis and the young age of presentation [387, 388]. Scarce compliance and intolerance to local or systemic steroids due to side effects, contribute to significantly limit the successes of the medical therapies [376].

Pathogenesis and clinics: Both variants of open-angle and angle closure glaucoma have been described in children with uveitis [376, 382, 387]. Open-angle glaucoma in uveitis establishes as a consequence of mechanical obstructive processes at the anterior chamber and subsequent enhanced resistance to the AH drainage, generally rooted to the massive inflammation occurring in the TM, that leads to accumulation of debris and immune materials, along with a chronic remodeling in the TM and SC, escalating in scarring and collapse of these structures [376, 382, 383, 389].

Some studies have demonstrated that patients with uveitis present a disruption of the blood-aqueous barrier deriving from the inflammation, that substantially leads to an increase level of proteins in the AH in uveitic eyes, linked with an impaired AH drainage and IOP elevation [390, 391]. Alternatively, a chronic employment of topical or systemic steroids for the long-term treatment of the uveitis, can be also a trigger of open-angle glaucoma, preventing the IOP control via an accumulation of extracellular matrices in the TM and thereby obstructing the AH facility and ultimately exacerbating the rise of IOP [369, 389].

Angle closure occurs as a result of extensive posterior synechiae, that guide to pupillary block or as a consequence of peripheral anterior synechiae, not generating pupillary block, but eliciting the formation of iris bombe, with the presence of fibrin membrane over the pupil, and rotation of the ciliary body [6, 376, 387].

From a clinical view, uveitic conditions present usually bilaterally, affecting both eyes concomitantly or involving at the beginning only one eye, and then rapidly afflicting the partner eye in few months. In active uveitic phases, the slit-lamp examination allows the detection of mild to moderate degree of fine anterior chamber cells, with or without non-granulomatous precipitates or endothelial inflammatory deposits [383].

Importantly, JIA-related uveitis is classified as a chronic non-granulomatous anterior uveitis, often asymptomatic in early stages, and typically accompanied by the development of cataract, band-shaped keratopathy and secondary glaucoma [383]. Of note, due to the pathophysiology of chronic anterior uveitis, specifically in JIA-uveitis, glaucoma is suggested to originate from trabecular scarring and sclerosis caused by chronic trabeculitis, and it is generally challenging to differentiate from steroid-induced glaucoma [376]. The slit-lamp examination can display in some cases the presence of granulomatous precipitates, and eventually, via a fundus evaluation, a posterior segment involvement, although these findings are a less typical presentation of active JIA-uveitis [392]. Additionally, in case of severe massive inflammation, ocular hypotony may manifest, as a result of a sudden ciliary body dysfunction [382]. Remarkably, while early stages often show on gonioscopy an open angle, in long-standing cases through the establishment of anterior synechiae, an angle closure can be observed, eventually together with pupillary block caused by posterior synechiae [382].

Figure 2.11 provides an overview on the pathogenetic events occurring in childhood uveitic glaucoma in JIA.

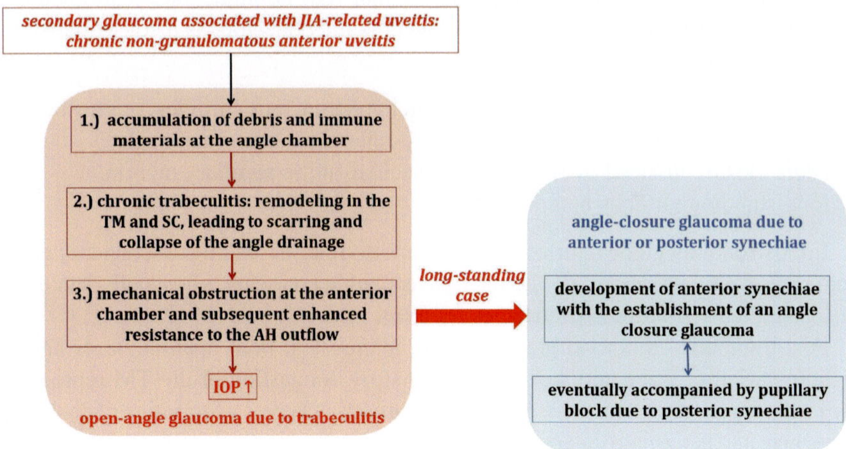

Fig. 2.11 *Scheme on uveitic glaucomatous pathogenesis in children.* AH: aqueous humor; IOP: intraocular pressure; JIA: juvenile idiopathic arthritis; SC: Schlemm's canal; TM: trabecular meshwork

Post-traumatic Glaucoma

Generalities: Penetrating or blunt craniofacial traumas can involve the eye and lead to traumatic optic nerve neuropathy and to secondary glaucoma [6, 393, 394]. Given the relative high frequency of pediatric ocular traumas, with around 3.3–5.7 million children suffering ocular injuries yearly, while hospitalization is annually required in approximatively 160,000–280,000 of individuals < 15 years of age, it is nost surprising noting that pediatric ocular traumas are a significant cause of monocular vision loss [395]. Remarkably, about 20% of childhood glaucomas are secondary to globe injuries [396]. A noteworthy investigation conducted by Kalamkar and Mukherjee, retrospectively analyzed 5-year hospital data of 205 pediatric eyes from children $\leq$ 16 years, concluding that a post-traumatic rise of IOP establishes in around 15% of pediatric eyes, more commonly in case of closed globe injury than open globe injury, while a pharmaceutic treatment is required in 63% eyes, and a surgical intervention in 37% of cases [397]. From a prognostic perspective, the visual acuity was poor in eyes with open globe injury, as a result of a posterior eye segment involvement [397].

Pathogenesis and clinics: Pathogenetic processes contributing to post-traumatic glaucomas in children differ depending on the type of trauma, being substantially subdivided into close/blunt or open/penetrating globe injury [396].

In case of open or penetrating globe trauma, IOP is, immediately after injury, firstly low, while after wound closure, glaucoma may develop, as a consequence of structural changings in form of [396]:

- blockage of TM through blood cells from hyphema, lens particles, or ghost cells;
- inflammatory debris leading to synechiae-related closure of the angle;
- angle closure induced by iris bombe synechiae at the pupillary margin;
- long-standing vitreous hemorrhage.

In close or blunt globe injuries, possible reported causes leading to secondary glaucoma are uveitic processes, hyphema, rebleed, angle recession, ghost cell glaucoma, dislocated lens, vitreous hemorrhages [6, 396].

Post-traumatic childhood glaucoma can manifest in both open-angle or angle-closure variants. Trabeculitis or an inflammatory congestion of the TM represents the primary pathomechanism in open-angle variants, whereas a formation of posterior synechiae and peripheral anterior synechiae are involved in the development of angle-closure forms [394]. Clinically, in both close and open globe injury, the slit lamp examination, along with the IOP measurement, is fundamental as a diagnostic tool.

Of note, a retrospective case analysis of 472 pediatric patients with traumatic hyphema, showed that over one-third of the injured eye resulted in blindness, highlighting the importance of preventing such evolution through an improved diagnostic process and prompt management of the possible consequences of the ocular trauma [398].

Figure 2.12 offers a schematic overview on the pathogenetic events in both penetrating and blunt traumas leading to secondary glaucomas in children.

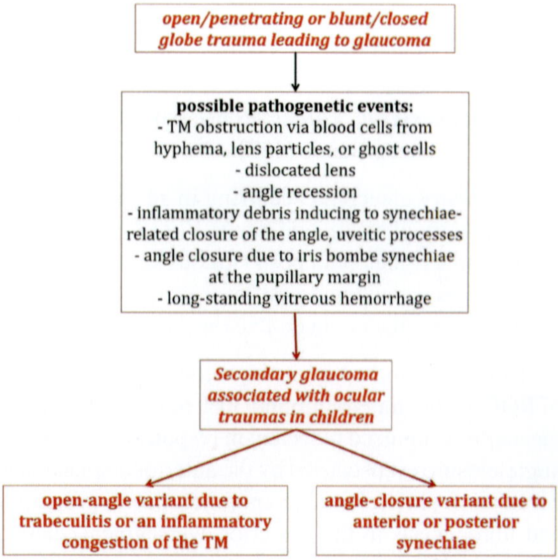

Fig. 2.12 *Scheme on post-traumatic glaucomatous pathogenesis in children.* TM: trabecular meshwork

Glaucoma Associated with Retinopathy of Prematurity

Generalities: Retinopathy of prematurity (ROP) is a developmental vascular proliferative disorder involving the retina and defined by an abnormal capillary growth in preterm newborns, globally representing a major risk factor for visual impairment and blindness in infants and young children [399]. Children affected by ROP are at higher risk to develop secondary glaucoma [400, 401]. The development of secondary glaucoma in ROP is predominantly due to angle-closure in eyes with cicatricial ROP [6].

A 19-year prospective study conducted by Senthil and colleagues in an Indian tertiary eye care institute, reported that on a total of approx. 6.000 children afflicted by ROP, circa 1.36% (82 eyes out of 6.000 children) of cases developed secondary glaucoma, with the majority presenting advanced stages of ROP (stage IV and V) [402]. Reported types of glaucoma were angle-closure in 47.6% of cases, open angle 42.7% of cases and neovascular in 9.8% [403].

Prematurity represents a risk factor for the occurrence of secondary glaucoma. In fact, the normal trabeculogenesis is entirely complete only late in gestation, posing the risk of structural vulnerability in preterm infants for the development of angle-closure glaucoma in a context of immature and dysfunctional TM [403]. Additionally, anterior segment abnormalities described in premature children, comprise among others, reduced anterior chamber depth, anteriorly displaced iris, as well as augmented lens thickness [404–406]. Eyes affected by ROP show narrower anterior chamber angles than full-term children [406]. However, ROP is a curable disorder, with potential positive visual outcomes, if not left untreated. The development of complications such as glaucoma represents an important driver of morbidity, and therefore, ROP requires a protracted follow-up [407]. The establishment of glaucoma certainly decreases future prospects for improved patient outcomes [408]. In fact, despite management and control of IOP, visual acuity improvements in these patients are substantially scarce [407, 409].

Pathogenesis and clinics: ROP-associated glaucomas can be caused by different triggers and backgrounds [407]:

1. secondary glaucoma occurring in advanced stages of ROP
2. secondary glaucoma post-anti-VEGF injection to treat ROP
3. secondary glaucoma post-vitreous surgery to treat ROP
4. secondary glaucoma post-laser therapy to treat ROP
5. secondary glaucoma co-existing with PCG in ROP.

The predominant type is the secondary glaucoma manifesting in advanced stages of ROP, accounting for around 30% of glaucomas in ROP [401, 407]. In this context, the major recognized mechanism responsible of the glaucomatous pathogenesis is an angle-closure event caused by the anterior displacement of iris-lens diaphragm due to contraction of retrolental membranes, due to processes of fibrovascular proliferation and fibrogenesis in the posterior eye segment, classic in the development of ROP [404, 407, 410]. In addition, other proposed pathogenetic events are neovascular glaucoma, pupillary block due to pupil dilation for fundus evaluation, and ciliary block glaucoma [411–414].

Clinically, any subtype of glaucoma shows through the slit-lamp examination corneal edema, Haab's striae, and enlarged corneal diameter [407]. Gonioscopic examinations show a shallow and flat anterior chamber in cases of closed angles, for example associated with neovascularization or retinal detachment, whereas it presents in cases of post-vitrectomy or coexisting primary trabeculodysgenesis [407].

Figure 2.13 schematically illustrates the pathogenesis of secondary glaucoma occurring in advanced stages of ROP.

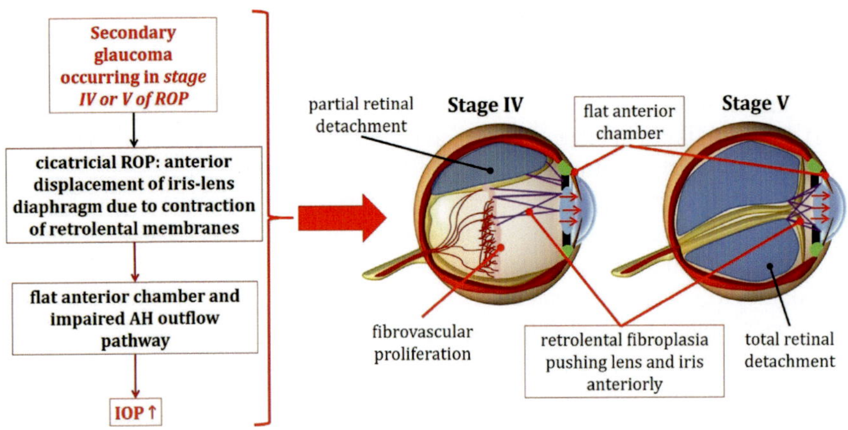

Fig. 2.13 *Scheme on the glaucomatous etiopathogenesis in advanced stages of ROP.* AH: aqueous humor; IOP: intraocular pressure

Steroid-Induced Glaucoma

Generalities: A recognized definition of steroid responsiveness is a clinically significant IOP elevation corresponding to > 10 mmHg over the baseline, that in long-term causes a glaucomatous optic neuropathy [415, 416]. Infants are at higher risk of being steroid responders, with a more rapid onset of secondary glaucoma than adults, higher frequency and worse severity [417–420]. Children under 10 years old show more rapid and severe elevations in IOP, possibly as a consequence of the incomplete degree of maturity of the drainage angle and the TM [416, 421]. Ang et al. reported that infants on long-term oral corticosteroids with severe, mixed-type of vernal keratoconjunctivitis and corneal involvement present a higher risk to develop corticosteroid response [422]. Another large investigation on 1259 cases of childhood glaucoma over a timeframe of 5 years, assessed that out of 59 children afflicted by steroid-induced glaucoma, 51 patients received topical steroids to treat vernal keratoconjunctivitis, concluding the necessity to consider steroid-sparing agents to manage vernal keratoconjunctivitis and monitor these subjects closely for glaucoma [423]. Topical steroid application is the most frequent formula employed in the clinical practice and hereby the most associated with elevation of IOP in children [417]. Importantly, the kind of corticosteroid employed as well as the treatment duration are critical factors for the development of glaucoma [424]. For example, Dexamethasone eye drops are more likely to induce glaucoma than prednisolone and fluoromethalone [424, 425]. The IOP response is typically age and dose dependent, being a higher and earlier peak of IOP associated with higher frequency of application and younger patient age [6].

Altogether, given the poor prognosis with possible evolution to irreversible visual loss in children, where possible it is recommended to discontinuing the corticosteroid therapy and eventually switch to steroid sparing medications [6, 423].

Pathogenesis and clinics: Given the lipophilic features of most corticosteroids, they permeate the epithelia and penetrate in the eye, till to the AH, already after 5–30 min of local administration [426]. Glucocorticoid receptors (GR) are expressed in the human TM [416, 427].

They are present in two isoforms, the GRα and the GRß. GRα binds glucocorticoids with high affinity and is the major biological receptor responsible of the steroid transcriptional effects, whereas GRβ does not interact with glucocorticoids and serves as negative regulator of the glucocorticoid activity [427]. A higher GRα/GRβ ratio is believed to explain the steroid responsiveness, particularly in patients with glaucoma [416]. Steroid-induced glaucoma mainly originates from augmented resistance to AH outflow [419]. In the TM cells, glucocorticoids elicit fibrogenesis and enhanced deposition of extracellular matrix, responsible of the augmented resistance of an AH drainage via the TM [427].

More specifically, the TM resistance is due to an upregulation of fibronectin, glycosaminoglycans, elastin, collagen, and laminin within the angle drainage [428, 429]. Additionally, dedicated in vitro investigations have demonstrated that a phagocytic activity in the TM is reduced through a downregulation of enzymes, such as proteases [430–432]. Taken together, structural changes in the TM, increased deposition of extracellular matrix material, and a reduced protease activity lead to an enhanced resistance to the AH facility, ultimately causing raised IOP and secondary glaucoma.

Clinically, it is noteworthy underscoring that topical drugs linked with a higher elevation in IOP are difluprednate, dexamethasone, betamethasone, and prednisolone acetate, whereas a lower rise in IOP has been reported with fluorometholone and loteprednol, with topical steroids tend to more often cause glaucoma whereas systemic steroids more often drive to cataract [416]. The steroid-induced elevation of IOP is reversible after approximatively 2–4 weeks of discontinuous therapy, unless irreversible structural changes occurred in the TM, which anyway tend to establish after a long-term therapy over one year [416].

Studies by Armaly and Becker in the 1960s assessed that around 5–6% of the general population can show a significant increase in IOP after the employment of topical ocular steroids and therefore may be considered high responders [433–435]. However, particular relevant in the clinical practice is the evidence that at least 30% of children afflicted by vernal keratoconjunctivitis may manifest unilateral visual loss deriving from an indiscriminate use of steroids, posing a critical importance for an extensive and constant ocular examination in these pediatric patients [416].

Figure 2.14 provides a scheme on the pathogenesis of steroid-induced glaucoma in children.

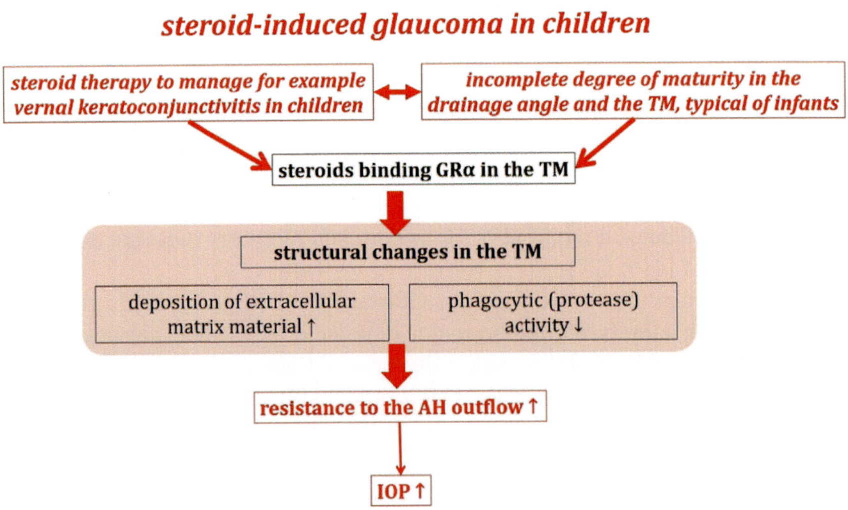

Fig. 2.14 *Scheme on the pathogenesis of steroid-induced glaucoma in children.* AH: aqueous humor; GR: glucocorticoid receptor; IOP: intraocular pressure; TM: trabecular meshwork

2.3.2.4 Glaucoma Following Cataract Surgery

As per the 2016 CGRN study, glaucoma arising after cataract surgery accounts for 18% of all cases of childhood glaucoma. This positions it as the third leading cause of glaucoma in children, following primary forms and glaucoma associated with acquired conditions [30].

Epidemiology and prognosis: Childhood cataract stands as one of the more frequent curable causes of severe visual impairment in children, being responsible of around 10–15% of pediatric blindness worldwide in individuals enrolled in schools [436]. A serious postoperative complication of pediatric cataract intervention is represented by glaucoma following cataract surgery (GFCS), previously also known as aphakic or pseudophakic glaucoma [437, 438]. Remarkably, GFCS is a major cause of blindness after successful pediatric cataract surgery [439, 440].

Depending on different follow-up durations and performed surgeries, and as a result of a substantial lack of unified diagnostic criteria for GFCS among the diverse studies, the incidence of this condition largely varies, ranging from 2 to 32% of cases [437, 441–444]. However, according to the infant aphakia treatment study (IATS), a large clinical trial including 114 children affected by unilateral congenital cataract, in the age of 1–6 months at surgery, the incidence of GFCS amounts to approximatively 22% after 10 years of follow-up [445].

A more recent epidemiological investigation in an Australian tertiary referral center assessed that on a total of 320 eyes in 216 children undergoing cataract surgery, glaucoma developed in 11.9% of eyes, with an average time to onset from surgery of 3.2 years, and a mean age of diagnosis of 4.58 years, further being microcornea the only adverse characteristic significantly associated with an increased risk of secondary glaucoma [446]. Several studies have examined and assessed numerous risk factors for GFCS [442, 444, 447–450]:

- age at lensectomy,
- intraocular lens (IOL) implantation
- type of cataract
- primary posterior capsulotomy with anterior vitrectomy
- preexisting ocular abnormalities such as microcornea
- additional intraocular surgery (reintervention)
- family history of congenital cataract or GFCS.

Regarding the timing of lensectomy, it is important to note that while early cataract intervention leads to improved visual outcomes, the risk of developing postoperative glaucoma is higher in younger children, particularly in infants below 9 months of age [451]. Despite the elevated risk of glaucoma following cataract surgery in younger individuals, delaying lensectomy is not advisable. The heightened risk of early intervention needs to be weighed against the imperative to minimize the duration of visual deprivation, thus preventing amblyopia—a condition significantly more challenging to manage than glaucoma [437, 438].

In clinical practice, diagnosing glaucoma following cataract surgery (GFCS) is notably challenging, and its manifestation can occur several years after the surgical procedure. Therefore, the consistent observation of children who have undergone cataract intervention is crucial for early detection and ongoing monitoring [6]. Thus, due to the challenging in early diagnosis and treatment initiation, GFCS is often related to a poor prognosis [441]. The first-line therapy for most cases of GFCS is pharmacological, while surgical intervention is typically indicated in case of angle-closure forms, being however an optimal surgical approach subject of discussion [441, 452, 453].

Pathogenesis and clinics: GFCS can develop as open-angle or also as angle-closure variant. Of note, the late-stage open-angle glaucoma is the major form of GFCS [454], whereas, through the progress of the pediatric surgery, a significant decrease of the rate of angle-closure variant of GFCS could be recorded [455], thereby becoming currently extremely rare [456]. Depending on the type of glaucomas, there exist different pathogenetic events that occur in case of angle-closure or in case of open-angle. Angle-closure has been associated with microcornea and sulcus/iris-placed IOLs, being further typically linked with a protracted postoperative inflammation or with uveitis, as a result of a formation of iris bombe following posterior synechiae or pupillary block [437, 451].

The pathophysiological process underlying the open-angle variant has been explained through two possible theories: the chemical and the mechanical hypotheses [437, 441].

According to the chemical theory, the impact of inflammatory material from the vitreous as well as retained lens epithelial cells after surgery, which may impair the morphology and function of the TM [457–459].

Specifically, it has been proposed that interleukin-4, alpha-B crystallin and VEGF, released from residual lens epithelial cells detectable in the anterior chamber after cataract surgery, may trigger structural and functional changes in the TM, altering its gene expression [458, 460, 461].

Furthermore, studies also underlined that an early lensectomy as well as an early and prolonged postoperative employment of high-dose steroids may also lead to structural alterations in the TM, being linked with an impairment of the physiological maturation of the angle chamber [453, 462, 463].

However, topical steroids are commonly employed in clinical practice for a duration of 1–2 months postoperatively. It is important to note that the majority of open-angle glaucoma following cataract surgery (GFCS) typically manifests many years after the surgical procedure. This raises uncertainties about the effective influence of topical steroids in the development of GFCS [437, 464–466].

According to the mechanical theory, through the lensectomy occurs a critical collapse of the TM deriving from a loss of ciliary body support and contraction, thereby leading to reduced trabecular functionality and decreased AH drainage [437, 441, 454].

Clinically, based on cataract type, GFCS is classified into 3 categories: congenital idiopathic cataract, congenital cataract associated with ocular anomalies/systemic disease and no previous glaucoma, and acquired cataract with no previous glaucoma [5]. Gonioscopy is fundamental to identify the variant of GFCS, that is subdivided into open angle, when the angle is for $\geq$ 50% open, and in angle closure when the angle is for < 50% open. Notably, the angle closure form typically occurs within 1 year after intervention, while the open angle variant generally develop several years after lensectomy [437, 465, 466]. Figure 2.15 shows a scheme on the pathogenesis of GFCS in children.

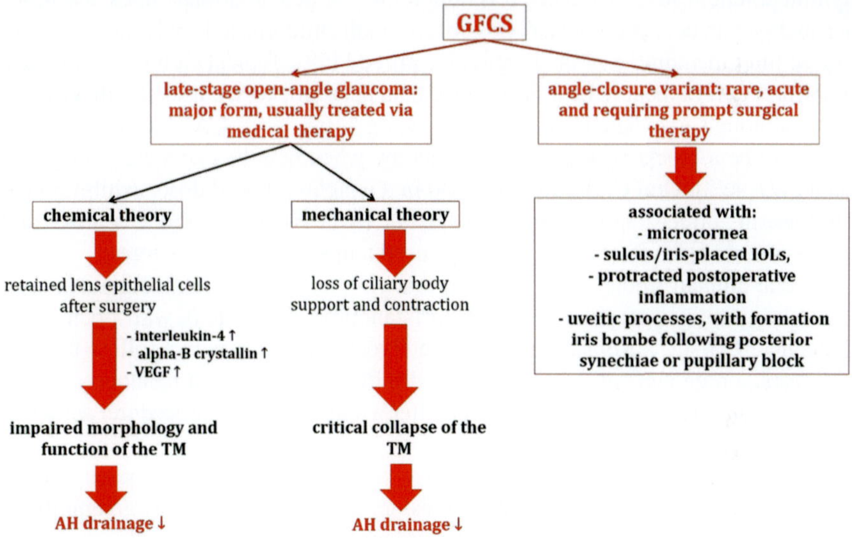

Fig. 2.15 *Scheme on the pathogenesis of glaucoma* following cataract surgery *in children.* AH: aqueous humor; GFCS: glaucoma following cataract surgery; IOL: intraocular lens; TM: trabecular meshwork; VEGF: vascular endothelial growth factor

2.4 Therapeutic Options in Childhood Glaucoma

2.4.1 Conservative Treatment Options

Medical intervention plays a crucial role in the management of childhood glaucoma, serving as both a temporary measure before surgery and as adjunctive therapy following partially successful surgical procedures [467]. However, as a standalone primary treatment, especially in PCG, medical therapy is rarely sufficient [6]. Beta-blockers, typically the first-line therapy, are employed unless contraindications such as asthma or prematurity are present. It is preferred to use the lowest dose (0.1% or 0.25%) and frequency.

Evidence suggests using beta-blockers with caution in premature and small infants, as bradycardia, bronchospasm and hypoglycemia have been reported [468]. To limit potential adverse effects, it is important to adhere to dosage times, use nasolacrimal system occlusion, if at all possible in small children, and apply the minimum dose or limit the number of medications required [468]. Topical carbonic anhydrase inhibitors (CAI) appear to be less effective than beta-blockers, but seem safe systemically, although associated with local irritation [469, 470]. CAI are useful as an adjunct to beta-blockers or as first line therapy when beta-blockers are contraindicated [471, 472]. Oral CAIs, administered in a weight-adjusted dose, exhibit potent IOP lowering effects in children. However, due to the risk of metabolic acidosis and other systemic side effects, they are often used temporarily before surgery.

Several clinical studies have reported that children with childhood glaucoma of mixed origin mixed respond less well to latanoprost than adults with open-angle glaucoma [473–477]. Remarkably, in an interventional study with a follow-up time of 3 years, a high percentage of children with PCG who received latanoprost alone and/or in combination with dorzolamide after a single surgical procedure, achieved a significant reduction in IOP [469].

Importantly, the α_2-adrenoceptor agonist, brimonidine, must be avoided in children due to the risk of bradycardia, hypotension, and apnea, which may go unnoticed in children who may be unable to express symptoms readily [478, 479].

Administration of pilocarpine to lower IOP in childhood glaucoma is not recommended, because the compound may promote cataract formation and myopia [480–482]. Additionally, in some anatomical variations, like in Weill-Marchesani syndrome, administration of pilocarpine may induce severe pupillary block [483]. However, in cases of PCG and glaucoma following cataract surgery, pre- and postoperative pilocarpine 1% may enhance angle accessibility and reduce the risk of anterior synechiae after angle surgery.

Importantly, compliance and adherence issues are greater and more complex in children on antiglaucoma medications than in adults.

2.4.2 Surgical Approaches

Childhood glaucoma presents a significant surgical challenge, especially in terms of its management. Surgery stands as the primary treatment modality and is often unavoidable throughout a child's life. The initial surgical intervention chosen typically represents the child's optimal opportunity for long-term success. Specialized procedures should ideally be conducted by trained surgeons in high-volume centers to ensure sufficient surgical experience and safe anesthesia practices. Notably, glaucoma surgeries in children carry a heightened risk of complications compared to adult cases. A lack of familiarity with buphthalmic eyes is associated with increased complications, necessitating meticulous modification and execution of surgical techniques to minimize adverse outcomes.

Various surgical procedures with distinct indications, advantages, and disadvantages are available. Referral centers with ample volume ensure skilled surgery and safe anesthesia, leading to potentially favorable success rates. The primary goal of surgery is to eliminate or bypass aqueous flow obstruction, and achieving a delicate balance between increased success and reduced complications is paramount. This equilibrium is attained through surgeon modification and the development of a technique that is both safe and effective in the hands of the surgeon. All operations pose technical challenges and potential complications, underscoring the importance of meticulous attention to detail.

The prognosis for childhood glaucoma was historically grim until Otto Barkan, employing direct gonioscopy with a specially designed lens, introduced goniotomy [484, 485]. This technique, aimed at incising the angle, revolutionized the outlook for congenital glaucoma, particularly PCG. Despite its historical impact, goniotomy faced limitations in cases with hazy corneas where angle structures were not clearly visible. A subsequent breakthrough occurred in 1960 with trabeculotomy, independently described by Redmond Smith and Hermann Burian [486, 487]. Trabeculotomy offered advantages in cases with unclear corneas, and modifications, such as Harms trabeculotome, further enhanced its utility. Endoscopic goniotomy was introduced to enable the procedure in the presence of corneal haze.

Recognizing the importance of the extent of angle incision, circumferential suture trabeculotomy was proposed in 1995 by Beck and Lynch [488]. This technique, using a blunted 6–0 prolene or an illuminated microcatheter, allows a circumferential incision in one session, potentially improving safety and technical ease.

Some authors advocate circumferential trabeculotomy as it treats the entire angle in a single session, eliminating the need for repeated surgeries.

Several studies have reported that goniotomy alone could control more than half of PCG eyes, and with additional filtering surgery, over three-fourths of cases achieved control [15, 489, 490].

Despite the prevalence of childhood glaucoma, the number of randomized controlled trials in the field has seen only marginal growth in the last decade. A recent Cochrane review, examining 16 randomized controlled trials or quasi-randomized controlled trials comparing surgical interventions for PCG, found limited evidence

[491]. For example, trials comparing combined trabeculotomy and trabeculectomy with trabeculotomy showed little to no difference in mean intraocular pressure (IOP) and surgical success at one year postoperatively. Trials comparing viscotrabeculotomy to conventional trabeculotomy also did not reveal significant differences in mean IOP and surgical success at six months postoperatively.

In contrast, trials comparing microcatheter-assisted 360-degree circumferential trabeculotomy to conventional trabeculotomy suggested potential advantages for the microcatheter group, indicating lower mean IOP at six months and a higher likelihood of surgical success at 12 months [491].

The remaining nine trials covered diverse surgical interventions, including comparisons like combined trabeculotomy and trabeculectomy versus combined trabeculotomy and trabeculectomy with sclerectomy, various suturing techniques and adjuvant use in combined trabeculotomy and trabeculectomy, combined trabeculotomy and trabeculectomy versus Ahmed valve implant in previously failed surgeries, combined trabeculotomy and trabeculectomy with trabeculectomy, trabeculotomy versus goniotomy, and different types of goniotomy. Unfortunately, none of the trials reported on quality of life or economic data, and several had limitations in study design, implementation, and reporting, leaving the reliability and applicability of the evidence unclear [491].

The lack of long-term data on the outcomes of these interventions is a notable concern, given the potentially lifelong consequences of childhood glaucoma. Future studies should incorporate measurement of quality of life metrics with a medium- to long-term follow-up to provide more comprehensive insights.

2.5 Future Directions and Concluding Remarks

Childhood glaucoma stands as a significant global cause of infantile blindness, presenting challenges for patients and healthcare systems alike. The substantial decline in patients' quality of life and the economic burdens on societies underscore the urgency of addressing this condition. The diverse and heterogeneous nature of childhood glaucoma, often misdiagnosed or detected belatedly, raises concerns regarding timely treatment initiation and effective management.

From a pathophysiological perspective, childhood glaucoma is commonly linked to developmental anomalies in the angle structures of the anterior eye segment, stemming from neural crest cells. Anomalies during embryogenesis, involving specific genes, lead to various types of glaucoma. Hence, the d the manifestations of childhood glaucoma vary clinically, categorized by age of onset, severity, and response to therapy.

A systematic classification and and a clear diagnostic algorithm have proven beneficial for physicians in differential diagnosis and categorization, while researchers benefit from standardized investigations with univocal parameters. Advancements in early screening and innovative ophthalmological imaging methods hold the potential to expedite the diagnostic process.

The management of childhood glaucoma is intricate, given the young age of patients, their reduced adherence, and the complexity of surgical procedures. Pediatric patients often undergo multiple general anesthesia procedures and numerous surgical interventions aimed at controlling IOP. Even those not requiring surgery are subjected to constant monitoring and often to pharmacological therapy. Additionally, managing nystagmus and amblyopia is crucial. Importantly, early unsuccessful angle surgery, along with nystagmus and anterior eye segment dysgenesis, serve as predictors of poor prognosis in children with glaucoma.

In summary, the current work provides insight into the diagnostic, pathophysiological, clinical, and, therapeutic facets of childhood glaucomas. The objective is to offer an updated overview to aid research efforts in combating this debilitating disease, a leading cause of irreversible visual loss in children worldwide. Addressing concerns related to early diagnosis and the complexity of current surgical therapies, future research may focus on advanced imaging procedures to enhance childhood glaucoma screening. Clinical investigations should strive to improve the current success rates of surgical interventions, minimizing postoperative adverse effects. Through ongoing scientific and clinical endeavors, research aims to improve visual outcomes for children with glaucoma, enabling them to lead satisfactory social and working lives.

References

1. Ruan Y, Buonfiglio F, Gericke A. Adrenoceptors in the eye—physiological and pathophysiological relevance. Handb Exp Pharmacol. 2023. https://doi.org/10.1007/164_2023_702.
2. Buonfiglio F, Pfeiffer N, Gericke A. Immunomodulatory and antioxidant drugs in glaucoma treatment. Pharmaceuticals (Basel). 2023;16(9). https://doi.org/10.3390/ph16091193.
3. Kingman S. Glaucoma is second leading cause of blindness globally. Bull World Health Organ. 2004;82(11):887–8.
4. Quigley HA, Broman AT. The number of people with glaucoma worldwide in 2010 and 2020. Br J Ophthalmol. 2006;90(3):262–7. https://doi.org/10.1136/bjo.2005.081224.
5. Weinreb RN, Grajewski AL, Papadopoulos M, Grigg J, Freedman S. Childhood glaucoma. Kugler Publications; 2013.
6. Karaconji T, Zagora S, Grigg JR. Approach to childhood glaucoma: a review. Clin Experiment Ophthalmol. 2022;50(2):232–46. https://doi.org/10.1111/ceo.14039.
7. Shen R, Li VSW, Wong MOM, Chan PPM. Pediatric glaucoma-from screening, early detection to management. Children (Basel). 2023;10(2). https://doi.org/10.3390/children10020181.
8. Bhattacharjee H, Das K, Borah RR, Guha K, Gogate P, Purukayastha S, et al. Causes of childhood blindness in the northeastern states of India. Indian J Ophthalmol. 2008;56(6):495.
9. Dorairaj SK, Bandrakalli P, Shetty C, Misquith D, Ritch R. Childhood blindness in a rural population of southern India: prevalence and etiology. Ophthalmic Epidemiol. 2008;15(3):176–82.
10. Durnian J, Cheeseman R, Kumar A, Raja V, Newman W, Chandna A. Childhood sight impairment: a 10-year picture. Eye. 2010;24(1):112–7.

11. Aponte EP, Diehl N, Mohney BG. Incidence and clinical characteristics of childhood glaucoma: a population-based study. Arch Ophthalmol. 2010;128(4):478–82. https://doi.org/10.1001/archophthalmol.2010.41.
12. Papadopoulos M, Cable N, Rahi J, Khaw PT, Investigators BES. The British infantile and childhood glaucoma (BIG) eye study. Invest Ophthalmol Vis Sci. 2007;48(9):4100–6.
13. Alanazi FF, Song JC, Mousa A, Morales J, Al Shahwan S, Alodhayb S, et al. Primary and secondary congenital glaucoma: baseline features from a registry at King Khaled Eye Specialist Hospital, Riyadh, Saudi Arabia. Am J Ophthal. 2013;155(5):882–9. e1.
14. Lopes NLV, Gracitelli CP, Moura CRd. Creation of a childhood glaucoma registry database. Arquivos Brasileiros de Oftalmologia. 2018;81:271–5.
15. MacKinnon JR, Giubilato A, Elder JE, Craig JE, Mackey DA. Primary infantile glaucoma in an Australian population. Clin Experiment Ophthalmol. 2004;32(1):14–8.
16. Taylor RH, Ainsworth JR, Evans AR, Levin AV. The epidemiology of pediatric glaucoma: the Toronto experience. J aapos. 1999;3(5):308–15. https://doi.org/10.1016/s1091-8531(99)70028-5.
17. Jaafar M. Care of the infantile glaucoma patient. Ophthalmology annual. 1988;7:15–37.
18. Dandona L, Williams JD, Williams BC, Rao GN. Population-based assessment of childhood blindness in southern India. Arch Ophthalmol. 1998;116(4):545–6.
19. Gencik A, Gencikova A, Ferák V. Population genetical aspects of primary congenital glaucoma. I. Incidence, prevalence, gene frequency, and age of onset. Hum Genet. 1982;61(3):193–7. https://doi.org/10.1007/bf00296440.
20. Chong C, McGhee CN, Dai SH. Causes of childhood low vision and blindness in New Zealand. Clin Experiment Ophthalmol. 2019;47(2):165–70.
21. Gilbert C, Canovas R, Hagan M, Rao S, Foster A. Causes of childhood blindness: results from west Africa, south India and Chile. Eye. 1993;7(1):184–8.
22. Kong L, Fry M, Al-Samarraie M, Gilbert C, Steinkuller PG. An update on progress and the changing epidemiology of causes of childhood blindness worldwide. Journal of American Association for Pediatric Ophthalmology and Strabismus. 2012;16(6):501–7.
23. Mezer E, Chetrit A, Kalter-Leibovici O, Kinori M, Ben-Zion I, Wygnanski-Jaffe T. Trends in the incidence and causes of severe visual impairment and blindness in children from Israel. Journal of American Association for Pediatric Ophthalmology and Strabismus. 2015;19(3):260–5. e1.
24. Tabbara KF, Badr IA. Changing pattern of childhood blindness in Saudi Arabia. Br J Ophthalmol. 1985;69(4):312.
25. Aghayeva FA, Schuster AK, Diel H, Chronopoulos P, Wagner FM, Grehn F, et al. Childhood glaucoma registry in Germany: initial database, clinical care and research (pilot study). BMC Res Notes. 2022;15(1):32. https://doi.org/10.1186/s13104-022-05921-8.
26. Liu D, Huang L, Mukkamala L, Khouri AS. The economic burden of childhood glaucoma. J Glaucoma. 2016;25(10):790–7. https://doi.org/10.1097/ijg.0000000000000412.
27. Ben-Zion I, Tomkins O, Moore DB, Helveston EM. Surgical results in the management of advanced primary congenital glaucoma in a rural pediatric population. Ophthalmology. 2011;118(2):231–5. e1.
28. McLaughlin DE, Semrov A, Munshi H, Patel AJ, Rahi J, Grajewski AL. The impact of childhood glaucoma on psychosocial functioning and quality of life: a review of the literature. Eye (Lond). 2023;37(15):3157–73. https://doi.org/10.1038/s41433-023-02492-1.
29. Thau A, Lloyd M, Freedman S, Beck A, Grajewski A, Levin AV. New classification system for pediatric glaucoma: implications for clinical care and a research registry. Curr Opin Ophthalmol. 2018;29(5):385–94.
30. Hoguet A, Grajewski A, Hodapp E, Chang TC. A retrospective survey of childhood glaucoma prevalence according to Childhood Glaucoma Research Network classification. Indian J Ophthalmol. 2016;64(2):118–23. https://doi.org/10.4103/0301-4738.179716.
31. Neustein RF, Bruce BB, Beck AD. Primary congenital glaucoma versus glaucoma following congenital cataract surgery: comparative clinical features and long-term outcomes. Am J Ophthalmol. 2016;170:214–22. https://doi.org/10.1016/j.ajo.2016.08.012.

32. Greenberg MB, Osigian CJ, Cavuoto KM, Chang TC. Clinical management outcomes of childhood glaucoma suspects. PLoS ONE. 2017;12(9): e0185546. https://doi.org/10.1371/journal.pone.0185546.
33. Zagora SL, Funnell CL, Martin FJ, Smith JE, Hing S, Billson FA, et al. Primary congenital glaucoma outcomes: lessons from 23 years of follow-up. Am J Ophthalmol. 2015;159(4):788–96. https://doi.org/10.1016/j.ajo.2015.01.019.
34. Bayoumi NH. Fellow eye in unilateral primary congenital glaucoma. J Curr Glaucoma Pract. 2017;11(1):28–30. https://doi.org/10.5005/jp-journals-10008-1217.
35. Kaur S, Kaushik S, Singh PS. Traumatic glaucoma in children. J Curr Glaucoma Pract. 2014;8(2):58–62. https://doi.org/10.5005/jp-journals-10008-1162.
36. Sarohia GS, Elsayed M, Solarte CE, Hornby SJ, Brookes J, Chang TCP, et al. Outcome measures in childhood glaucoma: a systematic review of randomized controlled trials. Graefes Arch Clin Exp Ophthalmol. 2023;261(9):2625–39. https://doi.org/10.1007/s00417-023-06061-w.
37. Qiao C-y, Wang L-h, Xin T, Tao W, Yang D-y, Wang N-l. Epidemiology of hospitalized pediatric glaucoma patients in Beijing Tongren Hospital. Chinese Med. J. 2009;122(10):1162–6.
38. Bouhenni RA, Ricker I, Hertle RW. Prevalence and clinical characteristics of childhood glaucoma at a tertiary care Children's hospital. J Glaucoma. 2019;28(7):655–9. https://doi.org/10.1097/ijg.0000000000001259.
39. Lopes NL, Gracitelli CPB, Rolim-de-Moura C. Childhood glaucoma profile in a Brazilian tertiary care center using childhood glaucoma research network classification. J Glaucoma. 2021;30(2):129–33. https://doi.org/10.1097/ijg.0000000000001712.
40. Mokbel TH, El Hefney EM, Hagras SM, AA AL, Badawi AE, Kasem MA, et al. Childhood glaucoma profile in Dakahelia, Egypt: a retrospective study. Int J Ophthalmol. 2018;11(4):674–80. https://doi.org/10.18240/ijo.2018.04.23.
41. Papadopoulos M, Vanner EA, Grajewski AL. International study of childhood glaucoma. Ophthalmol Glaucoma. 2020;3(2):145–57. https://doi.org/10.1016/j.ogla.2019.12.007.
42. Leite A, Rolim-de-Moura C. Referral reasons for evaluating childhood glaucoma in a tertiary service. Arq Bras Oftalmol. 2022;85(5):465–71. https://doi.org/10.5935/0004-2749.20220067.
43. Flemmons MS, Hsiao YC, Dzau J, Asrani S, Jones S, Freedman SF. Icare rebound tonometry in children with known and suspected glaucoma. J aapos. 2011;15(2):153–7. https://doi.org/10.1016/j.jaapos.2010.11.022.
44. Grigorian F, Grigorian AP, Olitsky SE. The use of the iCare tonometer reduced the need for anesthesia to measure intraocular pressure in children. J aapos. 2012;16(6):508–10. https://doi.org/10.1016/j.jaapos.2012.07.004.
45. Kageyama M, Hirooka K, Baba T, Shiraga F. Comparison of ICare rebound tonometer with noncontact tonometer in healthy children. J Glaucoma. 2011;20(1):63–6. https://doi.org/10.1097/IJG.0b013e3181d12dc4.
46. Lundvall A, Svedberg H, Chen E. Application of the ICare rebound tonometer in healthy infants. J Glaucoma. 2011;20(1):7–9. https://doi.org/10.1097/IJG.0b013e3181d1d1ef.
47. Dahlmann-Noor AH, Puertas R, Tabasa-Lim S, El-Karmouty A, Kadhim M, Wride NK, et al. Comparison of handheld rebound tonometry with Goldmann applanation tonometry in children with glaucoma: a cohort study. BMJ Open. 2013;3(4). https://doi.org/10.1136/bmjopen-2012-001788.
48. Rao A, Kumar M, Prakash B, Varshney G. Relationship of central corneal thickness and intraocular pressure by iCare rebound tonometer. J Glaucoma. 2014;23(6):380–4. https://doi.org/10.1097/IJG.0b013e318279b819.
49. Hohberger B, Sommerfeld C, Lucio M, Bergua A. ICare Pro: age dependent effect of central corneal thickness on intraocular pressure in glaucoma and ocular hypertension patients. Curr Eye Res. 2020;45(6):668–74. https://doi.org/10.1080/02713683.2019.1696977.
50. Bradfield YS, Melia BM, Repka MX, Kaminski BM, Davitt BV, Johnson DA, et al. Central corneal thickness in children. Arch Ophthalmol. 2011;129(9):1132–8. https://doi.org/10.1001/archophthalmol.2011.225.

51. Lopes JE, Wilson RR, Alvim HS, Shields CL, Shields JA, Calhoun J, et al. Central corneal thickness in pediatric glaucoma. J Pediatr Ophthalmol Strabismus. 2007;44(2):112–7. https://doi.org/10.3928/01913913-20070301-05.
52. Lopez JP, Freedman SF, Muir K, Duncan L, Stephens D, Atenafu E, et al. Central corneal thickness in children and adolescents with pediatric glaucoma and eye disorders at risk of developing glaucoma. J Pediatr Ophthalmol Strabismus. 2011;48(2):108–16. https://doi.org/10.3928/01913913-20100518-03.
53. Wygnanski-Jaffe T, Barequet IS. Central corneal thickness in congenital glaucoma. Cornea. 2006;25(8):923–5. https://doi.org/10.1097/01.ico.0000225712.62511.1c.
54. Lupinacci AP, da Silva Jordão ML, Massa G, Arieta CE, Costa VP. Central corneal thickness in children with congenital cataract and children with surgical aphakia: a case-control study. Br J Ophthalmol. 2009;93(3):337–41. https://doi.org/10.1136/bjo.2008.137596.
55. Chen TC, Walton DS, Bhatia LS. Aphakic glaucoma after congenital cataract surgery. Arch Ophthalmol. 2004;122(12):1819–25. https://doi.org/10.1001/archopht.122.12.1819.
56. Webb TR, Matarin M, Gardner JC, Kelberman D, Hassan H, Ang W, et al. X-linked megalocornea caused by mutations in CHRDL1 identifies an essential role for ventroptin in anterior segment development. Am J Hum Genet. 2012;90(2):247–59. https://doi.org/10.1016/j.ajhg.2011.12.019.
57. Shen L, You QS, Xu X, Gao F, Zhang Z, Li B, et al. Scleral and choroidal thickness in secondary high axial myopia. Retina. 2016;36(8):1579–85. https://doi.org/10.1097/iae.0000000000000947.
58. Sampaolesi R. Ocular echometry, a new parameter in the diagnosis and prevention of the development of congenital glaucoma. Bull Mem Soc Fr Ophtalmol. 1983;95:401–9.
59. Bach A, Villegas VM, Gold AS, Shi W, Murray TG. Axial length development in children. Int J Ophthalmol. 2019;12(5):815–9. https://doi.org/10.18240/ijo.2019.05.18.
60. Sampaolesi R. Corneal diameter and axial length in congenital glaucoma. Can J Ophthalmol. 1988;23(1):42–4.
61. Law SK, Bui D, Caprioli J. Serial axial length measurements in congenital glaucoma. Am J Ophthalmol. 2001;132(6):926–8. https://doi.org/10.1016/s0002-9394(01)01183-7.
62. Kiefer G, Schwenn O, Grehn F. Correlation of postoperative axial length growth and intraocular pressure in congenital glaucoma–a retrospective study in trabeculotomy and goniotomy. Graefes Arch Clin Exp Ophthalmol. 2001;239(12):893–9. https://doi.org/10.1007/s00417-001-0377-3.
63. Hylton C, Giangiacomo A, Beck A. 34 - Childhood Glaucomas. In: Shaarawy TM, Sherwood MB, Hitchings RA, Crowston JG, editors. Glaucoma (Second Edition). W.B. Saunders; 2015. p. 387–400.
64. Normal Chamber Angle in Newborns and Children. In: Sampaolesi R, Sampaolesi JR, Zárate J, editors. The Glaucomas: Volume I - Pediatric Glaucomas. Berlin, Heidelberg: Springer Berlin Heidelberg; 2009. p. 99–106.
65. Kaginalkar A, Gupta S, Gupta V. Childhood Glaucoma: Gonioscopy. In: Gupta S, Mahalingam K, Gupta V, editors. Childhood glaucoma: a case based color and video atlas. Singapore: Springer Nature Singapore; 2023. p. 43–54.
66. Sharma R, Sharma A, Arora T, Sharma S, Sobti A, Jha B, et al. Application of anterior segment optical coherence tomography in glaucoma. Surv Ophthalmol. 2014;59(3):311–27. https://doi.org/10.1016/j.survophthal.2013.06.005.
67. Edawaji BSA, Gottlob I, Proudlock FA. Anterior chamber measurements in healthy children: a cross-sectional study using optical coherence tomography. Transl Vis Sci Technol. 2021;10(6):13. https://doi.org/10.1167/tvst.10.6.13.
68. Gupta V, Chaurasia AK, Gupta S, Gorimanipalli B, Sharma A, Gupta A. In vivo analysis of angle dysgenesis in primary congenital, juvenile, and adult-onset open angle glaucoma. Invest Ophthalmol Vis Sci. 2017;58(13):6000–5. https://doi.org/10.1167/iovs.17-22695.
69. Gupta V, Jha R, Srinivasan G, Dada T, Sihota R. Ultrasound biomicroscopic characteristics of the anterior segment in primary congenital glaucoma. J aapos. 2007;11(6):546–50. https://doi.org/10.1016/j.jaapos.2007.06.014.

70. Janssens R, van Rijn LJ, Eggink CA, Jansonius NM, Janssen SF. Ultrasound biomicroscopy of the anterior segment in patients with primary congenital glaucoma: a review of the literature. Acta Ophthalmol. 2022;100(6):605–13. https://doi.org/10.1111/aos.15082.
71. Singh A, Mahalingam K, Gupta S. Fundus Evaluation in Childhood Glaucoma. In: Gupta S, Mahalingam K, Gupta V, editors. Childhood Glaucoma: A Case Based Color and Video Atlas. Singapore: Springer Nature Singapore; 2023. p. 55–64.
72. Agarwal K, Vinekar A, Chandra P, Padhi TR, Nayak S, Jayanna S, et al. Imaging the pediatric retina: an overview. Indian J Ophthalmol. 2021;69(4):812–23. https://doi.org/10.4103/ijo.IJO_1917_20.
73. Erraguntla V, MacKeen LD, Atenafu E, Stephens D, Buncic JR, Budning AS, et al. Assessment of change of optic nerve head cupping in pediatric glaucoma using the RetCam 120. J Am Ass Pediatric Ophthal Strabismus. 2006;10(6):528–33.
74. Kaur R, Singh H, Samria S, Kumar N, Parachuri N, Sharma R, et al. MII RetCam assisted smartphone-based fundus imaging (MSFI)—A boon for paediatric retinal imaging. Eye. 2020;34(8):1307–9. https://doi.org/10.1038/s41433-020-0822-3.
75. Sharma A, Goyal A, Bilong Y, Shah P, Banker A, Kumar N, et al. Comparison of a smartphone-based photography method with indirect ophthalmoscopic assessment in referable retinopathy of prematurity: a smart retinopathy of prematurity model pilot study. Ophthalmology Retina. 2019;3(10):911–2.
76. Goyal A, Gopalakrishnan M, Anantharaman G, Chandrashekharan DP, Thachil T, Sharma A. Smartphone guided wide-field imaging for retinopathy of prematurity in neonatal intensive care unit–a Smart ROP (SROP) initiative. Indian J Ophthalmol. 2019;67(6):840.
77. Shen R, Li VSW, Wong MOM, Chan PPM. Pediatric glaucoma—from screening, early detection to management. Children. 2023. https://doi.org/10.3390/children10020181.
78. Kitaguchi Y, Hayakawa R, Kawashima R, Matsushita K, Tanaka H, Kawasaki R, et al. Deep-learning approach to detect childhood glaucoma based on periocular photograph. Sci Rep. 2023;13(1):10141. https://doi.org/10.1038/s41598-023-37389-2.
79. Harju M, Saari J, Kurvinen L, Vesti E. Reversal of optic disc cupping in glaucoma. Br J Ophthalmol. 2008;92(7):901–5. https://doi.org/10.1136/bjo.2007.135350.
80. Ghasia FF, El-Dairi M, Freedman SF, Rajani A, Asrani S. Reproducibility of spectral-domain optical coherence tomography measurements in adult and Pediatric Glaucoma. J Glaucoma. 2015;24(1):55–63. https://doi.org/10.1097/IJG.0b013e31829521db.
81. Lever M, Halfwassen C, Unterlauft JD, Bechrakis NE, Manthey A, Böhm MRR. The paediatric glaucoma diagnostic ability of optical coherence tomography: a comparison of macular segmentation and peripapillary retinal nerve fibre layer thickness. Biology. 2021;10(4):260.
82. Shoji T, Sato H, Ishida M, Takeuchi M, Chihara E. Assessment of glaucomatous changes in subjects with high myopia using spectral domain optical coherence tomography. Invest Ophthalmol Vis Sci. 2011;52(2):1098–102. https://doi.org/10.1167/iovs.10-5922.
83. Rao A, Sahoo B, Kumar M, Varshney G, Kumar R. Retinal nerve fiber layer thickness in children <18 years by spectral-domain optical coherence tomography. Semin Ophthalmol. 2013;28(2):97–102. https://doi.org/10.3109/08820538.2012.760626.
84. Goh JP, Koh V, Chan YH, Ngo C. Macular ganglion cell and retinal nerve fiber layer thickness in children with refractive errors—an optical coherence tomography study. J Glaucoma. 2017;26(7):619–25. https://doi.org/10.1097/ijg.0000000000000683.
85. Shah SD, Haq A, Toufeeq S, Tu Z, Edawaji B, Abbott J, et al. Reliability and recommended settings for pediatric circumpapillary retinal nerve fiber layer imaging using hand-held optical coherence tomography. Translational Vision Science & Technology. 2020;9(7):43-.
86. Lee H, Purohit R, Patel A, Papageorgiou E, Sheth V, Maconachie G, et al. In vivo foveal development using optical coherence tomography. Invest Ophthalmol Vis Sci. 2015;56(8):4537–45.
87. Go MS, Barman NR, Kelly MP, House RJ, Rotruck JC, El-Dairi MA, et al. Overhead mounted optical coherence tomography in childhood glaucoma evaluation. J Glaucoma. 2020;29(9):742–9.
88. Pilat AV, Shah S, Sheth V, Purohit R, Proudlock FA, Abbott J, et al. Detection and characterisation of optic nerve and retinal changes in primary congenital glaucoma using hand-held optical coherence tomography. BMJ Open Ophthalmol. 2019;4(1).

89. Rolando M, Capris P, Gandolfo E, Burtolo C, Calabria GA, Zingirian M. Perimetry in Congenital and Infantile Glaucoma. In: Greve EL, Leydhecker W, Raitta C, editors. Second European Glaucoma Symposium, Helsinki, May 1984. Dordrecht: Springer, Netherlands; 1985. p. 65–8.
90. Sinha G, Patil B, Sihota R, Gupta V, Nayak B, Sharma R, et al. Visual field loss in primary congenital glaucoma. J aapos. 2015;19(2):124–9. https://doi.org/10.1016/j.jaapos.2014.12.008.
91. Patel DE, Walters BC, Russell-Eggitt I, Rahi JS, Cumberland P. OPTIC study: feasibility and reliability of perimetry in children with glaucoma. Investigative Ophthalmology & Visual Science. 2016;57(12):3935-.
92. Patel DE, Cumberland PM, Walters BC, Abbott J, Brookes J, Edmunds B, et al. Study of Optimal Perimetric Testing In Children (OPTIC): developing consensus and setting research priorities for perimetry in the management of children with glaucoma. Eye. 2022;36(6):1281–7. https://doi.org/10.1038/s41433-021-01584-0.
93. Meire FM, Bleeker-Wagemakers EM, Oehler M, Gal A, Delleman JW. X-linked megalocornea. Ocular findings and linkage analysis. Ophthalmic Paediatr Genet. 1991;12(3):153–7. https://doi.org/10.3109/13816819109029398.
94. Meire FM. Megalocornea. Clinical and genetic aspects Doc Ophthalmol. 1994;87(1):1–121. https://doi.org/10.1007/bf01676641.
95. Roche O, Dureau P, Uteza Y, Dufier JL. Congenital megalocornea. J Fr Ophtalmol. 2002;25(3):312–8.
96. Skuta GL, Sugar J, Ericson ES. Corneal endothelial cell measurements in megalocornea. Arch Ophthalmol. 1983;101(1):51–3. https://doi.org/10.1001/archopht.1983.01040010053007.
97. Sakuta H, Suzuki R, Takahashi H, Kato A, Shintani T, Iemura S, et al. Ventroptin: a BMP-4 antagonist expressed in a double-gradient pattern in the retina. Science. 2001;293(5527):111–5. https://doi.org/10.1126/science.1058379.
98. Liu T, Li B, Zheng XF, Jiang SD, Zhou ZZ, Xu WN, et al. Chordin-Like 1 improves osteogenesis of bone marrow mesenchymal stem cells through enhancing BMP4-SMAD pathway. Front Endocrinol (Lausanne). 2019;10:360. https://doi.org/10.3389/fendo.2019.00360.
99. Pfirrmann T, Emmerich D, Ruokonen P, Quandt D, Buchen R, Fischer-Zirnsak B, et al. Molecular mechanism of CHRDL1-mediated X-linked megalocornea in humans and in Xenopus model. Hum Mol Genet. 2015;24(11):3119–32. https://doi.org/10.1093/hmg/ddv063.
100. Davidson AE, Cheong SS, Hysi PG, Venturini C, Plagnol V, Ruddle JB, et al. Association of CHRDL1 mutations and variants with X-linked megalocornea, Neuhäuser syndrome and central corneal thickness. PLoS ONE. 2014;9(8): e104163. https://doi.org/10.1371/journal.pone.0104163.
101. Dudakova L, Tuft S, Cheong S-S, Skalicka P, Jedlickova J, Fichtl M, et al. Novel disease-causing variants and phenotypic features of X-linked megalocornea. Acta Ophthalmol. 2022;100(4):431–9. https://doi.org/10.1111/aos.15022.
102. Vithana EN, Morgan P, Sundaresan P, Ebenezer ND, Tan DT, Mohamed MD, et al. Mutations in sodium-borate cotransporter SLC4A11 cause recessive congenital hereditary endothelial dystrophy (CHED2). Nat Genet. 2006;38(7):755–7. https://doi.org/10.1038/ng1824.
103. Desir J, Abramowicz M. Congenital hereditary endothelial dystrophy with progressive sensorineural deafness (Harboyan syndrome). Orphanet J Rare Dis. 2008;3:28. https://doi.org/10.1186/1750-1172-3-28.
104. Ashar JN, Ramappa M, Vaddavalli PK. Paired-eye comparison of Descemet's stripping endothelial keratoplasty and penetrating keratoplasty in children with congenital hereditary endothelial dystrophy. Br J Ophthalmol. 2013;97(10):1247–9. https://doi.org/10.1136/bjophthalmol-2012-302602.
105. Patel SP, Parker MD. SLC4A11 and the pathophysiology of congenital hereditary endothelial dystrophy. Biomed Res Int. 2015;2015: 475392. https://doi.org/10.1155/2015/475392.
106. Aldave AJ, Han J, Frausto RF. Genetics of the corneal endothelial dystrophies: an evidence-based review. Clin Genet. 2013;84(2):109–19. https://doi.org/10.1111/cge.12191.
107. Paliwal P, Sharma A, Tandon R, Sharma N, Titiyal JS, Sen S, et al. Congenital hereditary endothelial dystrophy - mutation analysis of SLC4A11 and genotype-phenotype correlation in a North Indian patient cohort. Mol Vis. 2010;16:2955–63.

108. Hoguet A, Grajewski A, Hodapp E, Chang TCP. A retrospective survey of childhood glaucoma prevalence according to childhood glaucoma research network classification. Indian J Ophthalmol. 2016;64(2):118.
109. Sharafieh R, Child A, Sarfarazi M. Molecular genetics of primary congenital glaucoma. Oxford Monographs on Medical Genetics. 2012;61(1):295–310.
110. Mandal AK. Current concepts in the diagnosis and management of developmental glaucomas. Ind J Ophthalmol. 1993;41(2):51–70.
111. deLuise VP, Anderson DR. Primary infantile glaucoma (congenital glaucoma). Surv Ophthalmol. 1983;28(1):1–19.
112. Mandal AK, Chakrabarti D, Gothwal VK. Approach to primary congenital glaucoma: a perspective. Taiwan J Ophthalmol. 2023;13(4):451–60. https://doi.org/10.4103/tjo.TJO-D-23-00104.
113. Esfandiari H, Prager A, Hassanpour K, Kurup SP, Mets-Halgrimson R, Yoon H, et al. The long-term visual outcomes of primary congenital glaucoma. J Ophthalmic Vis Res. 2020;15(3):326–30. https://doi.org/10.18502/jovr.v15i3.7451.
114. Esfandiari H, Basith SST, Kurup SP, Mets-Halgrimson R, Hassanpour K, Yoon H, et al. Long-term surgical outcomes of ab externo trabeculotomy in the management of primary congenital glaucoma. J aapos. 2019;23(4):222.e1-.e5. https://doi.org/10.1016/j.jaapos.2019.05.008.
115. Genĉík A. Epidemiology and genetics of primary congenital glaucoma in Slovakia. Description of a form of primary congenital glaucoma in gypsies with autosomal-recessive inheritance and complete penetrance. Developments in ophthalmology. 1989;16:76–115.
116. Sarfarazi M, Stoilov I, Schenkman JB. Genetics and biochemistry of primary congenital glaucoma. Ophthalmology clinics of North America. 2003;16(4):543–54, vi.
117. Tamçelik N, Atalay E, Bolukbasi S, Çapar O, Ozkok A. Demographic features of subjects with congenital glaucoma. Indian J Ophthalmol. 2014;62(5):565.
118. Badawi AH, Al-Muhaylib AA, Al Owaifeer AM, Al-Essa RS, Al-Shahwan SA. Primary congenital glaucoma: an updated review. Saudi J Ophthalmol. 2019;33(4):382–8. https://doi.org/10.1016/j.sjopt.2019.10.002.
119. Al-Rajhi A, Awad A, Badeeb O, Bukhari A, Al-Qahtani S, Mulla I, et al. Causes of blindness in students attending schools for the blind in Saudi Arabia. Saudi J Ophthalmol. 2003;17(4):276–80.
120. Fung DS, Roensch MA, Kooner KS, Cavanagh HD, Whitson JT. Epidemiology and characteristics of childhood glaucoma: results from the dallas glaucoma registry. Clin Ophthalmol. 2013:1739–46.
121. de Silva DJ, Khaw PT, Brookes JL. Long-term outcome of primary congenital glaucoma. J Aapos. 2011;15(2):148–52. https://doi.org/10.1016/j.jaapos.2010.11.025.
122. Ling C, Zhang D, Zhang J, Sun H, Du Q, Li X. Updates on the molecular genetics of primary congenital glaucoma (Review). Exp Ther Med. 2020;20(2):968–77. https://doi.org/10.3892/etm.2020.8767.
123. Doshi M, Marcus C, Bejjani BA, Edward DP. Immunolocalization of CYP1B1 in normal, human, fetal and adult eyes. Exp Eye Res. 2006;82(1):24–32. https://doi.org/10.1016/j.exer.2005.04.016.
124. Stoilov I, Akarsu AN, Sarfarazi M. Identification of three different truncating mutations in cytochrome P4501B1 (CYP1B1) as the principal cause of primary congenital glaucoma (Buphthalmos) in families linked to the GLC3A locus on chromosome 2p21. Hum Mol Genet. 1997;6(4):641–7.
125. Moore DB, Tomkins O, Ben-Zion I. A review of primary congenital glaucoma in the developing world. Surv Ophthalmol. 2013;58(3):278–85.
126. Souzeau E, Dubowsky A, Ruddle JB, Craig JE. Primary congenital glaucoma due to paternal uniparental isodisomy of chromosome 2 and CYP1B1 deletion. Mol Genet Genomic Med. 2019;7(8): e774.
127. Faiq MA, Dada R, Qadri R, Dada T. CYP1B1-mediated pathobiology of primary congenital glaucoma. J Current Glaucoma Practice. 2015;9(3):77.
128. Khan AO. Genetics of primary glaucoma. Curr Opin Ophthalmol. 2011;22(5):347–55.

129. Zhao Y, Sorenson CM, Sheibani N. Cytochrome P450 1B1 and primary congenital glaucoma. J Ophthalmic Vis Res. 2015;10(1):60–7. https://doi.org/10.4103/2008-322x.156116.
130. Rauf B, Irum B, Khan SY, Kabir F, Naeem MA, Riazuddin S, et al. Novel mutations in LTBP2 identified in familial cases of primary congenital glaucoma. Mol Vis. 2020;26:14–25.
131. Suri F, Yazdani S, Elahi E. LTBP2 knockdown and oxidative stress affect glaucoma features including TGFβ pathways, ECM genes expression and apoptosis in trabecular meshwork cells. Gene. 2018;673:70–81. https://doi.org/10.1016/j.gene.2018.06.038.
132. Inoue T, Ohbayashi T, Fujikawa Y, Yoshida H, Akama TO, Noda K, et al. Latent TGF-β binding protein-2 is essential for the development of ciliary zonule microfibrils. Hum Mol Genet. 2014;23(21):5672–82.
133. Cascella R, Strafella C, Germani C, Novelli G, Ricci F, Zampatti S, et al. The genetics and the genomics of primary congenital glaucoma. Biomed Res Int. 2015;2015: 321291. https://doi.org/10.1155/2015/321291.
134. Wang S-L, Piao S-Y, Xu M-Y, Zhang W, Ma J-Q, Hao J, et al. Evaluating correlation between the ocular biometry and genetic variants of MYOC and ABCA1 with primary angle-closure glaucoma in a cohort from northern China. Int J Ophthalmol. 2019;12(8):1317.
135. Lines MA, Kozlowski K, Walter MA. Molecular genetics of Axenfeld-Rieger malformations. Hum Mol Genet. 2002;11(10):1177–87.
136. Nishimura DY, Swiderski RE, Alward WL, Searby CC, Patil SR, Bennet SR, et al. The forkhead transcription factor gene FKHL7 is responsible for glaucoma phenotypes which map to 6p25. Nat Genet. 1998;19(2):140–7. https://doi.org/10.1038/493.
137. Wang WH, McNatt LG, Shepard AR, Jacobson N, Nishimura DY, Stone EM, et al. Optimal procedure for extracting RNA from human ocular tissues and expression profiling of the congenital glaucoma gene FOXC1 using quantitative RT-PCR. Mol Vis. 2001;7:89–94.
138. Chakrabarti S, Kaur K, Rao KN, Mandal AK, Kaur I, Parikh RS, et al. The transcription factor gene FOXC1 exhibits a limited role in primary congenital Glaucoma. Invest Ophthalmol Vis Sci. 2009;50(1):75–83. https://doi.org/10.1167/iovs.08-2253.
139. Smith RS, Zabaleta A, Kume T, Savinova OV, Kidson SH, Martin JE, et al. Haploinsufficiency of the transcription factors FOXC1 and FOXC2 results in aberrant ocular development. Hum Mol Genet. 2000;9(7):1021–32. https://doi.org/10.1093/hmg/9.7.1021.
140. Siggs OM, Souzeau E, Pasutto F, Dubowsky A, Smith JEH, Taranath D, et al. Prevalence of FOXC1 variants in individuals with a suspected diagnosis of primary congenital glaucoma. JAMA Ophthalmol. 2019;137(4):348–55. https://doi.org/10.1001/jamaophthalmol.2018.5646.
141. Mauri L, Uebe S, Sticht H, Vossmerbaeumer U, Weisschuh N, Manfredini E, et al. Expanding the clinical spectrum of COL1A1 mutations in different forms of glaucoma. Orphanet J Rare Dis. 2016;11:1–12.
142. Vithana EN, Aung T, Khor CC, Cornes BK, Tay W-T, Sim X, et al. Collagen-related genes influence the glaucoma risk factor, central corneal thickness. Hum Mol Genet. 2011;20(4):649–58.
143. Dimasi DP, Chen JY, Hewitt AW, Klebe S, Davey R, Stirling J, et al. Novel quantitative trait loci for central corneal thickness identified by candidate gene analysis of osteogenesis imperfecta genes. Hum Genet. 2010;127:33–44.
144. Thomson BR, Souma T, Tompson SW, Onay T, Kizhatil K, Siggs OM, et al. Angiopoietin-1 is required for Schlemm's canal development in mice and humans. J Clin Invest. 2017;127(12):4421–36. https://doi.org/10.1172/jci95545.
145. Thurston G, Wang Q, Baffert F, Rudge J, Papadopoulos N, Jean-Guillaume D, et al. Angiopoietin 1 causes vessel enlargement, without angiogenic sprouting, during a critical developmental period. 2005.
146. Partanen J, Armstrong E, Mäkelä TP, Korhonen J, Sandberg M, Renkonen R, et al. A novel endothelial cell surface receptor tyrosine kinase with extracellular epidermal growth factor homology domains. Mol Cell Biol. 1992;12(4):1698–707.
147. Kizhatil K, Ryan M, Marchant JK, Henrich S, John SW. Schlemm's canal is a unique vessel with a combination of blood vascular and lymphatic phenotypes that forms by a novel developmental process. PLoS Biol. 2014;12(7): e1001912.

148. Dumont DJ, Fong GH, Puri MC, Gradwohl G, Alitalo K, Breitman ML. Vascularization of the mouse embryo: a study of flk-1, tek, tie, and vascular endothelial growth factor expression during development. Dev Dyn. 1995;203(1):80–92.
149. Dumont D, Yamaguchi T, Conlon R, Rossant J, Breitman M. Tek, a novel tyrosine kinase gene located on mouse chromosome 4, is expressed in endothelial cells and their presumptive precursors. Oncogene. 1992;7(8):1471–80.
150. Aspelund A, Tammela T, Antila S, Nurmi H, Leppänen V-M, Zarkada G, et al. The Schlemm's canal is a VEGF-C/VEGFR-3–responsive lymphatic-like vessel. J Clin Investig. 2014;124(9):3975–86.
151. Souma T, Tompson SW, Thomson BR, Siggs OM, Kizhatil K, Yamaguchi S, et al. Angiopoietin receptor TEK mutations underlie primary congenital glaucoma with variable expressivity. J Clin Investig. 2016;126(7):2575–87.
152. Kim J, Park D-Y, Bae H, Kim D, Lee C-k, Song S, et al. Impaired angiopoietin/Tie2 signaling compromises Schlemm's canal integrity and induces glaucoma. J Clin Invest. 2017;127(10):3877–96.
153. Thackaberry EA, Zhou Y, de Zafra CLZ, Fuh G, Lee CV, Sanowar S, et al. Rapid development of glaucoma via ITV nonselective ANGPT 1/2 antibody: a potential role for ANGPT/TIE2 signaling in primate aqueous humor outflow. Invest Ophthalmol Vis Sci. 2019;60(13):4097–108.
154. Thomson BR, Liu P, Onay T, Du J, Tompson SW, Misener S, et al. Cellular crosstalk regulates the aqueous humor outflow pathway and provides new targets for glaucoma therapies. Nat Commun. 2021;12(1):6072. https://doi.org/10.1038/s41467-021-26346-0.
155. Siggs OM, Souzeau E, Taranath DA, Dubowsky A, Chappell A, Zhou T, et al. Biallelic CPAMD8 variants are a frequent cause of childhood and juvenile open-angle glaucoma. Ophthalmology. 2020;127(6):758–66.
156. Gupta V, Somarajan BI, Kaur G, Gupta S, Singh R, Pradhan D, et al. Exome sequencing identifies procollagen-lysine 2-oxoglutarate 5-dioxygenase 2 mutations in primary congenital and juvenile glaucoma. Ind J Ophthalmol. 2021;69(10):2710.
157. Ferre-Fernández J-J, Aroca-Aguilar J-D, Medina-Trillo C, Bonet-Fernández J-M, Méndez-Hernández C-D, Morales-Fernández L, et al. Whole-exome sequencing of congenital glaucoma patients reveals hypermorphic variants in GPATCH3, a new gene involved in ocular and craniofacial development. Sci Rep. 2017;7(1):46175.
158. Labelle-Dumais C, Pyatla G, Paylakhi S, Tolman NG, Hameed S, Seymens Y, et al. Loss of PRSS56 function leads to ocular angle defects and increased susceptibility to high intraocular pressure. Disease models and Mechanisms. 2020;13(5):dmm042853.
159. Alsaif HS, Khan AO, Patel N, Alkuraya H, Hashem M, Abdulwahab F, et al. Congenital glaucoma and CYP1B1: an old story revisited. Hum Genet. 2019;138(8–9):1043–9. https://doi.org/10.1007/s00439-018-1878-z.
160. Abu-Amero KK, Osman EA, Mousa A, Wheeler J, Whigham B, Allingham RR, et al. Screening of CYP1B1 and LTBP2 genes in Saudi families with primary congenital glaucoma: genotype-phenotype correlation. Mol Vis. 2011;17:2911.
161. Yazdani S, Miraftabi A, Pakravan M, Ghahari E, Tousi BK, Sedigh M, et al. Phenotype and genotype correlation in Iranian primary congenital glaucoma patients. J Glaucoma. 2016;25(1):33–8.
162. Cardoso MS, Anjos R, Vieira L, Ferreira C, Xavier A, Brito C. CYP1B1 gene analysis and phenotypic correlation in Portuguese children with primary congenital glaucoma. Eur J Ophthalmol. 2015;25(6):474–7.
163. Berraho A, Serrou A, Fritez N, El Annas A, Bencherifa F, Gaboun F, et al. Genotype-phenotype correlation in Moroccan patients with primary congenital glaucoma. J Glaucoma. 2015;24(4):297–305.
164. Mandal AK, Chakrabarti D. Update on congenital glaucoma. Indian J Ophthalmol. 2011;59(Suppl1):S148.
165. El Sayed YM, Elhusseiny AM, Gawdat GI, Esmael AF, Elhilali HM. Childhood glaucoma profile in a tertiary centre in Egypt according to the childhood glaucoma research network

classification. PLoS ONE. 2023;18(1): e0279874. https://doi.org/10.1371/journal.pone.0279874.
166. Shohdy KS, Rashad WA, Fargoun MK, Urban P. The morphogen behind primary congenital glaucoma and the dream of targeting. Rom J Morphol Embryol. 2017;58(2):351–61.
167. Abdeen W, Esmael AF, Gawdat G, El-Fayoumi D. Anterior chamber angle features in primary congenital glaucoma infants using hand-held anterior segment-oct. Eye (Lond). 2022;36(6):1238–45. https://doi.org/10.1038/s41433-021-01583-1.
168. Jin SW, Ryu WY. Clinical Manifestations of Strabismus in Patients with Primary Congenital Glaucoma. Seminars in Ophthalmology. 2019;34(6):451–7. https://doi.org/10.1080/08820538.2019.1648689.
169. Gupta V, Bhandari A, Gupta S, Singh A, Gupta A. Consanguinity and severity of primary congenital glaucoma. J Am Ass Pediatric Ophthal Strabismus (JAAPOS). 2022;26(3):119.e1-.e5. https://doi.org/10.1016/j.jaapos.2022.01.010.
170. Mahalingam K, Gupta S. Primary Congenital Glaucoma. In: Gupta S, Mahalingam K, Gupta V, editors. Childhood glaucoma: a case based color and video atlas. Singapore: Springer Nature Singapore; 2023. p. 87–94.
171. Barkan O. Pathogenesis of Congenital Glaucoma: Gonioscopic and Anatomic Observation of the Angle of the Anterior Chamber in the Normal Eye and in Congenital Glaucoma. Am J Ophthalmol. 1955;40(1):1–11. https://doi.org/10.1016/0002-9394(55)92114-0.
172. Shue A, Wong MO, Freedman SF. Primary Congenital Glaucoma. In: Albert D, Miller J, Azar D, Young LH, editors. Albert and Jakobiec's principles and practice of ophthalmology. Cham: Springer International Publishing; 2020. p. 1–40.
173. Amini H, Fakhraie G, Abolmaali S, Amini N, Daneshvar R. Central corneal thickness in Iranian congenital glaucoma patients. Middle East Afr J Ophthalmol. 2012;19(2):194–8. https://doi.org/10.4103/0974-9233.95248.
174. Beck AD. Diagnosis and management of pediatric glaucoma. Ophthalmol Clin North Am. 2001;14(3):501–12. https://doi.org/10.1016/s0896-1549(05)70248-0.
175. Chang TC, Grajewski AL, Cavuoto KM. Evolving perspectives on congenital glaucoma. Current Ophthalmol Rep. 2015;3(2):85–90. https://doi.org/10.1007/s40135-015-0065-9.
176. Alward WL, Fingert JH, Coote MA, Johnson AT, Lerner SF, Junqua D, et al. Clinical features associated with mutations in the chromosome 1 open-angle glaucoma gene (GLC1A). N Engl J Med. 1998;338(15):1022–7. https://doi.org/10.1056/nejm199804093381503.
177. Kwun Y, Lee EJ, Han JC, Kee C. Clinical characteristics of juvenile-onset open angle glaucoma. Korean J Ophthalmol. 2016;30(2):127–33. https://doi.org/10.3341/kjo.2016.30.2.127.
178. Fingert JH. Penetrance of Myocilin mutations-who gets glaucoma? JAMA Ophthalmol. 2019;137(1):35–7. https://doi.org/10.1001/jamaophthalmol.2018.4470.
179. Ikeda H, Ishigooka H, Muto T, Tanihara H, Nagata M. Long-term outcome of trabeculotomy for the treatment of developmental glaucoma. Arch Ophthalmol. 2004;122(8):1122–8. https://doi.org/10.1001/archopht.122.8.1122.
180. Koraszewska-Matuszewska B, Samochowiec-Donocik E, Filipek E. Prognosis in juvenile glaucoma after trabeculectomy. Klin Oczna. 2002;104(2):115–8.
181. Selvan H, Singh A, Gupta V. Juvenile Onset Open-Angle Glaucoma. In: Gupta S, Mahalingam K, Gupta V, editors. Childhood glaucoma: a case based color and video atlas. Singapore: Springer Nature Singapore; 2023. p. 95–110.
182. Johnson AT, Drack AV, Kwitek AE, Cannon RL, Stone EM, Alward WL. Clinical features and linkage analysis of a family with autosomal dominant juvenile glaucoma. Ophthalmology. 1993;100(4):524–9.
183. Wiggs JL, Haines JL, Paglinauan C, Fine A, Sporn C, Lou D. Genetic linkage of autosomal dominant juvenile glaucoma to 1q21-q31 in three affected pedigrees. Genomics. 1994;21(2):299–303.
184. Gupta V, Somarajan BI, Gupta S, Chaurasia AK, Kumar S, Dutta P, et al. The inheritance of juvenile onset primary open angle glaucoma. Clin Genet. 2017;92(2):134–42. https://doi.org/10.1111/cge.12906.

185. Svidnicki PV, Braghini CA, Costa VP, Schimiti RB, de Vasconcellos JPC, de Melo MB. Occurrence of MYOC and CYP1B1 variants in juvenile open angle glaucoma Brazilian patients. Ophthalmic Genet. 2018;39(6):717–24. https://doi.org/10.1080/13816810.2018.1546405.
186. Han X, Souzeau E, Ong JS, An J, Siggs OM, Burdon KP, et al. Myocilin Gene Gln368Ter variant penetrance and association with glaucoma in population-based and registry-based studies. JAMA Ophthalmol. 2019;137(1):28–35. https://doi.org/10.1001/jamaophthalmol.2018.4477.
187. Jerndal T. Goniodysgenesis and hereditary juvenile glaucoma. A clinical study of a Swedish pedigree. Acta Ophthalmol Suppl. 1970;107:3–100.
188. Tawara A, Inomata H. Developmental immaturity of the trabecular meshwork in juvenile glaucoma. Am J Ophthalmol. 1984;98(1):82–97. https://doi.org/10.1016/0002-9394(84)90193-4.
189. Jerndal T. Congenital glaucoma due to dominant goniodysgenesis. A new concept of the heredity of glaucoma. Am J Hum Genet. 1983;35(4):645–51.
190. Gupta V, Gupta S, Dhawan M, Sharma A, Kapoor KS, Sihota R. Extent of asymmetry and unilaterality among juvenile onset primary open angle glaucoma patients. Clin Experiment Ophthalmol. 2011;39(7):633–8. https://doi.org/10.1111/j.1442-9071.2011.02522.x.
191. Stangos AN, Whatham AR, Sunaric-Megevand G. Primary viscocanalostomy for juvenile open-angle glaucoma. Am J Ophthalmol. 2005;140(3):490–6. https://doi.org/10.1016/j.ajo.2005.04.038.
192. Gupta V, James MK, Singh A, Kumar S, Gupta S, Sharma A, et al. Differences in optic disc characteristics of primary congenital glaucoma, juvenile, and adult onset open angle glaucoma patients. J Glaucoma. 2016;25(3):239–43. https://doi.org/10.1097/ijg.0000000000000154.
193. Yazdanpanah G, Bohm KJ, Hassan OM, Karas FI, Elhusseiny AM, Nonpassopon M, et al. Management of congenital aniridia-associated keratopathy: long-term outcomes from a tertiary referral center. Am J Ophthalmol. 2020;210:8–18. https://doi.org/10.1016/j.ajo.2019.11.003.
194. Landsend ECS, Lagali N, Utheim TP. Congenital aniridia – A comprehensive review of clinical features and therapeutic approaches. Surv Ophthalmol. 2021;66(6):1031–50. https://doi.org/10.1016/j.survophthal.2021.02.011.
195. van Velthoven AJH, Utheim TP, Notara M, Bremond-Gignac D, Figueiredo FC, Skottman H, et al. Future directions in managing aniridia-associated keratopathy. Surv Ophthalmol. 2023;68(5):940–56. https://doi.org/10.1016/j.survophthal.2023.04.003.
196. Ihnatko R, Eden U, Fagerholm P, Lagali N. Congenital aniridia and the ocular surface. Ocul Surf. 2016;14(2):196–206.
197. Grant WM, Walton DS. Progressive changes in the angle in congenital aniridia, with development of glaucoma. Trans Am Ophthalmol Soc. 1974;72:207–28.
198. Samant M, Chauhan BK, Lathrop KL, Nischal KK. Congenital aniridia: etiology, manifestations and management. Expert Rev Ophthalmol. 2016;11(2):135–44. https://doi.org/10.1586/17469899.2016.1152182.
199. Nelson LB, Spaeth GL, Nowinski TS, Margo CE, Jackson L. Aniridia A review. Survey of Ophthalmol. 1984;28(6):621–42.
200. Shaw MW, Falls HF, Neel JV. Congenital Aniridia. Am J Hum Genet. 1960;12(4 Pt 1):389.
201. Edén U, Iggman D, Riise R, Tornqvist K. Epidemiology of aniridia in Sweden and Norway. Acta Ophthalmol. 2008;86(7):727–9.
202. Edén U, Beijar C, Riise R, Tornqvist K. Aniridia among children and teenagers in Sweden and Norway. Acta Ophthalmologica. 2009;87(2):242
203. Landsend ES, Utheim ØA, Pedersen HR, Lagali N, Baraas RC, Utheim TP. The genetics of congenital aniridia—a guide for the ophthalmologist. Surv Ophthalmol. 2018;63(1):105–13.
204. Daruich A, Duncan M, Robert MP, Lagali N, Semina EV, Aberdam D, et al. Congenital aniridia beyond black eyes: From phenotype and novel genetic mechanisms to innovative therapeutic approaches. Prog Retin Eye Res. 2023;95: 101133. https://doi.org/10.1016/j.preteyeres.2022.101133.

205. Daruich A, Robert MP, Leroy C, De Vergnes N, Beugnet C, Malan V, et al. Foveal hypoplasia grading in 95 cases of congenital aniridia: correlation to phenotype and PAX6 genotype. Am J Ophthalmol. 2022;237:122–9.
206. Ma AS, Grigg JR, Jamieson RV. Phenotype-genotype correlations and emerging pathways in ocular anterior segment dysgenesis. Hum Genet. 2019;138(8–9):899–915. https://doi.org/10.1007/s00439-018-1935-7.
207. Lima Cunha D, Arno G, Corton M, Moosajee M. The spectrum of PAX6 mutations and genotype-phenotype correlations in the eye. Genes (Basel). 2019;10(12). https://doi.org/10.3390/genes10121050
208. Barkan O. Goniotomy for glaucoma associated with Aniridia. AMA Arch Ophthalmol. 1953;49(1):1–5.
209. Gramer E, Reiter C, Gramer G. Glaucoma and frequency of ocular and general diseases in 30 patients with aniridia: a clinical study. Eur J Ophthalmol. 2012;22(1):104–10.
210. Bobilev AM, Hudgens-Haney ME, Hamm JP, Oliver WT, McDowell JE, Lauderdale JD, et al. Early and late auditory information processing show opposing deviations in aniridia. Brain Res. 2019;1720: 146307.
211. Shimo N, Yasuda T, Kitamura T, Matsushita K, Osawa S, Yamamoto Y, et al. Aniridia with a heterozygous PAX6 mutation in which the pituitary function was partially impaired. Intern Med. 2014;53(1):39–42.
212. Grant MK, Bobilev AM, Branch A, Lauderdale JD. Structural and functional consequences of PAX6 mutations in the brain: implications for aniridia. Brain Res. 2021;1756: 147283.
213. Edén U, Riise R, Tornqvist K. Corneal involvement in congenital Aniridia. Cornea. 2010;29(10):1096–102.
214. Hingorani M. Molecular Genetics of Aniridia. eLS.
215. Prosser J, van Heyningen V. PAX6 mutations reviewed. Hum Mutat. 1998;11(2):93–108.
216. Schedl A, Ross A, Lee M, Engelkamp D, Rashbass P, van Heyningen V, et al. Influence of PAX6 gene dosage on development: overexpression causes severe eye abnormalities. Cell. 1996;86(1):71–82.
217. Davis N, Yoffe C, Raviv S, Antes R, Berger J, Holzmann S, et al. Pax6 dosage requirements in iris and ciliary body differentiation. Dev Biol. 2009;333(1):132–42. https://doi.org/10.1016/j.ydbio.2009.06.023.
218. Wang X, Shan X, Gregory-Evans CY. A mouse model of aniridia reveals the in vivo downstream targets of Pax6 driving iris and ciliary body development in the eye. Biochimica et Biophysica Acta (BBA)-Molecular Basis of Disease. 2017;1863(1):60–7.
219. Kroeber M, Davis N, Holzmann S, Kritzenberger M, Shelah-Goraly M, Ofri R, et al. Reduced expression of Pax6 in lens and cornea of mutant mice leads to failure of chamber angle development and juvenile glaucoma. Hum Mol Genet. 2010;19(17):3332–42.
220. Baulmann DC, Ohlmann A, Flügel-Koch C, Goswami S, Cvekl A, Tamm ER. Pax6 heterozygous eyes show defects in chamber angle differentiation that are associated with a wide spectrum of other anterior eye segment abnormalities. Mech Dev. 2002;118(1):3–17. https://doi.org/10.1016/S0925-4773(02)00260-5.
221. Cole JD, McDaniel JA, Nilak J, Ban A, Rodriguez C, Hameed Z, et al. Characterization of neural damage and neuroinflammation in Pax6 small-eye mice. Exp Eye Res. 2024;238: 109723. https://doi.org/10.1016/j.exer.2023.109723.
222. Ansari M, Rainger J, Hanson IM, Williamson KA, Sharkey F, Harewood L, et al. Genetic analysis of 'PAX6-Negative' individuals with Aniridia or gillespie syndrome. PLoS ONE. 2016;11(4): e0153757. https://doi.org/10.1371/journal.pone.0153757.
223. Perveen R, Lloyd IC, Clayton-Smith J, Churchill A, van Heyningen V, Hanson I, et al. Phenotypic variability and asymmetry of Rieger syndrome associated with PITX2 mutations. Invest Ophthalmol Vis Sci. 2000;41(9):2456–60.
224. Zhang X, Qin G, Chen G, Li T, Gao L, Huang L, et al. Variants in TRIM44 cause Aniridia by Impairing PAX6 expression. Hum Mutat. 2015;36(12):1164–7. https://doi.org/10.1002/humu.22907.

225. Hingorani M, Williamson KA, Moore AT, van Heyningen V. Detailed ophthalmologic evaluation of 43 individuals with PAX6 mutations. Invest Ophthalmol Vis Sci. 2009;50(6):2581–90. https://doi.org/10.1167/iovs.08-2827.
226. Adachi M, Dickens CJ, Hetherington J, Hoskins HD, Iwach AG, Wong PC, et al. Clinical experience of trabeculotomy for the surgical treatment of Aniridic glaucoma. Ophthalmology. 1997;104(12):2121–5. https://doi.org/10.1016/S0161-6420(97)30041-4.
227. Lahri B, Mahalingam K, Gupta S. Aniridia with Glaucoma. In: Gupta S, Mahalingam K, Gupta V, editors. Childhood glaucoma: a case based color and video atlas. Singapore: Springer Nature Singapore; 2023. p. 143–50.
228. Okamoto F, Nakano S, Okamoto C, Hommura S, Oshika T. Ultrasound biomicroscopic findings in aniridia. Am J Ophthalmol. 2004;137(5):858–62. https://doi.org/10.1016/j.ajo.2003.12.014.
229. Muzyka L, Winterhalter E, LoPresti MA, Scoville J, Bohnsack BL, Lam SK. Axenfeld-Rieger syndrome: a systematic review examining genetic, neurological, and neurovascular associations to inform screening. Heliyon. 2023;9(7): e18225. https://doi.org/10.1016/j.heliyon.2023.e18225.
230. Seifi M, Walter MA. Axenfeld-rieger syndrome. Clin Genet. 2018;93(6):1123–30. https://doi.org/10.1111/cge.13148.
231. Axenfeld T. Embryotoxon corneae posterius. Ber Deutsh Ophthalmol Gesellsch. 1920;42:301–2.
232. Rieger H. Dysgenesus mesodermalis corneae etiridis. Z Augenheilkd. 1935;86:333.
233. Shields MB. Axenfeld-rieger syndrome: a theory of mechanism and distinctions from the iridocorneal endothelial syndrome. Trans Am Ophthalmol Soc. 1983;81:736.
234. Shields MB, Buckley E, Klintworth GK, Thresher R. Axenfeld-Rieger syndrome. A spectrum of developmental disorders. Survey of Ophthal. 1985;29(6):387–409.
235. Khandwala NS, Ramappa M, Edward DP, Mocan MC. Axenfeld-Rieger syndrome in the pediatric population: a review. Taiwan J Ophthalmol. 2023;13(4):417–24. https://doi.org/10.4103/tjo.TJO-D-23-00089.
236. Panigrahi A, Gupta S, Gupta V. Axenfeld-Rieger Syndrome. In: Gupta S, Mahalingam K, Gupta V, editors. Childhood glaucoma: a case based color and video atlas. Singapore: Springer Nature Singapore; 2023. p. 113–24.
237. Michels K, Bohnsack BL. Ophthalmological manifestations of axenfeld-rieger syndrome: current perspectives. Clin Ophthalmol. 2023;17:819–28. https://doi.org/10.2147/opth.S379853.
238. Souzeau E, Siggs OM, Zhou T, Galanopoulos A, Hodson T, Taranath D, et al. Glaucoma spectrum and age-related prevalence of individuals with FOXC1 and PITX2 variants. Eur J Hum Genet. 2017;25(7):839–47.
239. Zepeda EM, Branham K, Moroi SE, Bohnsack BL. Surgical outcomes of Glaucoma associated with Axenfeld-Rieger syndrome. BMC Ophthalmol. 2020;20(1):172. https://doi.org/10.1186/s12886-020-01417-w.
240. Hjalt TA, Semina EV. Current molecular understanding of Axenfeld-Rieger syndrome. Expert Rev Mol Med. 2005;7(25):1–17.
241. Reis LM, Tyler RC, Volkmann Kloss BA, Schilter KF, Levin AV, Lowry RB, et al. PITX2 and FOXC1 spectrum of mutations in ocular syndromes. Eur J Hum Genet. 2012;20(12):1224–33.
242. French CR, Seshadri S, Destefano AL, Fornage M, Arnold CR, Gage PJ, et al. Mutation of FOXC1 and PITX2 induces cerebral small-vessel disease. J Clin Investig. 2014;124(11):4877–81.
243. French CR. Mechanistic insights into axenfeld-rieger syndrome from zebrafish foxc1 and Pitx2 mutants. Int J Mol Sci. 2021;22(18):10001.
244. Idrees F, Vaideanu D, Fraser SG, Sowden JC, Khaw PT. A review of anterior segment dysgeneses. Surv Ophthalmol. 2006;51(3):213–31.
245. Tanwar M, Dada T, Dada R. Axenfeld-Rieger syndrome associated with congenital glaucoma and cytochrome P4501B1 gene mutations. Case Reports in Medicine. 2010;2010.

246. Reis LM, Semina EV. Conserved genetic pathways associated with microphthalmia, anophthalmia, and coloboma. Birth Defects Res C Embryo Today. 2015;105(2):96–113.
247. Ma A, Yousoof S, Grigg JR, Flaherty M, Minoche AE, Cowley MJ, et al. Revealing hidden genetic diagnoses in the ocular anterior segment disorders. Genet Med. 2020;22(10):1623–32.
248. Evans AL, Gage PJ. Expression of the homeobox gene Pitx2 in neural crest is required for optic stalk and ocular anterior segment development. Hum Mol Genet. 2005;14(22):3347–59.
249. Bohnsack BL, Kasprick DS, Kish PE, Goldman D, Kahana A. A zebrafish model of axenfeld-rieger syndrome reveals that pitx2 regulation by retinoic acid is essential for ocular and craniofacial development. Invest Ophthalmol Vis Sci. 2012;53(1):7–22.
250. Seo S, Chen L, Liu W, Zhao D, Schultz KM, Sasman A, et al. Foxc1 and Foxc2 in the neural crest are required for ocular anterior segment development. Invest Ophthalmol Vis Sci. 2017;58(3):1368–77.
251. Hendee KE, Sorokina EA, Muheisen SS, Reis LM, Tyler RC, Markovic V, et al. PITX2 deficiency and associated human disease: insights from the zebrafish model. Hum Mol Genet. 2018;27(10):1675–95.
252. Minoux M, Rijli FM. Molecular mechanisms of cranial neural crest cell migration and patterning in craniofacial development. Development. 2010;137(16):2605–21.
253. Williams AL, Bohnsack BL. Neural crest derivatives in ocular development: discerning the eye of the storm. Birth Defects Res C Embryo Today. 2015;105(2):87–95. https://doi.org/10.1002/bdrc.21095.
254. Chen L, Gage PJ. Heterozygous Pitx2 null mice accurately recapitulate the ocular features of Axenfeld-Rieger syndrome and congenital glaucoma. Invest Ophthalmol Vis Sci. 2016;57(11):5023–30. https://doi.org/10.1167/iovs.16-19700.
255. Prem Senthil M, Knight LSW, Taranath D, Mackey DA, Ruddle JB, Chiang MY, et al. Comparison of anterior segment abnormalities in individuals with FOXC1 and PITX2 variants. Cornea. 2022;41(8):1009–15. https://doi.org/10.1097/ico.0000000000003020.
256. Zhou L, Wang X, An J, Zhang Y, He M, Tang L. Genotype-phenotype association of PITX2 and FOXC1 in Axenfeld-Rieger syndrome. Exp Eye Res. 2023;226: 109307. https://doi.org/10.1016/j.exer.2022.109307.
257. Wang X, Liu X, Huang L, Fang S, Jia X, Xiao X, et al. Mutation survey of candidate genes and genotype-phenotype analysis in 20 Southeastern Chinese Patients with Axenfeld-Rieger Syndrome. Curr Eye Res. 2018;43(11):1334–41. https://doi.org/10.1080/02713683.2018.1493129.
258. Khasnavis A, Fernandes M. Peters anomaly: An overview. Taiwan J Ophthalmol. 2023;13(4):434–42. https://doi.org/10.4103/tjo.TJO-D-23-00065.
259. Nischal KK. A new approach to the classification of neonatal corneal opacities. Curr Opin Ophthalmol. 2012;23(5):344–54. https://doi.org/10.1097/ICU.0b013e328356893d.
260. Arora M, Kaginalkar A, Tandon R. Peters Anomaly with Glaucoma. In: Gupta S, Mahalingam K, Gupta V, editors. Childhood glaucoma: a case based color and video atlas. Singapore: Springer Nature Singapore; 2023. p. 125–33.
261. Harissi-Dagher M, Colby K. Anterior segment dysgenesis: peters anomaly and sclerocornea. Int Ophthalmol Clin. 2008;48(2):35–42.
262. Kuper C, Kuwabara T, Stark WJ. The histopathology of Peters' anomaly. Am J Ophthalmol. 1975;80(4):653–60.
263. Peters A. Ueber angeborene defektbildung der descemetschen membran. Klin Monatsbl Augenheilkd. 1906;44:27–40.
264. Ozeki H, Shirai S, Nozaki M, Sakurai E, Mizuno S, Ashikari M, et al. Ocular and systemic features of Peters' anomaly. Graefes Arch Clin Exp Ophthalmol. 2000;238:833–9.
265. Kurilec JM, Zaidman GW. Incidence of peters anomaly and congenital corneal opacities interfering with vision in the United States. Cornea. 2014;33(8):848–50. https://doi.org/10.1097/ico.0000000000000182.
266. Traboulsi EI, Maumenee IH. Peters' anomaly and associated congenital malformations. Arch Ophthalmol. 1992;110(12):1739–42.

267. Vanathi M, Panda A, Vengayil S, Chaudhuri Z, Dada T. Pediatric keratoplasty. Surv Ophthalmol. 2009;54(2):245–71.
268. Chang J, Kim J, Kim S, Yu Y. Long-term clinical course and visual outcome associated with Peters' anomaly. Eye. 2012;26(9):1237–42.
269. Heon E, Barsoum-Homsy M, Cevrette L, Jacob JL, Milot J, Polemeno R, et al. Peters' anomaly. The spectrum of associated ocular and systemic malformations. Ophthalmic Paediatr Genet. 1992;13(2):137–43. https://doi.org/10.3109/13816819209087614.
270. Mayer UM. Peters' anomaly and combination with other malformations (series of 16 patients). Ophthalmic Paediatr Genet. 1992;13(2):131–5. https://doi.org/10.3109/13816819209087613.
271. van Schooneveld MJ, Delleman JW, Beemer FA, Bleeker-Wagemakers EM. Peters'-plus: a new syndrome. Ophthalmic Paediatr Genet. 1984;4(3):141–5. https://doi.org/10.3109/13816818409006113.
272. Spierer O, Cavuoto KM, Suwannaraj S, McKeown CA, Chang TC. Outcome of optical iridectomy in Peters anomaly. Graefes Arch Clin Exp Ophthalmol. 2018;256:1679–83.
273. Wowra B, Dobrowolski D, Parekh M, Wylęgała E. General treatment and ophthalmic management of Peters' Anomaly. J Clin Med. 2024;13(2). https://doi.org/10.3390/jcm13020532.
274. Huang C, O'Hara M, Mannis MJ. Primary pediatric keratoplasty: indications and outcomes. Cornea. 2009;28(9):1003–8.
275. Rezende RA, Uchoa UB, Uchoa R, Rapuano CJ, Laibson PR, Cohen EJ. Congenital corneal opacities in a cornea referral practice. Cornea. 2004;23(6):565–70.
276. Lowe MT, Keane MC, Coster DJ, Williams KA. The outcome of corneal transplantation in infants, children, and adolescents. Ophthalmology. 2011;118(3):492–7.
277. Frydman M, Weinstock AL, Cohen HA, Savir H, Varsano I. Autosomal recessive Peters anomaly, typical facial appearance, failure to thrive, hydrocephalus, and other anomalies: Further delineation of the Krause-Kivlin syndrome. Am J Med Genet. 1991;40(1):34–40.
278. Azuma N, Yamaguchi Y, Handa H, Hayakawa M, Kanai A, Yamada M. Missense mutation in the alternative splice region of the PAX6 gene in eye anomalies. Am J Human Genetics. 1999;65(3):656–63.
279. Reis LM, Semina EV. Genetics of anterior segment dysgenesis disorders. Curr Opin Ophthalmol. 2011;22(5):314.
280. Weh E, Reis LM, Happ HC, Levin AV, Wheeler PG, David KL, et al. Whole exome sequence analysis of Peters anomaly. Hum Genet. 2014;133:1497–511.
281. Vincent A, Billingsley G, Priston M, Glaser T, Oliver E, Walter M, et al. Further support of the role of CYP1B1 in patients with Peters anomaly. Mol Vis. 2006;12(1):506–10.
282. Thompson E, Winter R, Baraitser M. Kivlin syndrome and Peters'-Plus syndrome: are they the same disorder? Clin Dysmorphol. 1993;2(4):301–16.
283. Ürel Demir G, Lafci N, Dogan P, Şimşek Kiper P, Ütine G. Peters Plus syndrome: a recognizable clinical entity. Turkish J Pediatrics. 2020;62(1).
284. Weh E, Reis LM, Tyler RC, Bick D, Rhead WJ, Wallace S, et al. Novel B3GALTL mutations in classic Peters plus syndrome and lack of mutations in a large cohort of patients with similar phenotypes. Clin Genet. 2014;86(2):142–8. https://doi.org/10.1111/cge.12241.
285. Lesnik Oberstein SA, Kriek M, White SJ, Kalf ME, Szuhai K, den Dunnen JT, et al. Peters plus syndrome is caused by mutations in B3GALTL, a putative glycosyltransferase. Am J Hum Genet. 2006;79(3):562–6. https://doi.org/10.1086/507567.
286. Bhandari R, Ferri S, Whittaker B, Liu M, Lazzaro DR. Peters anomaly: review of the literature. Cornea. 2011;30(8):939–44.
287. Shigeyasu C, Yamada M, Mizuno Y, Yokoi T, Nishina S, Azuma N. Clinical features of anterior segment dysgenesis associated with congenital corneal opacities. Cornea. 2012;31(3):293–8. https://doi.org/10.1097/ICO.0b013e31820cd2ab.
288. Waring GO, Rodrigues MM, Laibson PR. Anterior chamber cleavage syndrome a stepladder classification. Survey of Ophthalmol. 1975;20(1):3–27. https://doi.org/10.1016/0039-6257(75)90034-X.

289. Townsend WM, Font RL, Zimmerman LE. Congenital corneal leukomas: 2. Histopathologic findings in 19 eyes with central defect in Descemet's membrane. Am J Ophthalmol 1974;77(2):192–206.
290. Almarzouki HS, Tayyib AA, Khayat HA, Alsulami RE, Alzahrani SM, Alkahtani AS, et al. Peters anomaly in twins: a case report of a rare incident with novel comorbidities. Case Rep Ophthalmol. 2017;7(3):464–70.
291. Kenyon KR. Mesenchymal dysgenesis in Peters' anomaly, sclerocornea and congenital endothelial dystrophy. Exp Eye Res. 1975;21(2):125–42.
292. Nischal K, Naor J, Jay V, MacKeen L, Rootman D. Clinicopathological correlation of congenital corneal opacification using ultrasound biomicroscopy. Br J Ophthalmol. 2002;86(1):62.
293. Majander AS, Lindahl PM, Vasara LK, Krootila K. Anterior segment optical coherence tomography in congenital corneal opacities. Ophthalmology. 2012;119(12):2450–7.
294. Sridhar U, Tripathy K. Iris Ectropion Syndrome. StatPearls. Treasure Island (FL): StatPearls Publishing Copyright © 2024, StatPearls Publishing LLC.; 2024.
295. Dowling JL Jr, Albert DM, Nelson LB, Walton DS. Primary glaucoma associated with iridotrabecular dysgenesis and ectropion uveae. Ophthalmology. 1985;92(7):912–21.
296. Ritch R, Forbes M, Hetherington J Jr, Harrison R, Podos SM. Congenital ectropion uveae with glaucoma. Ophthalmology. 1984;91(4):326–31.
297. Tanwar V, Mahalingam K, Gupta S. Congenital Ectropion Uveae with Glaucoma. In: Gupta S, Mahalingam K, Gupta V, editors. Childhood glaucoma: a case based color and video atlas. Singapore: Springer Nature Singapore; 2023. p. 135–41.
298. Wicherkiewicz B. Beitrag zur kenntniss des ectropion uveae congenitum. Albrecht von Graefes Archiv für Ophthalmologie. 1891;37:204–7.
299. Spiro G. Ein Fall von Ectropion uveae congenitum. Centralbl Prakt Augenheilkd. 1896;20:310–1.
300. Kolomeyer AM, Kim BJ. Bilateral, presumed congenital ectropion uveae in a patient with pathologic myopia. Am J Ophthalmol Case Rep. 2018;11:119–20. https://doi.org/10.1016/j.ajoc.2018.06.017.
301. Snehi S, Kaur M, Singh AK, Thattarattody F, Raj S, Pandav SS, et al. Unilateral advanced glaucoma in isolated congenital ectropion uveae with ipsilateral ptosis: a pictorial description of five children. Rom J Ophthalmol. 2022;66(2):125–31. https://doi.org/10.22336/rjo.2022.25.
302. Futterweit W, Ritch R, Teekhasaenee C, Nelson ES. Coexistence of Prader-Willi syndrome, congenital ectropion uveae with glaucoma, and factor XI deficiency. JAMA. 1986;255(23):3280–2.
303. Libov AJ, Maino DM. Prader-Willi syndrome. J Am Optom Assoc. 1994;65(5):355–9.
304. Edward DP, Morales J, Bouhenni RA, Patil J, Edward PR, Cummings TJ, et al. Congenital ectropion uvea and mechanisms of glaucoma in neurofibromatosis type 1: new insights. Ophthalmology. 2012;119(7):1485–94.
305. Kumar V, Kumar K, Chanana B, Rohatgi J, Gupta V. Congenital ectropion uveae with iris coloboma and telecanthus. Cont Lens Anterior Eye. 2011;34(3):147–8.
306. Lim FPM, Ho CL. Long-term treatment outcomes for congenital ectropion uveae with ptosis and glaucoma. J Am Association for Pediatric Ophthalmology Strabismus. 2020;24(6):369–71.
307. Quigley HA, Stanish FS. Unilateral congenital iris pigment epithelial hyperplasia associated with late-onset glaucoma. Am J Ophthalmol. 1978;86(2):182–4. https://doi.org/10.1016/s0002-9394(14)76809-6.
308. Kaushik S, Choudhary S, Kaur A, Srivastava P, Pokharel B, Akella M, et al. Neonatal-onset congenital ectropion Uveae may be caused by a distinct CYP1B1 pathologic variant. Am J Ophthalmol. 2022;239:54–65. https://doi.org/10.1016/j.ajo.2022.01.014.
309. Willcock C, Grigg J, Wilson M, Tam P, Billson F, Jamieson R. Congenital iris ectropion as an indicator of variant aniridia. Br J Ophthalmol. 2006;90(5):658–569. https://doi.org/10.1136/bjo.2005.089698.

310. Harasymowycz PJ, Papamatheakis DG, Eagle RC Jr, Wilson RP. Congenital Ectropion Uveae and Glaucoma. Arch Ophthalmol. 2006;124(2):271–3. https://doi.org/10.1001/archopht.124.2.271.
311. Mandal AK. Late-onset unilateral primary developmental glaucoma associated with iridotrabecular dysgenesis, congenital ectropion uveae and thickened corneal nerves: a new neural crest syndrome? Ophthalmic Surg Lasers. 1999;30(7):567–70.
312. Politi F, Sachs R, Barishak R. Neurofibromatosis and congenital glaucoma. A case report Ophthalmologica. 1977;176(3):155–9. https://doi.org/10.1159/000308708.
313. Wolter JR, Butler RG. Pigment spots of the iris and ectropion UVEAE. Am J Ophthalmol. 1963;56:964–73.
314. Sánchez-Espino LF, Ivars M, Antoñanzas J, Baselga E. Sturge-weber syndrome: a review of pathophysiology, genetics, clinical features, and current management approache. Appl Clin Genet. 2023;16:63–81. https://doi.org/10.2147/tacg.S363685.
315. Patokar A, Lohe V, Reche A, Sune R, Datkar D. A deep insight on psychological aspect in patients with Sturge-Weber syndrome. J Educ Health Promot. 2023;12:343. https://doi.org/10.4103/jehp.jehp_104_23.
316. Zallmann M, Leventer RJ, Mackay MT, Ditchfield M, Bekhor PS, Su JC. Screening for Sturge-Weber syndrome: a state-of-the-art review. Pediatr Dermatol. 2018;35(1):30–42.
317. Sturge WA. A case of partial epilepsy, apparently due to a lesion of one of the vaso-motor centers of the brain. Trans Clin Soc Lond. 1879;12:162–7.
318. Weber FP. Right-sided hemi-hypotrophy resulting from right-sided congenital spastic hemiplegia, with a morbid condition of the left side of the brain, revealed by radiograms. J Neurol Psychopathol. 1922;3(10):134.
319. Roach E. Neurocutaneous syndromes. Pediatr Clin North Am. 1992;39(4):591–620.
320. Formisano M, Abdolrahimzadeh B, Mollo R, Bruni P, Malagola R, Abdolrahimzadeh S. Bilateral diffuse choroidal hemangioma in Sturge Weber syndrome: a case report highlighting the role of multimodal imaging and a brief review of the literature. J Curr Ophthalmol. 2019;31(2):242–9. https://doi.org/10.1016/j.joco.2018.10.001.
321. Waelchli R, Aylett S, Robinson K, Chong W, Martinez A, Kinsler V. New vascular classification of port-wine stains: improving prediction of Sturge-Weber risk. Br J Dermatol. 2014;171(4):861–7.
322. Higueros E, Roe E, Granell E, Baselga E. Sturge-Weber syndrome: a review. Actas Dermo-Sifiliográficas (English Edition). 2017;108(5):407–17.
323. Singh AK, Keenaghan M. Sturge-weber syndrome. StatPearls. Treasure Island (FL): StatPearls Publishing
324. Ravindra AP, Mahalingam K, Gupta S. Sturge-Weber syndrome and associated syndromes with glaucoma. In: Gupta S, Mahalingam K, Gupta V, editors. Childhood glaucoma: a case based color and video atlas. Singapore: Springer Nature Singapore; 2023. p. 161–71.
325. Ciancimino C, Di Pippo M, Rullo D, Ruggeri F, Grassi F, Scuderi G, et al. An update on multimodal ophthalmological imaging of diffuse choroidal hemangioma in sturge-weber syndrome. Vision (Basel). 2023;7(4). https://doi.org/10.3390/vision7040064.
326. Hassanpour K, Nourinia R, Gerami E, Mahmoudi G, Esfandiari H. Ocular Manifestations of the sturge-weber syndrome. J Ophthalmic Vis Res. 2021;16(3):415–31. https://doi.org/10.18502/jovr.v16i3.9438.
327. Basler L, Sowka J. Sturge-Weber syndrome and glaucoma. Optometry—J Am Optometric Ass. 2011;82(5):306–9. https://doi.org/10.1016/j.optm.2010.11.015.
328. Yan H, Hu M, Cui Y, Li L, Liang T. Clinical characteristics of infants with port-wine stain and glaucoma secondary to Sturge-Weber Syndrome. BMC Ophthalmol. 2022;22(1):260. https://doi.org/10.1186/s12886-022-02476-x.
329. Anand R. Photodynamic therapy for diffuse choroidal hemangioma associated with Sturge Weber syndrome. Am J Ophthalmol. 2003;136(4):758–60.
330. Shirley MD, Tang H, Gallione CJ, Baugher JD, Frelin LP, Cohen B, et al. Sturge-Weber syndrome and port-wine stains caused by somatic mutation in GNAQ. N Engl J Med. 2013;368(21):1971–9.

331. Nakashima M, Miyajima M, Sugano H, Iimura Y, Kato M, Tsurusaki Y, et al. The somatic GNAQ mutation c. 548G> A (p. R183Q) is consistently found in Sturge–Weber syndrome. J Human Genet. 2014;59(12):691–3.
332. Huang L, Couto JA, Pinto A, Alexandrescu S, Madsen JR, Greene AK, et al. Somatic GNAQ mutation is enriched in brain endothelial cells in Sturge-Weber syndrome. Pediatr Neurol. 2017;67:59–63.
333. Van Trigt WK, Kelly KM, Hughes CCW. GNAQ mutations drive port wine birthmark-associated Sturge-Weber syndrome: A review of pathobiology, therapies, and current models. Front Hum Neurosci. 2022;16:1006027. https://doi.org/10.3389/fnhum.2022.1006027.
334. Thorpe J, Frelin LP, McCann M, Pardo CA, Cohen BA, Comi AM, et al. Identification of a mosaic activating mutation in GNA11 in atypical Sturge-Weber syndrome. J Invest Dermatol. 2021;141(3):685.
335. Mantelli F, Bruscolini A, La Cava M, Abdolrahimzadeh S, Lambiase A. Ocular manifestations of Sturge-Weber syndrome: pathogenesis, diagnosis, and management. Clin Ophthalmol. 2016;10:871–8. https://doi.org/10.2147/opth.S101963.
336. Arora KS, Quigley HA, Comi AM, Miller RB, Jampel HD. Increased choroidal thickness in patients with Sturge-Weber syndrome. JAMA ophthalmology. 2013;131(9):1216–9.
337. Phelps CD. The pathogenesis of glaucoma in Sturge-Weber syndrome. Ophthalmology. 1978;85(3):276–86. https://doi.org/10.1016/s0161-6420(78)35667-0.
338. Cibis GW, Tripathi RC, Tripathi BJ. Glaucoma in Sturge-Weber syndrome. Ophthalmology. 1984;91(9):1061–71. https://doi.org/10.1016/s0161-6420(84)34194-x.
339. Sharan S, Swamy B, Taranath DA, Jamieson R, Yu T, Wargon O, et al. Port-wine vascular malformations and glaucoma risk in Sturge-Weber syndrome. J Am Ass Pediatric Ophthalmol Strabismus. 2009;13(4):374–8.
340. Sullivan TJ, Clarke MP, Morin JD. The ocular manifestations of the Sturge-Weber syndrome. SLACK Incorporated Thorofare, NJ; 1992. p. 349–56.
341. Wu Y, Peng C, Huang L, Xu L, Ding X, Liu Y, et al. Somatic GNAQ R183Q mutation is located within the sclera and episclera in patients with Sturge-Weber syndrome. Br J Ophthalmol. 2022;106(7):1006–11. https://doi.org/10.1136/bjophthalmol-2020-317287.
342. Sujansky E, Conradi S. Outcome of Sturge-Weber syndrome in 52 adults. Am J Med Genet. 1995;57(1):35–45.
343. Sujansky E, Conradi S. Sturge-Weber syndrome: age of onset of seizures and glaucoma and the prognosis for affected children. J Child Neurol. 1995;10(1):49–58.
344. Lambiase A, Mantelli F, Mannino G, Recupero SM. An unusual case of acute glaucoma in Sturge-Weber syndrome. Eur J Ophthalmol. 2015;25(6):e103–5.
345. Maruyama I, Ohguro H, Nakazawa M. A case of acute angle-closure glaucoma secondary to posterior scleritis in patient with Sturge-Weber syndrome. Jpn J Ophthalmol. 2002;46(1):74–7. https://doi.org/10.1016/s0021-5155(01)00463-4.
346. Su WW. Acute primary angle-closure in Sturge-Weber syndrome. Am J Ophthalmol Case Rep. 2018;10:101–4. https://doi.org/10.1016/j.ajoc.2018.02.004.
347. Lee DH, Shin J, Seo JH, Byon IS, Jung JH, Lee JE. Mobile lens-induced angle closure glaucoma and rubeosis iridis in Sturge Weber syndrome. Int J Ophthalmol. 2015;8(5):1080–2. https://doi.org/10.3980/j.issn.2222-3959.2015.05.40.
348. Mwinula JH, Sagawa T, Tawara A, Inomata H. Anterior chamber angle vascularization in Sturge-Weber syndrome. Report of a case. Graefes Arch Clin Exp Ophthalmol. 1994;232(7):387–91. https://doi.org/10.1007/bf00186578.
349. Boltshauser E, Wilson J, Hoare R. Sturge-Weber syndrome with bilateral intracranial calcification. J Neurol Neurosurg Psychiatry. 1976;39(5):429.
350. Scott M, Neal AE. Congenital heart disease. Prim Care. 2021;48(3):351–66. https://doi.org/10.1016/j.pop.2021.04.005.
351. Hennekam RC, Stevens CA, Van de Kamp JJ. Etiology and recurrence risk in Rubinstein-Taybi syndrome. Am J Med Genet Suppl. 1990;6:56–64. https://doi.org/10.1002/ajmg.1320370610.

352. Rubinstein JH, Taybi H. Broad thumbs and toes and facial abnormalities. A possible mental retardation syndrome. Am J Dis Child. 1963;105:588–608. https://doi.org/10.1001/archpedi.1963.02080040590010.
353. Huang FR, Zhang AM, Xu J, Huang L. A clinical characteristics and genetic analysis of a case of Rubinstein-Taybi syndrome with glaucoma. Eur Rev Med Pharmacol Sci. 2021;25(3):1447–54. https://doi.org/10.26355/eurrev_202102_24852.
354. Rubinstein J. The broad thumbs syndrome. Progress report 1968, Birth Defects. 1969:25–41.
355. Rubinstein JH. Broad thumb-hallux (Rubinstein-Taybi) syndrome 1957–1988. Am J Med Genet Suppl. 1990;6:3–16. https://doi.org/10.1002/ajmg.1320370603.
356. Shaffer RN, Weiss DI. Congenital and pediatric glaucomas. (No Title). 1970.
357. Weiss D. Glaucoma and systemic disease. Clinical Ophthal. 1978;5:3–4.
358. DaCosta J, Brookes J. Infantile glaucoma in Rubinstein-Taybi syndrome. Eye (Lond). 2012;26(9):1270–1. https://doi.org/10.1038/eye.2012.123.
359. Quaranta L, Quaranta CA. Congenital glaucoma associated with Rubinstein-Taybi syndrome. Acta Ophthalmol Scand. 1998;76(1):112–3. https://doi.org/10.1034/j.1600-0420.1998.760122.x.
360. van Genderen MM, Kinds GF, Riemslag FC, Hennekam RC. Ocular features in Rubinstein-Taybi syndrome: investigation of 24 patients and review of the literature. Br J Ophthalmol. 2000;84(10):1177–84. https://doi.org/10.1136/bjo.84.10.1177.
361. Brei TJ, Burke MJ, Rubinstein JH. Glaucoma and findings simulating glaucoma in the Rubinstein-Taybi syndrome. J Pediatr Ophthalmol Strabismus. 1995;32(4):248–52. https://doi.org/10.3928/0191-3913-19950701-12.
362. Petrif F, Giles RH, Dauwerse HG, Saris JJ, Hennekam RC, Masuno M, et al. Rubinstein-Taybi syndrome caused by mutations in the transcriptional co-activator CBP. Nature. 1995;376(6538):348–51.
363. Roelfsema JH, White SJ, Ariyürek Y, Bartholdi D, Niedrist D, Papadia F, et al. Genetic heterogeneity in Rubinstein-Taybi syndrome: mutations in both the CBP and EP300 genes cause disease. Am J Human Genetics. 2005;76(4):572–80.
364. Bartholdi D, Roelfsema JH, Papadia F, Breuning MH, Niedrist D, Hennekam RC, et al. Genetic heterogeneity in Rubinstein-Taybi syndrome: delineation of the phenotype of the first patients carrying mutations in EP300. J Med Genet. 2007;44(5):327–33.
365. Hennekam R. Rubinstein-Taybi syndrome. Eur J Hum Genet. 2006;14(9):981–5.
366. Milani D, Manzoni FM, Pezzani L, Ajmone P, Gervasini C, Menni F, et al. Rubinstein-Taybi syndrome: clinical features, genetic basis, diagnosis, and management. Ital J Pediatr. 2015;41:4. https://doi.org/10.1186/s13052-015-0110-1.
367. Edelsten C, Reddy MA, Stanford MR, Graham EM. Visual loss associated with pediatric uveitis in english primary and referral centers. Am J Ophthalmol. 2003;135(5):676–80. https://doi.org/10.1016/s0002-9394(02)02148-7.
368. Cunningham J, Emmett T. Uveitis in children. Ocul Immunol Inflamm. 2000;8(4):251–61.
369. Päivönsalo-Hietanen T, Tuominen J, Matti SK. Uveitis in children: population-based study in Finland. Acta Ophthalmol Scand. 2000;78(1):84–8.
370. Kanski JJ. Uveitis in juvenile chronic arthritis: incidence, clinical features and prognosis. Eye. 1988;2(6):641–5.
371. Hettinga YM, Verhagen FH, van Genderen M, de Boer JH. Characteristics of childhood uveitis leading to visual impairment and blindness in the Netherlands. Acta Ophthalmol. 2014;92(8):798–804. https://doi.org/10.1111/aos.12491.
372. De Boer J, Wulffraat N, Rothova A. Visual loss in uveitis of childhood. Br J Ophthalmol. 2003;87(7):879–84.
373. Abd El Latif E, Mousa R, Tawfeeq Mahdi M, Mahmoud Amin A, Mohammed Ahmed Ali M, Abdelhamid NE, et al. Etiology of Pediatric Uveitis in a Tertiary Pediatric Eye Hospital in Egypt. Ocular Immunology and Inflammation. 2023;31(10):1978–83. https://doi.org/10.1080/09273948.2022.2117201.
374. Paroli MP, Speranza S, Marino M, Pirraglia M, Pivetti-Pezzi P. Prognosis of juvenile rheumatoid arthritis-associated uveitis. Eur J Ophthalmol. 2003;13(7):616–21.

375. Da Mata AP, Foster CS. Ahmed valve and uveitic glaucoma. Int Ophthalmol Clin. 1999;39(1):155–67.
376. Kaur S, Kaushik S, Pandav SS. Pediatric uveitic glaucoma. J Current Glaucoma Practice. 2013;7(3):115.
377. Djodeyre MR, Calvo JP, Gomez JA. Clinical evaluation and risk factors of time to failure of Ahmed glaucoma valve implant in pediatric patients. Ophthalmology. 2001;108(3):614–20.
378. Morad Y, Donaldson CE, Kim YM, Abdolell M, Levin AV. The Ahmed drainage implant in the treatment of pediatric glaucoma. Am J Ophthalmol. 2003;135(6):821–9.
379. Holland GN, Stiehm ER. Special considerations in the evaluation and management of uveitis in children. Am J Ophthalmol. 2003;135(6):867–78.
380. Dietlein T. Glaucoma and uveitis. Causes of and treatment options for increased intraocular pressure in cases of inflammatory ophthalmology. Der Ophthalmologe: Zeitschrift der Deutschen Ophthalmologischen Gesellschaft. 2003;100(11):991–1006; quiz 7.
381. Hettinga YM, de Groot-Mijnes JDF, Rothova A, de Boer JH. Infectious involvement in a tertiary center pediatric uveitis cohort. Br J Ophthalmol. 2015;99(1):103–7.
382. Rani D, Mahalingam K, Gupta S, Venkatesh P. Uveitic Glaucoma. In: Gupta S, Mahalingam K, Gupta V, editors. Childhood glaucoma: a case based color and video atlas. Singapore: Springer Nature Singapore; 2023. p. 203–11.
383. van Meerwijk CLLI, Jansonius NM, Los LI. Uveitic glaucoma in children: a systematic review on surgical outcomes. J Ophthalmic Inf Infect. 2022;12(1):35. https://doi.org/10.1186/s12348-022-00313-2.
384. Muñoz-Negrete FJ, Moreno-Montañés J, Hernández-Martínez P, Rebolleda G. Current approach in the diagnosis and management of uveitic glaucoma. BioMed Res Int. 2015;2015.
385. Abu Samra K, Maghsoudlou A, Roohipoor R, Valdes-Navarro M, Lee S, Foster CS. Current treatment modalities of JIA-associated uveitis and its complications: literature review. Ocul Immunol Inflamm. 2016;24(4):431–9.
386. Sung VC, Barton K. Management of inflammatory glaucomas. Curr Opin Ophthalmol. 2004;15(2):136–40.
387. Iannucci V, Manni P, Mecarelli G, Giammaria S, Giovannetti F, Lambiase A, et al. Childhood Uveitic glaucoma: complex management in a fragile population. Appl Sci. 2023;13(4):2205.
388. Kalogeropoulos D, Kalogeropoulos C, Moschos MM, Sung V. The Management of Uveitic Glaucoma in Children. Turk J Ophthalmol. 2019;49(5):283–93. https://doi.org/10.4274/tjo.galenos.2019.36589.
389. Kalogeropoulos D, Sung VC. Pathogenesis of uveitic glaucoma. J Current Glaucoma Pract. 2018;12(3):125.
390. Peretz WL, Tomasi TB. Aqueous humor proteins in uveitis: Immunoelectrophoretic and gel diffusion studies on normal and pathological human aqueous humor. Arch Ophthalmol. 1961;65(1):20–3.
391. Ladas JG, Yu F, Loo R, Davis JL, Coleman AL, Levinson RD, et al. Relationship between aqueous humor protein level and outflow facility in patients with uveitis. Invest Ophthalmol Vis Sci. 2001;42(11):2584–8.
392. Vitale AT, Graham E, de Boer JH. Juvenile idiopathic arthritis-associated uveitis: clinical features and complications, risk factors for severe course, and visual outcome. Ocul Immunol Inflamm. 2013;21(6):478–85.
393. Buonfiglio F, Böhm EW, Pfeiffer N, Gericke A. Oxidative stress: a suitable therapeutic target for optic nerve diseases? Antioxidants. 2023;12(7):1465.
394. Selvan H, Khokhar SK, Gupta S. Post-Traumatic Glaucoma. In: Gupta S, Mahalingam K, Gupta V, editors. Childhood glaucoma: a case based color and video atlas. Singapore: Springer Nature Singapore; 2023. p. 213–26.
395. Abbott J, Shah P. The epidemiology and etiology of pediatric ocular trauma. Surv Ophthalmol. 2013;58(5):476–85.
396. Kaur S, Kaushik S, Pandav SS. Traumatic glaucoma in children. J Current Glaucoma Practice. 2014;8(2):58.

397. Kalamkar C, Mukherjee A. Incidence, clinical profile, and short-term outcomes of post-traumatic glaucoma in pediatric eyes. Indian J Ophthalmol. 2019;67(4):509–14. https://doi.org/10.4103/ijo.IJO_655_18.
398. Ashaye AO. Traumatic hyphaema: a report of 472 consecutive cases. BMC Ophthalmol. 2008;8:24. https://doi.org/10.1186/1471-2415-8-24.
399. Zhang L, Buonfiglio F, Fieß A, Pfeiffer N, Gericke A. Retinopathy of Prematurity—Targeting Hypoxic and Redox Signaling Pathways. Antioxidants. 2024;13(2):148.
400. Lenis TL, Ledesma Vicioso N, Reddy V, Kovacs KD, Van Tassel SH, Orlin A. Case report: glaucoma in an infant with retinopathy of prematurity. Front Pediatr. 2021;9: 786327. https://doi.org/10.3389/fped.2021.786327.
401. Bremer DL, Rogers DL, Good WV, Tung B, Hardy RJ, Fellows R. Glaucoma in the early treatment for retinopathy of prematurity (ETROP) study. J Am Ass Pediatric Ophthal Strabismus. 2012;16(5):449–52. https://doi.org/10.1016/j.jaapos.2012.06.011.
402. Senthil S, Balijepalli P, Mohamed A, Rani PK, Nayak S, Garudadri C, et al. Management outcomes of secondary glaucoma due to retinopathy of prematurity: a 19-year prospective study at a tertiary eye care Institute. The Indian Twin Cities ROP Screening (ITCROPS) Database Report Number 8. PLoS One. 2020;15(9):e0238633. https://doi.org/10.1371/journal.pone.0238633.
403. Hosaka F, Rodríguez-Vázquez JF, Abe H, Murakami G, Fujimiya M, Ohguro H. Qualitative changes in fetal trabecular meshwork fibers at the human iridocorneal angle. Anatomy & Cell Biology. 2013;46(1):49–56.
404. Hittner HM, Rhodes LM, McPherson AR. Anterior segment abnormalities in cicatricial retinopathy of prematurity. Ophthalmology. 1979;86(5):803–16.
405. Wu W-C, Lin R-I, Shih C-P, Wang N-K, Chen Y-P, Chao A-N, et al. Visual acuity, optical components, and macular abnormalities in patients with a history of retinopathy of prematurity. Ophthalmology. 2012;119(9):1907–16.
406. Chang SH, Lee Y-S, Wu S-C, See L-C, Chung C-C, Yang M-L, et al. Anterior chamber angle and anterior segment structure of eyes in children with early stages of retinopathy of prematurity. Am J Ophthalmol. 2017;179:46–54.
407. Shaikh N, Tewari R, Chandra P. Glaucoma in Retinopathy of Prematurity. In: Gupta S, Mahalingam K, Gupta V, editors. Childhood glaucoma: a case based color and video atlas. Singapore: Springer Nature Singapore; 2023. p. 227–34.
408. Chandra P, Tewari R, Salunkhe N, Kumawat D, Chaurasia AK, Gupta V. Short-term incidence and management of glaucoma after successful surgery for stage 4 retinopathy of prematurity. Indian J Ophthalmol. 2019;67(6):917–21. https://doi.org/10.4103/ijo.IJO_33_18.
409. Hartnett ME, Gilbert MM, Hirose T, Richardson TM, Katsumi O. Glaucoma as a cause of poor vision in severe retinopathy of prematurity. Graefes Arch Clin Exp Ophthalmol. 1993;231(8):433–8. https://doi.org/10.1007/BF02044227.
410. Pollard ZF. Secondary angle-closure glaucoma in cicatricial retrolental fibroplasia. Am J Ophthalmol. 1980;89(5):651–3.
411. Kushner BJ. Ciliary block glaucoma in retinopathy of prematurity. Arch Ophthalmol. 1982;100(7):1078–9.
412. Wu S-C, Lee Y-S, Wu W-C, Chang SHL. Acute angle-closure glaucoma in retinopathy of prematurity following pupil dilation. BMC Ophthalmol. 2015;15(1):96. https://doi.org/10.1186/s12886-015-0099-7.
413. Smith J, Shivitz I. Angle-closure glaucoma in adults with cicatricial retinopathy of prematurity. Arch Ophthalmol. 1984;102(3):371–2.
414. Michael AJ, Pesin SR, Katz LJ, Tasman WS. Management of late-onset angle-closure glaucoma associated with retinopathy of prematurity. Ophthalmology. 1991;98(7):1093–8.
415. Roberti G, Oddone F, Agnifili L, Katsanos A, Michelessi M, Mastropasqua L, et al. Steroid-induced glaucoma: Epidemiology, pathophysiology, and clinical management. Surv Ophthalmol. 2020;65(4):458–72.

416. Varshney T, Dudani P, Gupta V. Steroid-Induced Glaucoma. In: Gupta S, Mahalingam K, Gupta V, editors. Childhood glaucoma: a case based color and video atlas. Singapore: Springer Nature Singapore; 2023. p. 235–43.
417. Fan DS, Ng JS, Lam DS. A prospective study on ocular hypertensive and antiinflammatory response to different dosages of fluorometholone in children. Ophthalmology. 2001;108(11):1973–7. https://doi.org/10.1016/s0161-6420(01)00781-3.
418. Fan DS, Yu CB, Chiu TY, Wong CY, Ng JS, Pang CP, et al. Ocular-hypertensive and anti-inflammatory response to rimexolone therapy in children. Arch Ophthalmol. 2003;121(12):1716–21. https://doi.org/10.1001/archopht.121.12.1716.
419. Lam CS, Umi Kalthum MN, Norshamsiah MD, Bastion M. Case series of children with steroid-Induced glaucoma. Malays Fam Physician. 2018;13(3):32–7.
420. Nuyen B, Weinreb RN, Robbins SL. Steroid-induced glaucoma in the pediatric population. J Am Ass Pediatric Ophthalmol Strabismus (JAAPOS). 2017;21(1):1–6. https://doi.org/10.1016/j.jaapos.2016.09.026.
421. Kwok AK, Lam DS, Ng JS, Fan DS, Chew S-J, Tso MO. Ocular-hypertensive response to topical steroids in children. Ophthalmology. 1997;104(12):2112–6.
422. Ang M, Ti S-E, Loh R, Farzavandi S, Zhang R, Tan D, et al. Steroid-induced ocular hypertension in Asian children with severe vernal keratoconjunctivitis. Clin Ophthalmol. 2012:1253–8.
423. Gupta S, Shah P, Grewal S, Chaurasia AK, Gupta V. Steroid-induced glaucoma and childhood blindness. Br J Ophthalmol. 2015;99(11):1454–6. https://doi.org/10.1136/bjophthalmol-2014-306557.
424. Cantrill HL, Palmberg PF, Zink HA, Waltman SR, Podos SM, Becker B. Comparison of in vitro potency of corticosteroids with ability to raise intraocular pressure. Am J Ophthalmol. 1975;79(6):1012–7.
425. Mindel JS, Tavitian HO, Smith H, Walker EC. Comparative ocular pressure elevation by medrysone, fluorometholone, and dexamethasone phosphate. Arch Ophthalmol. 1980;98(9):1577–8.
426. McGhee CN, Dean S, Danesh-Meyer H. Locally administered ocular corticosteroids: benefits and risks. Drug Saf. 2002;25:33–55.
427. Patel PD, Kodati B, Clark AF. Role of glucocorticoids and glucocorticoid receptors in glaucoma pathogenesis. Cells. 2023;12(20). https://doi.org/10.3390/cells12202452.
428. Wordinger RJ, Clarka AF. Effects of glucocorticoids on the trabecular meshwork: towards a better understanding of glaucoma. Prog Retin Eye Res. 1999;18(5):629–67.
429. Clark AF, Wordinger RJ. The role of steroids in outflow resistance. Exp Eye Res. 2009;88(4):752–9.
430. Dibas A, Yorio T. Glucocorticoid therapy and ocular hypertension. Eur J Pharmacol. 2016;787:57–71. https://doi.org/10.1016/j.ejphar.2016.06.018.
431. Shan SW, Do CW, Lam TC, Kong RPW, Li KK, Chun KM, et al. New insight of common regulatory pathways in human trabecular meshwork cells in response to dexamethasone and prednisolone using an integrated quantitative proteomics: SWATH and MRM-HR mass spectrometry. J Proteome Res. 2017;16(10):3753–65.
432. Tektas O-Y, Lütjen-Drecoll E. Structural changes of the trabecular meshwork in different kinds of glaucoma. Exp Eye Res. 2009;88(4):769–75.
433. Armaly MF. Statistical attributes of the steroid hypertensive response in the clinically normal eye. I. the demonstration of three levels of response. Invest Ophthalmol. 1965;4:187–97.
434. Becker B, Hahn KA. Topical corticosteroids and heredity in primary open-angle glaucoma. Am J Ophthalmol. 1964;57:543–51. https://doi.org/10.1016/0002-9394(64)92500-0.
435. Becker B. Intraocular pressure response to topical corticosteroids. Invest Ophthalmol. 1965;4:198–205.
436. Brandt JD, Shankar SP. Glaucoma following cataract surgery in children—finally, a clue. JAMA Ophthalmol. 2023;141(9):880–1. https://doi.org/10.1001/jamaophthalmol.2023.3804.
437. Zhang Y, Song Y, Zhou Y, Bai B, Zhang X, Chen W. A comprehensive review of pediatric glaucoma following cataract surgery and progress in treatment. The Asia-Pacific J Ophthalmol. 2023;12(1):94–102. https://doi.org/10.1097/apo.0000000000000586.

438. Lawrence MG, Kramarevsky NY, Christiansen SP, Wright MM, Young TL, Summers CG. Glaucoma following cataract surgery in children: surgically modifiable risk factors. Trans Am Ophthalmol Soc. 2005;103:46–55.
439. Mataftsi A. Incidence of and risk factors for postoperative glaucoma and its treatment in paediatric cataract surgery. Pediatric Cataract. 2016;57:40–8.
440. Jamerson EC, Solyman O, Yacoub MS, Abushanab MMI, Elhusseiny AM. Angle surgery in Pediatric glaucoma following cataract surgery. Vision. 2021;5(1):9.
441. Simons AS, Casteels I, Grigg J, Stalmans I, Vandewalle E, Lemmens S. Management of childhood glaucoma following cataract surgery. J Clin Med. 2022;11(4). https://doi.org/10.3390/jcm11041041.
442. Rabiah PK. Frequency and predictors of glaucoma after pediatric cataract surgery. Am J Ophthalmol. 2004;137(1):30–7.
443. Chen TC, Chen PP, Francis BA, Junk AK, Smith SD, Singh K, et al. Pediatric glaucoma surgery: a report by the American Academy of Ophthalmology. Ophthalmology. 2014;121(11):2107–15.
444. Swamy BN, Billson F, Martin F, Donaldson C, Hing S, Jamieson R, et al. Secondary glaucoma after paediatric cataract surgery. Br J Ophthalmol. 2007;91(12):1627–30.
445. Freedman SF, Beck AD, Nizam A, Vanderveen DK, Plager DA, Morrison DG, et al. Glaucoma-related adverse events at 10 years in the infant aphakia treatment study: a secondary analysis of a randomized clinical trial. JAMA ophthalmology. 2021;139(2):165–73.
446. Wood A, Lim B, Matthews J, Karaconji T, Zagora SL, Jamieson RV, et al. Prevalence of glaucoma following paediatric cataract surgery in an Australian tertiary referral centre. Clin Ophthalmol. 2023;17:2171–9. https://doi.org/10.2147/opth.S400512.
447. Kim J-A, Lee S-Y, Park KH, Yu YS, Jeoung JW. Incidence and risk factors for glaucoma development after bilateral congenital cataract surgery in microphthalmic eyes. Am J Ophthalmol. 2019;208:265–72.
448. Solebo AL, Rahi JS. Glaucoma following cataract surgery in the first 2 years of life: frequency, risk factors and outcomes from IoLunder2. Br J Ophthalmol. 2020;104(7):967–73.
449. Kuhli-Hattenbach C, Lüchtenberg M, Kohnen T, Hattenbach L-O. Risk factors for complications after congenital cataract surgery without intraocular lens implantation in the first 18 months of life. Am J Ophthalmol. 2008;146(1):1–7. e1.
450. Mataftsi A, Haidich A-B, Kokkali S, Rabiah PK, Birch E, Stager DR, et al. Postoperative glaucoma following infantile cataract surgery: an individual patient data meta-analysis. JAMA Ophthalmol. 2014;132(9):1059–67.
451. Balasubramaniam N, Mahalingam K, Gupta S. Postsurgical Glaucoma. In: Gupta S, Mahalingam K, Gupta V, editors. Childhood glaucoma: a case based color and video atlas. Singapore: Springer Nature Singapore; 2023. p. 191–201.
452. Traboulsi EI, Utz VM. Practical management of pediatric ocular disorders and strabismus. Springer; 2016.
453. Mandal AK, Netland PA. Glaucoma in aphakia and pseudophakia after congenital cataract surgery. Indian J Ophthalmol. 2004;52(3):185–98.
454. Daniel MC, Dubis AM, Theodorou M, Quartilho A, Adams G, Brookes J, et al. Childhood Lensectomy is associated with static and dynamic reduction in Schlemm canal size: a biomechanical hypothesis of glaucoma after Lensectomy. Ophthalmology. 2019;126(2):233–41. https://doi.org/10.1016/j.ophtha.2018.08.031.
455. Tatham A, Odedra N, Tayebjee S, Anwar S, Woodruff G. The incidence of glaucoma following paediatric cataract surgery: a 20-year retrospective study. Eye (Lond). 2010;24(8):1366–75. https://doi.org/10.1038/eye.2010.46.
456. Smolar LO, Ayalon A, Ela-Dalman N, Moisseiev E. Acute angle closure in an aphakic infant: Case report and review of the literature. Am J Ophthalmol Case Rep. 2019;15: 100459.
457. Asrani S, Freedman S, Hasselblad V, Buckley EG, Egbert J, Dahan E, et al. Does primary intraocular lens implantation prevent "aphakic" glaucoma in children? J Am Ass Pediatric Ophthalmol Strabismus. 2000;4(1):33–9.

458. Michael I, Shmoish M, Walton DS, Levenberg S. Interactions between trabecular meshwork cells and lens epithelial cells: a possible mechanism in infantile aphakic glaucoma. Invest Ophthalmol Vis Sci. 2008;49(9):3981–7.
459. Kirwan C, O'Keefe M. Paediatric aphakic glaucoma. Acta Ophthalmol Scand. 2006;84(6):734–9. https://doi.org/10.1111/j.1600-0420.2006.00733.x.
460. Michael I, Walton DS, Levenberg S. Infantile aphakic glaucoma: a proposed etiologic role of IL-4 and VEGF. J Pediatr Ophthalmol Strabismus. 2011;48(3):98–107.
461. Xu H, Zhu L, Wang Y, Bao Y. Effect of exogenous alpha-B crystallin on the structures and functions of trabecular meshwork cells. J Ophthalmol. 2018;2018.
462. Lam DS, Fan DS, Ng JS, Yu CB, Wong CY, Cheung AY. Ocular hypertensive and anti-inflammatory responses to different dosages of topical dexamethasone in children: a randomized trial. Clin Experiment Ophthalmol. 2005;33(3):252–8. https://doi.org/10.1111/j.1442-9071.2005.01022.x.
463. Abdelmassih Y, Beaujeux P, Dureau P, Edelson C, Caputo G. Incidence and risk factors of glaucoma following pediatric cataract surgery with primary implantation. Am J Ophthalmol. 2021;224:1–6.
464. Mills MD, Robb RM, Simon JW. Glaucoma following childhood cataract surgery/discussion. SLACK Incorporated Thorofare, NJ; 1994. p. 355–61.
465. Freedman SF, Lynn MJ, Beck AD, Bothun ED, Örge FH, Lambert SR. Glaucoma-related adverse events in the first 5 years after unilateral cataract removal in the infant Aphakia treatment study. JAMA Ophthalmol. 2015;133(8):907–14. https://doi.org/10.1001/jamaophthalmol.2015.1329.
466. Kang KD, Yim HB, Biglan AW. Comparison of delayed-onset glaucoma and early-onset glaucoma after infantile cataract surgery. Korean J Ophthalmol. 2006;20(1):41–6.
467. Papadopoulos M, Cable N, Rahi J, Khaw PT. The british infantile and childhood glaucoma (BIG) eye study. Invest Ophthalmol Vis Sci. 2007;48(9):4100–6. https://doi.org/10.1167/iovs.06-1350.
468. Lingham G, Thakur S, Safi S, Gordon I, Evans JR, Keel S. A systematic review of clinical practice guidelines for childhood glaucoma. BMJ Open Ophthalmol. 2022;7(1): e000933. https://doi.org/10.1136/bmjophth-2021-000933.
469. Quaranta L, Biagioli E, Riva I, Galli F, Poli D, Rulli E, et al. The glaucoma Italian pediatric study (GIPSy): 3-year results. J Glaucoma. 2018;27(10):856–63. https://doi.org/10.1097/ijg.0000000000001038.
470. Ott EZ, Mills MD, Arango S, Getson AJ, Assaid CA, Adamsons IA. A randomized trial assessing dorzolamide in patients with glaucoma who are younger than 6 years. Arch Ophthalmol. 2005;123(9):1177–86. https://doi.org/10.1001/archopht.123.9.1177.
471. Coppens G, Stalmans I, Zeyen T, Casteels I. The safety and efficacy of glaucoma medication in the pediatric population. J Pediatr Ophthalmol Strabismus. 2009;46(1):12–8. https://doi.org/10.3928/01913913-20090101-05.
472. Talbot AW, Russell-Eggitt I. Pharmaceutical management of the childhood glaucomas. Expert Opin Pharmacother. 2000;1(4):697–711. https://doi.org/10.1517/14656566.1.4.697.
473. Enyedi LB, Freedman SF, Buckley EG. The effectiveness of latanoprost for the treatment of pediatric glaucoma. J aapos. 1999;3(1):33–9. https://doi.org/10.1016/s1091-8531(99)70092-3.
474. Yang CB, Freedman SF, Myers JS, Buckley EG, Herndon LW, Allingham RR. Use of latanoprost in the treatment of glaucoma associated with Sturge-Weber syndrome. Am J Ophthalmol. 1998;126(4):600–2. https://doi.org/10.1016/s0002-9394(98)00129-9.
475. Altuna JC, Greenfield DS, Wand M, Liebmann JM, Taglia DP, Kaufman PL, et al. Latanoprost in glaucoma associated with Sturge-Weber syndrome: benefits and side-effects. J Glaucoma. 1999;8(3):199–203.
476. Ong T, Chia A, Nischal KK. Latanoprost in port wine stain related paediatric glaucoma. Br J Ophthalmol. 2003;87(9):1091–3. https://doi.org/10.1136/bjo.87.9.1091.
477. Urban B, Bakunowicz-Lazarczyk A, Mrugacz M, Oziebło-Kupczyk M. The effectiveness of latanoprost for the treatment of pediatric glaucoma. Klin Oczna. 2004;106(1–2 Suppl):243–4.

478. Ghaffari Z, Zakariaei Z, Ghazaeian M, Jafari R, Ezoddin N, Yousefi Nouraee H, et al. Adverse effects of brimonidine eye drop in children: A case series. J Clin Pharm Ther. 2021;46(5):1469–72. https://doi.org/10.1111/jcpt.13401.
479. Rahman MQ, Ramaesh K, Montgomery DM. Brimonidine for glaucoma. Expert Opin Drug Saf. 2010;9(3):483–91. https://doi.org/10.1517/14740331003709736.
480. Zimmerman TJ, Wheeler TM. Miotics: side effects and ways to avoid them. Ophthalmology. 1982;89(1):76–80. https://doi.org/10.1016/s0161-6420(82)34866-6.
481. Kanski JJ. Miotics. Br J Ophthalmol. 1968;52(12):936–7. https://doi.org/10.1136/bjo.52.12.936.
482. Tong L, Cui D, Zeng J. Effects of topical pilocarpine on ocular growth and refractive development in rabbits. Eur J Ophthalmol. 2021;31(4):2107–15. https://doi.org/10.1177/1120672120934962.
483. Wright KW, Chrousos GA. Weill-Marchesani syndrome with bilateral angle-closure glaucoma. J Pediatr Ophthalmol Strabismus. 1985;22(4):129–32. https://doi.org/10.3928/0191-3913-19850701-04.
484. Barkan O. Technic of goniotomy for congenital glaucoma. Arch Ophthal. 1949;41(1):65–82. https://doi.org/10.1001/archopht.1949.00900040068008.
485. Barkan O. Goniotomy knife and surgical contact glass. AMA Arch Ophthalmol. 1950;44(3):431–3. https://doi.org/10.1001/archopht.1950.00910020440013.
486. Smith R. A new technique for opening the canal of Schlemm. Preliminary report Br J Ophthalmol. 1960;44(6):370–3. https://doi.org/10.1136/bjo.44.6.370.
487. Burian HM. A case of Marfan's syndrome with bilateral glaucoma. With description of a new type of operation for developmental glaucoma (trabeculotomy ab externo). Am J Ophthalmol. 1960;50:1187–92.
488. Beck AD, Lynch MG. 360 degrees trabeculotomy for primary congenital glaucoma. Arch Ophthalmol. 1995;113(9):1200–2. https://doi.org/10.1001/archopht.1995.01100090126034.
489. Morgan KS, Black B, Ellis FD, Helveston EM. Treatment of congenital glaucoma. Am J Ophthalmol. 1981;92(6):799–803. https://doi.org/10.1016/s0002-9394(14)75633-8.
490. Turaçh ME, Aktan G, Idil A. Medical and surgical aspects of congenital glaucoma. Acta Ophthalmol Scand. 1995;73(3):261–3. https://doi.org/10.1111/j.1600-0420.1995.tb00281.x.
491. Gagrani M, Garg I, Ghate D. Surgical interventions for primary congenital glaucoma. Cochrane Database Syst Rev. 2020;8(8):Cd008213. https://doi.org/10.1002/14651858.CD008213.pub3.

Chapter 3
Congenital Corneal Opacities

Ken K. Nischal and Sarah Zwingelberg

Abstract Corneal disease is among the most important causes of visual impairment in children worldwide. Congenital and infantile corneal opacities have a narrow therapeutic window for intervention due to the risk of amblyopia, and are often complex. The causes and clinical presentation of congenital corneal opacities are varied. The correct diagnosis should be made early and appropriate interdisciplinary involvement established as necessary. The most important carers for the affected child are his/her parents and close cooperation between the parents and the clinical team involved is therefore essential. The ophthalmic workup of patients with congenital corneal opacities includes a thorough history with subsequent clinical examination, often performed under general anesthesia and supported by new imaging modalities such as linear ultrasound, high frequency ultrasound and optical coherence tomography. The structured classification of congenital corneal opacities provides the basis for targeted therapy and should be focused on whether the disease is due to a primary corneal disorder or if the corneal disease is due to secondary corneal disorders.. However, in children, ophthalmologic surgery is surgically more demanding and the prognosis is generally worse. Surgical procedures include e.g. phototherapeutic keratectomy, optical iridectomy, and lamellar, penetrating, and autokeratoplasty procedures. Newer techniques of selective endothelial removal and the use of simple limbal epithelial transplant are also part of the armamentarium for the surgeon. An equally important part of therapy is represented by conservative treatment with bandage lenses, glasses, contact lenses, and occlusion if necessary. The present work provides an overview of evaluation including clinical, diagnostic molecular of congenital corneal opacities and discusses current treatment.

Keywords Congenital · Infantile · Corneal opacity · Dystrophy · Dysgenesis · Keratoconus · Brittle cornea · Genetics · Diagnostics · Keratoplasty · DALK · DSAEK DMEK · PKP · Crosslinking · PTK

Parts of this chapter are taken from: Zwingelberg S. B. "Diagnosis and Surgical Therapy of Infantile Corneal Opacities", In Clinical Practice, https://doi.org/10.1007/978-3-031-47141-4, ISBN: 978-3-031-47140-7, Springer Verlag, 2024.

I. Broekaert et al., *Infantile Anterior Segment Disorders*,
https://doi.org/10.1007/978-3-031-68558-3_3

3.1 Introduction

Corneal blindness is one of the most important causes of severe visual impairment in children worldwide [1, 2].

Visual acuity plays an essential role in the global development of a child's neuro-behavior and thus the long-term quality of life of the patient and family members [3, 4]. Therefore, early detection and treatment of visual acuity function threatening pathologies is particularly important to avoid or refractory deprivational amblyopia.

Corneal opacities in children can be acquired or congenital. The etiologies of congenital corneal opacity (CCO) in children are diverse, and the incidences are highly variable depending on the region in the world the child inhabits.

When deciding on the operation, many peculiarities of the child's situation must be taken into account to determine the optimal supply for the child. Pre-operative diagnostics and post-operative therapy require therefore close interdisciplinary cooperation between pediatrics, human genetics and ophthalmology, as well as neurophysiology.

The aims of corneal surgical care for children are

- The fastest possible improvement in the optical and refractive properties of the cornea.
- The lowest possible follow-up effort to minimize the number of anesthetic examinations or revision procedures under anesthesia.
- Minimizing the surgical trauma through e.g. lamellar transplantation to minimize the risk of secondary increased intraocular pressure, rejection or wound dehiscence.

Based on a literature search on "Pubmed" and own clinical examples, this book offers an up-to-date structured overview and guide to the clinical, diagnostic, and genetic evaluation and therapy of the most important primary and secondary corneal opacities.

The following factors must be taken into account when making an decision for an operation

- The cause and exact location of corneal opacity
- The presence of co-existing ocular comorbidities
- Systemic status of child with respect to anesthesia and any postoperative investigations
- Social circumstances of the child and their affect on post-operative therapy, and compliance for occlusion therapy if needed
- The effect of any surgery on disruption of visual development especially in the amblyogenic period.

3.2 Anatomy, Physiology, Metabolism and Embryology of the Cornea

To understand the pathology of infantile corneal opacities, it is important to look at the anatomy and physiology, as well the metabolism and embryology of the cornea in further detail.

The cornea forms the transparent, curved anterior part of the eye, lubricated by the tear film, and it performs a large part of the refraction of light. It assumes an important function within visual ability. With its physiological refractive power of approx. 43D, it is the eye structure that is most involved in the refraction of light, accounting for 70% [5, 6]. However, the refractive power of + 43D only emerges because there is aqueous humor behind the cornea. If there were air in the eye chambers, the cornea would be a minus lens (diverging lens), because it is thinner in the center than at the edge [7].

The transparency of the cornea allows light to transmit to the receptors located in the retina, while acting as a protector for all subsequent layers. The required shape, clarity and resistance are made possible by the complex anatomical structure [8]. The translucent cornea is convex in shape and forms a depression within the less convex sclera. The transition to the sclera is formed by the limbus [9, 10].

The smallest disturbances and opacities can affect the refractive power and thus influence the sharpness of the image.

3.2.1 Anatomy of the Cornea

The diameter of the cornea is 11.5 mm (vertically 9–11 mm, horizontally 11–12, 5 mm) in adults and 9.5 mm (8–10 mm) in infants. Below 10 mm, it is called microcornea, and above 13 mm macro- or megalocornea [7–12]. The radius of this curvature is about 7.7 mm. It shows a central thickness of 520–550 μm and peripherally 640–700 μm.

If the horizontal radius differs from the vertical radius, it is called astigmatism. The cornea can be deformed by externally applied pressure, for example from hard contact lenses, and then needs days to regain its original shape after prolonged wear.

The human cornea comprises six layers (compare Fig. 3.1): the epithelial layer (1 in the figure), Bowman's membrane (2), the stroma (3), Descemet's membrane (4) and the endothelial cell layer (5). In a 2013 study, the sixth is defined as a 15 μm thick layer between the stroma and Descemet's membrane (pre-Descemet layer of Dua), which comprises five to eight lamellae of collagen type 1 bundles [13].

The cornea is physiologically free of vessels (avascular), and its supply is primarily by diffusion from the aqueous humor. The absence of vessels results in a slow regeneration as well as an immunological special position, which influences the transplantability [7, 9, 10, 14].

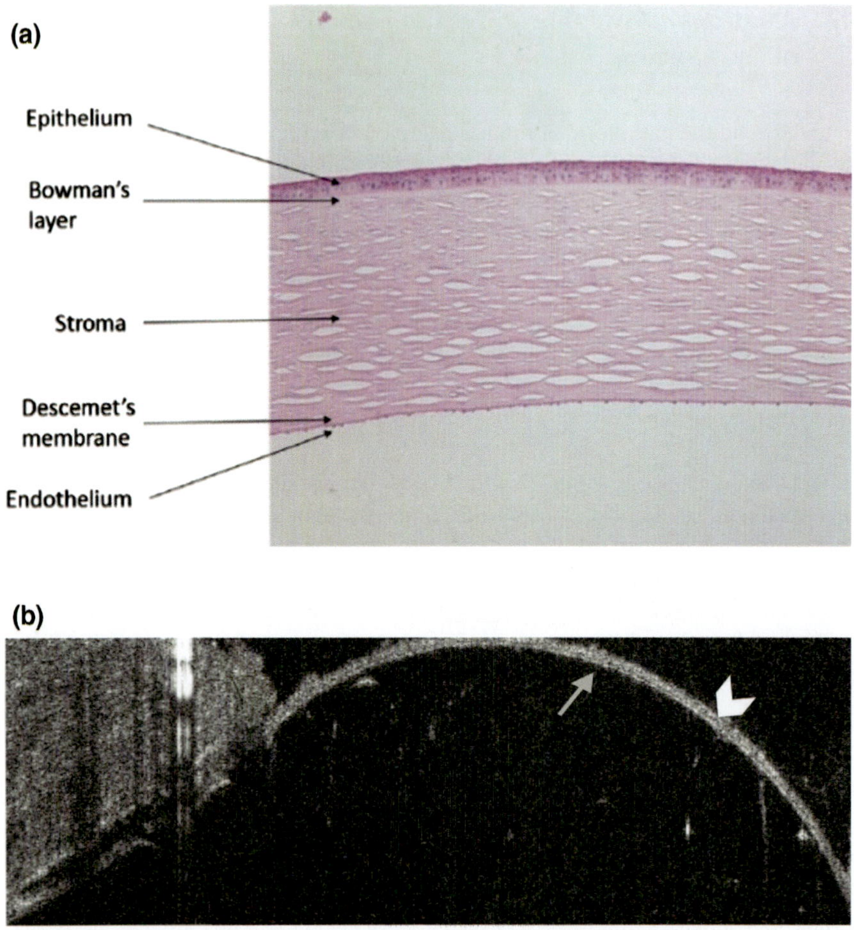

Fig. 3.1 a: Overview of the anatomy of the human cornea with the Dua layer, which is between the stroma and Descemet's membrane. b: OCT of a DALK after viscodissection to remove stroma in a 11yr old child. Descemet Membrane (white arrow) with Pre-DM layer of DUA (white chevron)

- **Epithelium**

The surface [9] of the cornea comprises five to six layers of non-keratinizing squamous epithelium. The epithelium is 40–60 μm thick on average, while the thickness increasing towards the limbus. Attached to its cell appendages is the tear film [7, 10, 12, 15].

In a healthy state, it is characterized by its rapid regenerative capacity, as a diffusion barrier to the tear film and as protection against external pathogens as well as mechanical damage [7, 9, 15–17]. The epithelium regenerates within seven days and usually heals without scarring. The presence of corneal stem cells in the area of the corneal limbus is a prerequisite for regeneration [7, 9, 15]. The diffusion barrier and protective function are enabled by the epithelial cell association.

The superficial epithelial cells are connected by tight junctions, which prevent the invasion of microorganisms [6, 15]. Their desmosomes on the anterior and lateral walls and basal hemidesmosome anchorages with the basement membrane make the corneal epithelium resistant to mechanical stress (e.g. eye rubbing) [6, 10, 17, 18]. The protective function is complemented by free nerve endings, which trigger the eyelid closure reflex and cause symptoms when injured [19, 20].

- **Bowman's membrane**

The basement membrane connects the epithelium with the 8–14 μm thick Bowman membrane (lamina limitans anterior). This second layer is acellular, and it comprises randomly arranged collagen fibrils as well as proteoglycans produced by the adjacent stroma. It is not capable of self-regeneration but shows strong resistance to damage. Once injured, it heals only with scarring [6, 7, 9, 10, 12, 15, 17].

- **Stroma**

The third layer, the 450–550 μm thick corneal stroma (substantia propria), occupies the largest part[132] of the cornea (approx. 90%). It comprises 250–400 perpendicular corneal lamellae (each approx. 5–6 μm), which are mainly composed of parallel collagen fibrils (each 25–35 nm) of connective tissue type I and V (type I, VI and XII) [7].

Interposed between the fibrils are two groups of proteoglycans as part of the extracellular matrix, the dermatan sulfate proteoglycans and the keratan sulfate proteoglycans. They act like spacers between fibrils and bind water. Since the posterior stroma has a lower proportion of dermatan sulfate, it shows a stronger tendency to swell with excess water in the event of endothelial insufficiency [20].

Between the lamellae are keratocytes, which are responsible for the production of the fibrils and are mainly located in the anterior part of the stroma [6, 7, 10, 15, 18, 21].

Keratocytes are fixed cells resembling fibrocytes of connective tissue. They have an elongated shape and possess long, branched processes. These cells are interconnected by protoplasmic bridges and form a syncytium. This is a cell association in which the cells are in cytoplasmic connection. This means that no boundaries are visible between them.

Under normal circumstances, keratocytes rarely divide. The turnover rate is about 2–3 years. When the cornea is injured to the stroma, the keratocytes proliferate and migrate into the damaged tissue, where they transform into fibroblasts and produce collagens and proteoglycans.

Thus, the wound is closed with scar formation. In addition, the fibrocytes constantly produce collagen, securing the basic substance of the stroma.

The migratory cells can appear in different forms (reticulocytes, macrophages, lymphocytes, etc.). In case of inflammation, these cells migrate towards the affected area and ensure an effective defense. In the limbal area, the lamellae intertwine and merge into the opaque, white sclera.

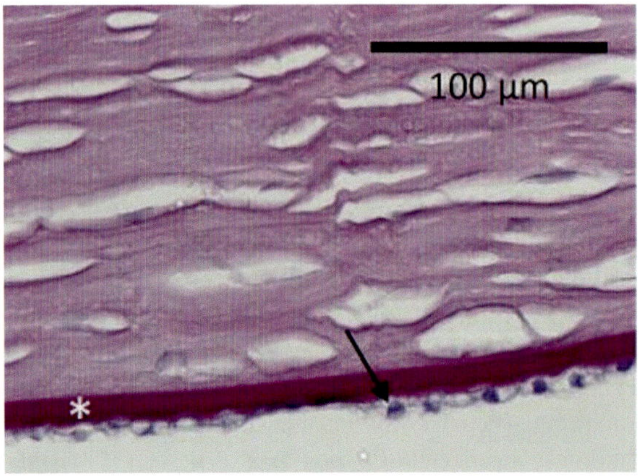

Fig. 3.2 Cross-sectional view of the cornea (arrow: endothelium, asterisk: Descemet's membrane)

The tight cellular structure allows the stroma to have strength and transparency. A high elasticity results from a water content of about 80% [10, 19, 22–24].

The end of the corneal stroma is formed by the Descemet's membrane and the corneal endothelium. Interposed between them is the pre-Descemet's membrane, a layer of interwoven collagen fibrils [12].

- **Pre-Descemet layer of Dua**

The Dua layer is a fine yet very resilient membrane, about 15 μm thick, located between the stroma and Descemet's membrane. Despite its small thickness, it is very tear-resistant and can withstand a pressure load of up to 2 bar [25].

- **Descemet's membrane**

Descemet's membrane (lamina limitans posterior) is the 5–10 μm thin fourth corneal layer (compare Fig. 3.2).

It can be ultrastructurally divided into an anterior banded layer (ABL) and a posterior non-banded layer (PNBL). The ABL is about 3 μm thick and is formed prenatally.

The PNBL is produced by endothelial cells throughout life. Its diameter increases during life (from about 3 μm in 20-year-olds to about 10 μm in 80-year-olds) [7, 9, 15, 21, 26, 27].

Descemet's membrane is transparent, homogeneous, and mainly comprises type VIII collagen fibrils and laminin. The collagen fibrils form a regular, two-dimensional hexagonal grid.

This makes Descemet's membrane the most resistant elastic membrane in the entire cornea. As a protective layer for the endothelium, Descemet's membrane effectively counteracts infection, mechanical and chemical injury, and enzymatic destruction. Injuries heal only with scarring.

- **Endothelium**

The approximately 4 μm thick, single-layer endothelium comprises approximately 400,000 hexagonal endothelial cells and forms the innermost layer of the cornea [9, 10, 18]. The endothelial cells originate from the neural crest. Its main function is to ensure transparency. It is in direct contact with the aqueous humor on the inside. The transfer of solutes, nutrients as well as water from there towards the cornea is passively limited by tight junctions between the cells. Like the epithelium, the endothelium performs a barrier function [10, 28].

In addition, the endothelial cells possess ion pumps (sodium–potassium ATPase) that, when sufficient in number (approximately 2500 cells/mm^2), actively pump excess water out of the cornea into the aqueous humor, thereby maintaining the physiological water content. The pumps are supported by transmembrane proteins (aquaporins) and sodium-borate co-transporters (SLC4A11). The endothelium is not capable of regeneration. Dead cells lose their shape and migrate within the cornea (migration). The loss is compensated by enlargement (polymegatism) and remodeling (polymorphism) of the remaining cells. More severe loss of endothelial cells to a value of less than 400–700 cells/mm^2 with accompanying loss of tight junctions may result in endothelial insufficiency, so that the pumping function of the remaining cells is no longer sufficient. This is followed by decompensation of the endothelium, and hydration leads to stromal and epithelial edema as well as severe visual impairment [10, 20, 22, 26, 29–32].

A physiological decrease In endothelial cell number is observed with age. average endothelial cell density of children is 3500 cells/mm^2, in adults 2400 cells/mm^2 and decreases by approximately 0.3–0.6% per year (compare Figs. 3.3 and 3.4a, b) [7, 20, 26, 33–35].

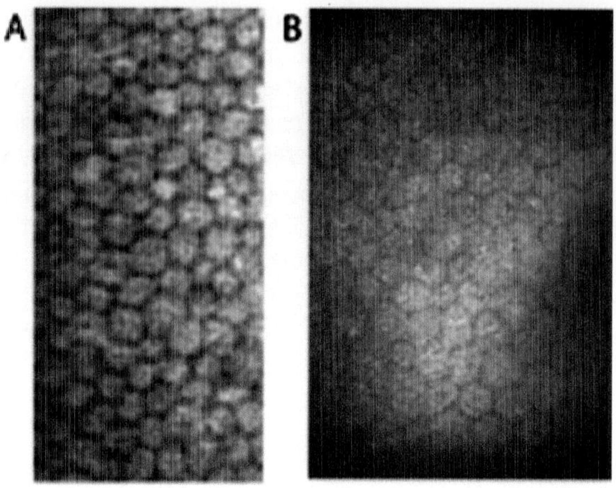

Fig. 3.3 Healthy endothelium in A) specular microscopy and B) confocal microscopy

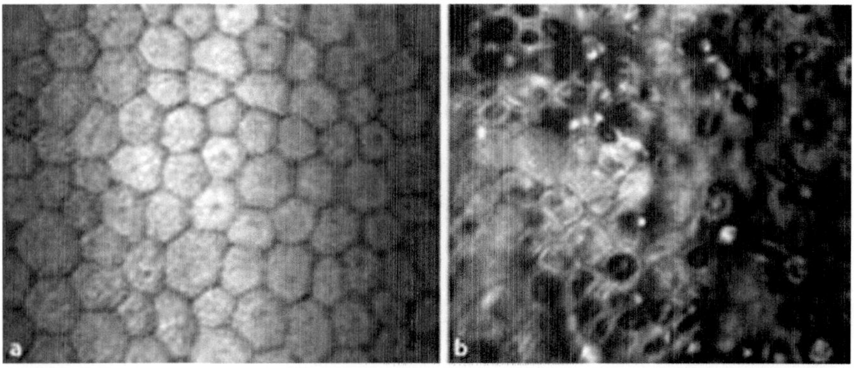

Fig. 3.4 A) Healthy endothelium versus. B) damaged endothelium in endothelial corneal diseases

3.2.2 Physiology of the Cornea

The transparency of the cornea is due to a regular ultrastructural arrangement of its components of collagens and proteoglycans and a strictly defined water content of the stroma. When the water content of the corneal stroma is disturbed, for example by swelling, the regular arrangement is lost and light scattering increases. In extreme cases, light scattering causes complete whitening of the cornea. The water content is actively regulated by the endothelial cell layer with oxygen consumption.

3.2.2.1 Tearfilm

Most of the tear film is secreted by the lacrimal gland and drains into the nasal cavity via the angle of the eye and the tear duct. The entire tear film is composed of two different types of tear layer, the preocular and the precorneal tear film.

The preocular tear film coats the cornea and conjunctiva within the palpebral fissure. The precorneal tear film, on the other hand, only covers the surface of the cornea. On the ocular surface, the precorneal tear fluid forms a three-layer tear film. Microscopic blebs appear when blinking, which temporarily reduce visual acuity. After around 0.5–1.5 s, they dissolve (depending on the consistency of the film) and any thickening caused by blinking is evened out. After about 5 s, the film breaks up and again creates irregularities, which improves visual performance again.

3.2.2.2 Corneal Metabolism

The outer layers of the cornea are supplied with nutrients and oxygen by the tear fluid, the inner layers by the aqueous humor and the marginal loop network.

Deficits in the energy metabolism immediately lead to edema in the cornea and reduced epithelial regeneration. The cornea is therefore dependent on a constant and good supply of nutrients and on the complete removal of metabolic waste products.

Metabolism mainly requires glucose (dextrose) and oxygen, which must be supplied from the outside. Metabolic end products are mainly water, carbon dioxide and lactate (lactic acid). Substances needed for metabolism from the tear film and aqueous humor must be brought into the cornea by diffusion, since it is avascular. Similarly, metabolic end products must be carried out of the cornea by diffusion. Only the marginal loop network as a peripheral vascular system in the limbal area is able to supply the periphery of the cornea with glucose and oxygen directly. Further, the substances reach the cornea only by diffusion. In case of possible injuries of the marginal loop network and its complete failure in the nutritional participation of the cornea, meanwhile, does not lead to the cornea's inability to function. It is believed that the contribution to the nutrition of the cornea is extremely small. The tear fluid provides the largest amount of oxygen, entering the tear film from the atmosphere when the eyelids are open and diffusing into the tear film from the vessels of the marginal loop and conjunctiva when the eyelids are closed.

While very little glucose is present in the tear film (about 0.2 μmol/g water), little dissolved oxygen exists in the aqueous humor. This is just sufficient to supply the most posterior region of the cornea. On the other hand, the aqueous humor contains the largest amount of glucose (about 6.5 μmol/g water).

For the cornea, the degradation of glucose is crucial for energy supply. Degradation occurs in three pathways with the participation of numerous enzymes. One pathway proceeds in the absence of oxygen, i.e. anaerobic, two pathways require the presence of oxygen, they proceed aerobically:

In the absence of oxygen, glucose is broken down by the anaerobic glycolysis pathway. The process is also called the Embden-Meyerhof cycle. This process leads in several stages via pyruvic acid to lactate or lactic acid.

The lactic acid is then transported away via the aqueous humor. In case of glucose deficiency, glycogen stored in the epithelium is resorted to. It is estimated that about 55% of the glucose available to the cornea is broken down via this pathway [9]. However, only two moles of energy-rich ATP are generated per mole of glucose. Thus, the energy yield is relatively low.

The hexose monophosphate pathway yields varying amounts of energy that is stored in the form of ATP. With one mole of energy-rich ATP per mole of glucose, the hexose monophosphate pathway is probably the least productive, but about 35% of all glucose is converted via it.

In the presence of oxygen, the lactate produced via aerobic glycolysis is completely converted to carbon dioxide and water. This process is known as the citric acid cycle. During the aerobic breakdown of glucose (citric acid cycle), 36 mol of ATP are generated per mole of glucose. However, only about 15% of the metabolized glucose takes this path.

It can therefore be seen that the oxygen supply is decisive for energy utilization.

In the absence of oxygen, glucose is only incompletely broken down to lactate. This then accumulates in the cornea and inhibits or interrupts the conversion to water and carbon dioxide. This leads to swelling of the cornea, a resulting disturbance of the regular arrangement of the fibrils in the stroma and ultimately to opacification in the cornea.

3.2.2.3 Innervation of the Cornea

The cornea is innervated by sensitive nerve branches of the ophthalmic nerve, which are not myelinated in the cornea. About 70–80 nerve trunks radiate into the cornea.

The epithelial axons, not accompanied by Schwann cells, are parallel to the basement membrane in an invagination of the basal plasmalemma of the basal cells. Most axons terminate here. However, some nerves extend further into the epithelium almost to the surface. Interestingly, the less abundant nerve fibers in the stroma also respond to external stimuli, as do the nerves in the epithelium. Thus, the nerves in the stroma are able to replace the protective function of the nerves in the epithelium when they are lost. Because a symbiotic relationship exists between the nerves and the corneal epithelium, epithelial stress or trauma causes changes in corneal neurology. Damage to the nerves triggers an epithelial reaction. Innervation is a prerequisite for the corneal reflex, the involuntary eyelid closure with increased production of lacrimal fluid, after mechanical corneal irritation. Furthermore, the corneal nerves release growth factors which, like an intact tear film, are essential for regular renewal of the epithelial layer (Fig. 3.5).

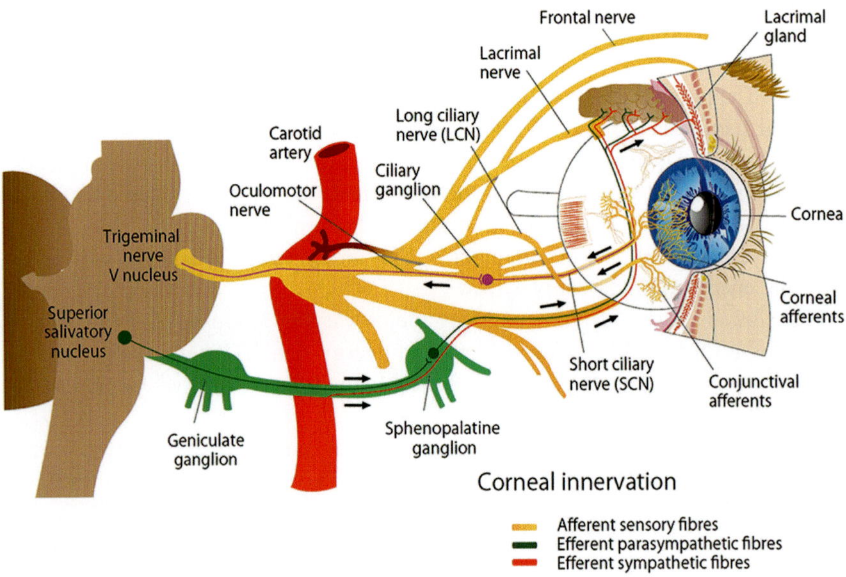

Fig. 3.5 Innervation of the Cornea

3.2.3 *Embryology*

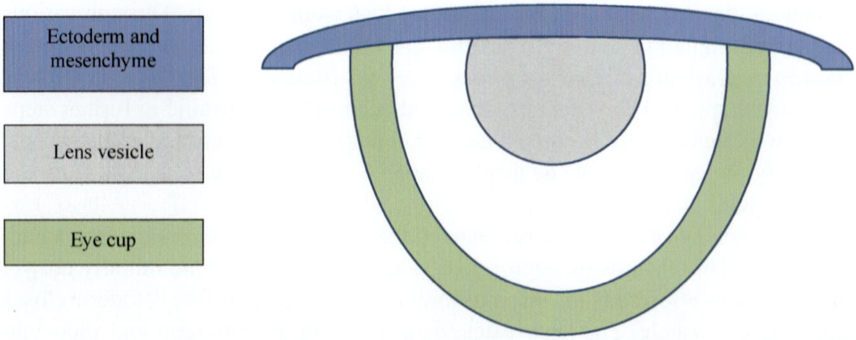

Already at the end of gastrulation the first course for the development of the eye is set. This is still the case at an early stage of embryonic development, when the formation of the three germ layers entoderm, mesoderm and ectoderm (inner layer, middle layer, outer layer) comes to an end.

In the eye, as in the other sense organs, the ectoderm is the essential germ layer from which the structures develop. In humans, these first steps occur from day 17 of gestation.

The development of the shoe sole-shaped neural plate on the gastrula, from which first the neural tube and from it later the brain and spinal cord arise, is triggered (induced) by the underlying mesoderm, and it comes to the formation first of a uniform eye field on this flap.

The genes *Rx1*, *Six3*, and *Pax6* are essential for the initiating steps. During neural tube formation, the eye field divides into two outer eye domains, controlled by the gene Sonic hedgehog (Shh), which is activated in a midline between these two domains and represses Pax6. Failure to express it at this crucial site results in the development of cyclopia [36]. Failure to activate (express) the aforementioned switch genes results in the loss of eye formation [37].

- **Ocular vesicle and lens placode**

Subsequently, around the beginning of the second month of pregnancy in humans, a bilateral protrusion of the anterior neural tube occurs at the eye fields and their outgrowth as optic vesicles from the diencephalon, [12] called the ocular peduncle. According to this, the excitation arriving here first reaches the diencephalon, and processing takes place in the cerebrum.

The protrusion of the ocular vesicles is based on individual cell migration. The protein Rx3 provides molecular signposts to the eye precursor cells. They provide these cells with information on how to move from the center of the brain towards the eye field, where larger accumulations of these cells occur [38, 39].

The outgrowing optical vesicle interacts with the outer layer and, as a new important induction step, triggers the formation of the lens placode there, a thickening of this ectoderm and indentation of the eye pit.

Without the vesicle, no thickening and no lens would develop. Through various mesodermal signaling and signals from the optic vesicle, the surface ectoderm becomes increasingly primed for prospective lens formation. The tissue is initially designated competent for lens formation and becomes lens-specific in further steps [40]. The tissue can only become lens after contact with the vesicle and its signals. Thus, only the epidermis of the head is capable of responding to signals from the optical vesicle.

The thickening of the ectoderm leads to the reshaping of the vesicle into a cup, the eye cup. This ensures by appropriate induction signals that the initially not yet transparent lens is formed [41]. After its initial formation, the surface ectoderm closes again over the vesicle. The lens vesicle detaches from the ectoderm and sinks into the depths.

- **Lens and cornea**

The early lens, the lens vesicle arising from the lens placode, is initially a hollow ball of surrounding cells. Each of these cells contains a nucleus with chromosomes and DNA. The anterior side faces the outside, the posterior side faces the inside of the eye. The cells are surrounded by a capsule with proteinaceous material.

In a first step, from the fifth week in humans, the posterior cells extend into the cavity. They form primary lens fibers, the later lens nucleus. The layering around the central nucleus always occurs from the lens equator [42]. During elongation, these fibers form several proteins, the crystallins. These fill the cavity of the lens and later form its main components with three types and 90% share of all proteins of the lens [43]. First they form the lens fibers. Subsequently, the lens fiber cells degrade their nucleus as well as other organelles, including the energy centers (mitochondria). This drastically reduces cell metabolism and minimizes light scattering. This process does not lead to programmed cell death (apoptosis), as is usually the case. Due to this process, the lens cells cannot and do not renew themselves until death.

The anterior cells remain as a single layer of cells on the outer surface of the lens (lens epithelium), even in the fully developed lens. They continue to divide, giving rise to secondary lens fibers at the upper and lower ends from the seventh week in humans. These lens fibers become very long and overlay the lens in concentric rings onion-skin-like in many layers [44]. For this purpose, new secondary lens fibers constantly grow from the mentioned positions at the top and bottom around the lens, displacing the previously formed secondary lens fibers inward, while new secondary lens fibers are always generated, which grow equally around the lens. Continuously, the anterior outer layer forms replenishment material for this process by cell division. Continuous formation of new rings allows the lens to grow [45]. Throughout the period of prenatal lens development, a vascular network containing blood vessels is spread over it posteriorly and laterally, the tunica vasculosa lentis, which disappears only shortly after birth.

The formation of new secondary lens fibers continues throughout the life of the organism. During this process, the lens no longer enlarges significantly, but it increases in density. The developed lens contains a nucleus of early cells. With increasing age, the elasticity of the lens decreases and it increasingly loses the ability to accommodate. The finished lens is the only organic tissue comprising completely transparent living cells.

The next process after lens induction is another induction, this time of the lens with the surface ectoderm. There it leads to a new thickening, the cornea [41].

In contrast to the cells of the lens, corneal cells have an extremely short life span and renew themselves weekly even after birth. The cornea is heavily permeated with nerves. The anterior rim of the cup becomes the pupil.

The cornea is formed by transformation of the surface ectoderm into anterior epithelium. The choroid, sclera develops from the mesodermal mesenchyme of the head area. With the formation of the sclera, the formation of blood vessels can begin, which cross the retina.

> **Notes**
>
> - Only the epithelium originates from the embryonic ectoderm, the remaining corneal layers develop from the mesoderm.
> - The endothelial cells originate from the neural crest. The mean corneal diameter of a newborn is 9.5 mm.
> - Corneal growth is completed by the end of the second year of life. An adult has an average corneal diameter of 11.5 mm (< 10 = microcornea, > 13 = macrocornea).

3.3 Clinical History, Examination and Further Diagnostics

3.3.1 Clinical History

Since the examination of young patients is often a challenge, the thorough collection of clinical history holds strong importance. Among the signs noticed by parents that may indicate corneal opacity are photophobia and blepharospasm, nystagmus, strabismus, epiphora, eye rubbing, increased screaming, and “clouding” or “graying” of the cornea.

In addition to a history of the presenting problem, a family history, including a family pedigree, pregnancy history (including possible infections, medication intake of the mother) and birth history (possible trauma/pincer birth, gestational age, weight at birth, premature retinopathy) should be taken [51].

The clarification of the social environment is also very important for the planning of the treatment, with respect to associated steps such as compliance of topical drop use, insertion/change of contact lenses, occlusion therapy, the avoidance of eye rubbing, the coordination of follow-up appointments, and the effect of all the family unit [46, 52].

The additional examination of parents, siblings and other biological relatives can provide important additional information here. In this context, genetic testing can provide further basic important information for the finding of the correct diagnosis and thus contribute significantly to the improvement of the therapy of ocular as well as systemic pathology. However accurate deep phenotyping is essential for accurate phenotype-genotype correlation. For this anterior segment imaging is essential [50–52].

> **Note: Signs of corneal opacity in children may include**
>
> - Photophobia
> - Blepharospasm
> - Epiphora
> - Eye rubbing
> - Increased crying
> - "Opacity" or "graying" of the cornea
> - Nystagmus
> - Strabismus.

3.3.2 Examination and Further Diagnostics

The examination of visual function including refraction, and ocular motility must always be carried out as standard. The presence of nystagmus in children over 6 weeks of age should be assessed. Fixation behavior to light can give an induction of visual function. Any obvious red reflex should be looked for with a direct ophthalmoscope. It is always important to check for dysmorphic facial features that may point to an underlying systemic condition.

Assessment of the cornea, includes detecting laterality (unilateral vs bilateral), location of the opacity (central vs eccentric vs complete). While an orienting examination on the awake patient is usually quite possible, the further examination immediately after food intake on the calmer or even sleeping patient can be helpful [46].

If possible, a (hand) slit lamp microscopy (with and without fluorescein), an indirect ophthalmoscopy, a measurement of the intraocular pressure e.g. by means of rebound tonometry and—if necessary in case of corneal opacity—a sonography (A and B image measurement) should be carried out (compare Fig. 3.6).

Since rebound tonometry is practicable in children with the diseases described here, but is often also prone to errors, palpation of the intraocular pressure is essential as a cross-check [47]. The use of axial length can be very helpful to assess if there

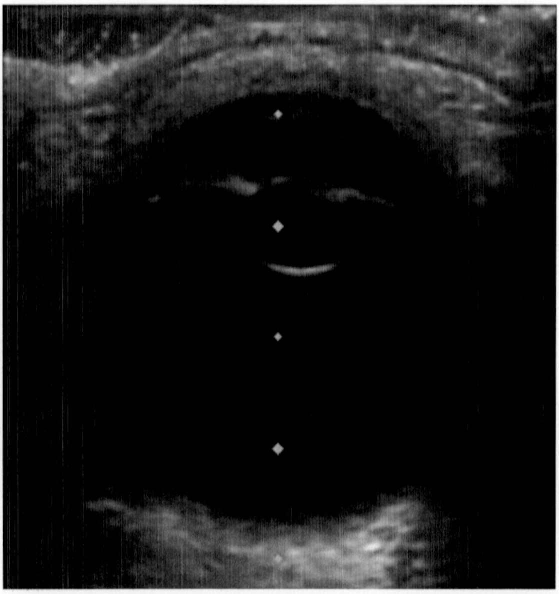

Fig. 3.6 Linear Ultrasound allows evaluation of the globe and also shows that in this cases of opaque cornea due to Posterior Polymorphous Dystrophy (PPCD)

might be glaucoma e.g. in a newborn the axial length should be 16.5 mm—if it is found to be > 18mm then the chances of glaucoma are high.

If a macroscopic photo or even a slit lamp microscopic image is possible and successful, the examiner can then assess the pathology in greater detail without further burden on the young patient. Images using optical coherence tomography (currently swept-source OCT) as well as intraoperative microscope-integrated OCT devices (MI-OCT) can provide even more information [1, 2, 4, 48, 49].

The OCT is a contactless and high-resolution procedure and can now be carried out within a few seconds. The evaluation of those tomographic data enables assessing the cornea including the severity and depth of the opacity, the astigmatism, the corneal thickness, the anterior chamber depth as well as an assessment of the underlying structures of the eye, including the chamber angle, iris and lens with possible adhesions (compare Fig. 3.7).

Examination techniques with direct eye contact such as gonioscopy, ultrasound biomicroscopy (UBM) and pachymetry or tonometric methods (e.g. Schiötz or Goldmann tonometry) are often difficult and represent an additional burden for the little patient. Ultimately, the detailed examination of the newborn or child, including further diagnostics, often requires general anesthesia and can be planned after weighing up the risk of anesthesia. Under anesthesia UBM is a very useful tool to assess the overall anterior segment (compare Fig. 3.8).

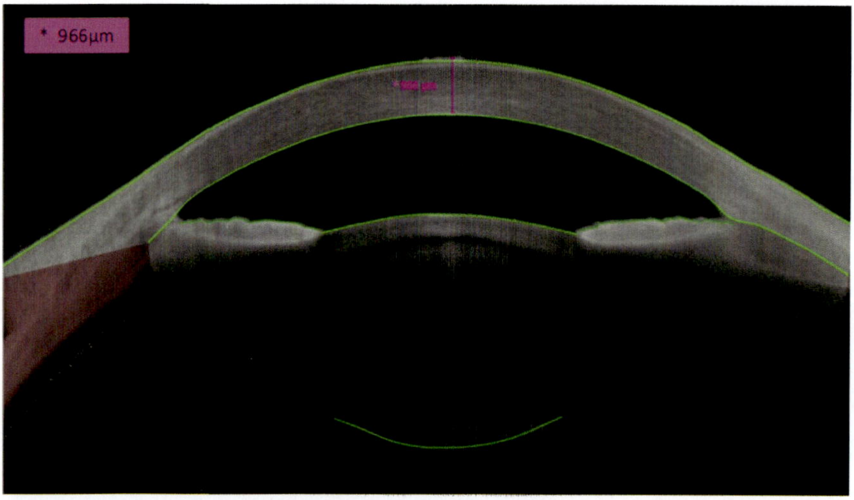

Fig. 3.7 Swept-source OCT image in a one-year-old child with CHED: a close to 1000 μm thick cornea with central stromal corneal opacity. The OCT shows a regular chamber angle and scleral spur without evidence of any synechiae. The lens appears age-appropriate and clear

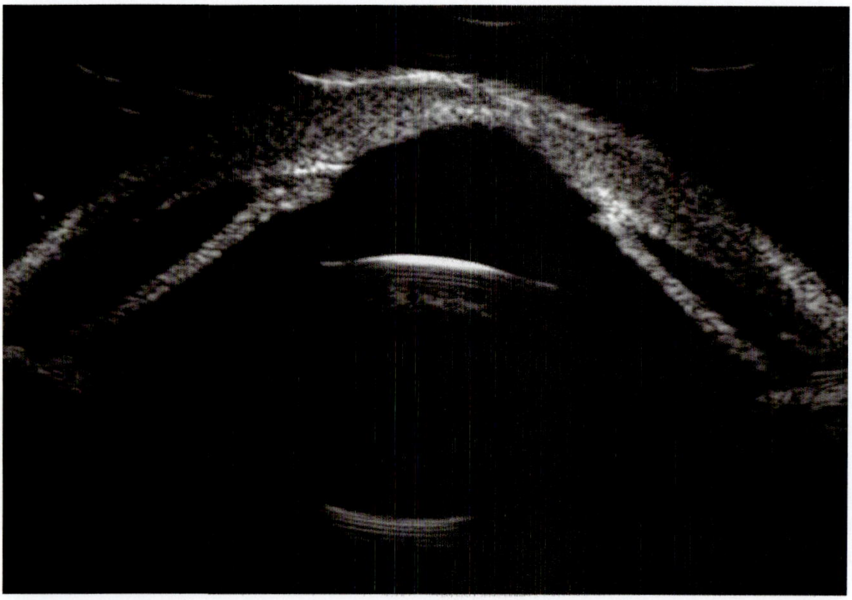

Fig. 3.8 High frequency ultrasound (UBM) of a child with iridocorneal adhesions and excavation of central cornea

➢ **Notes**

- The additional examination of parents, siblings, and other caregivers can provide important additional information.
- In this context, genetic testing can provide further fundamental important information for the correct diagnosis and can thus contribute significantly to the improvement of the therapy, both of ocular and systemic pathology.
- The development of new, genotype-specific therapies therefore plays an increasingly important role.

➢ **Overview**

Important examinations in the child to determine diagnosis

- Fixation behavior
- Light reaction
- Presence of a possible nystagmus?
- Fundus reflex
- In case of corneal opacities: Which layer is affected?
- Are other ocular structures affected?
- Measurement of intraocular pressure e.g. by rebound tonometry
- Taking macroscopic images or even a slit lamp microscopic image
- If possible, performance of optical coherence tomography
- If necessary, sonography (A- and B-scan measurement)
- If necessary, anesthesia examination.

3.4 Clinical Features and Genetics

The causes and the clinical features of congenital and childhood corneal opacity are diverse. A possible subdivision of congenital corneal opacity is the subdivision according to Nischal [53, 54]. This classification divides between primary and secondary corneal diseases (compare Table 3.1). In the upcoming chapters, primary and secondary infantile corneal opacities will be discussed individually in further detail.

Table 3.1 Summary table of primary and secondary infantile corneal opacities

Primary corneal disease	Corneal dystrophies	➢ Posterior polymorphic corneal dystrophy (PPCD)
		➢ Congenital hereditary endothelial dystrophy (CHED)
		➢ Congenital hereditary stromal dystrophy (CHSD)
		➢ X-linked endothelial corneal dystrophy (XECD)
	Corneal structure defects due to dermoids	
	CYP1B1 Cytopathy	
	Peripheral sclerocornea	
Secondary corneal disease: developmental abnormalities of the anterior segment	Irido-corneal dysgenesia	➢ Peters anomaly ➢ Aniridia ➢ Coloboma
	Irido-trabecular dysgenesia	➢ Axenfeld Rieger Syndrome (ARS) ➢ Embryotoxon posterius ➢ Aniridia
	Ectasia of the anterior segment:	➢ Keratoconus
	Brittle cornea syndrome (BCS)	
	Microcornea	
	Primary congenital glaucoma	
	Intracorneal cyst	
Secondary corneal disease: Acquired corneal disease	Metabolic disease	➢ Mucolipidosis
		➢ LCAT deficiency
		➢ Tyrosinemia type 2
		➢ Liposomal storage diseases
		➢ Fabry's disease
	Trauma	
	Infectious keratitis	➢ Viral and bacterial infections ➢ Infections due to funghi and protozoa

3.5 Primary Corneal Disease

In primary corneal diseases, a distinction is made between dystrophies, dermoids, peripheral sclerocornea and CYP1B1 cytopathy.

3.5.1 Corneal Dystrophies

The corneal dystrophies and thus also the associated congenital and childhood dystrophies are described in the current IC3D classification [3, 4].

Most of the corneal dystrophies usually affect visual acuity only beyond the amblyopia-relevant age. In the following, we will discuss in further detail selected dystrophies for which operative treatment may be indicated in the early childhood.

3.5.1.1 Epithelial and Subepithelial Dystrophies in Childhood

- **Epithelial recurrent erosive dystrophy (ERED)**

Epithelial recurrent erosive dystrophy also known as Franceschetti corneal dystrophy, is an autosomal dominant inherited dystrophy. It is caused by a mutation in the *COL17A1* gene on chromosome 10, q25.1. The ERED shows its onset in childhood and can occur spontaneously or by minor trauma, as well as by dust or smoke corneal erosions. Clinically, ERCD manifests with conjunctival redness, photophobia, and epiphora. Rarely, reduced visual acuity is present.

- **Subepithelial mucinous erosive dystrophy (SMCD)**

Subepithelial mucinous erosive dystrophy usually begins in the first decade of life and presents clinically with recurrent erosions of the cornea. These become less frequent during puberty, although there is often an increasing loss of visual acuity, resulting in bilateral opacities and haze over the entire cornea. Deposits of glycosaminoglycans (chondroitin and dermatan sulfate) are found particularly centrally. The disease is inherited in an autosomal dominant manner.

- **Lisch epithelial corneal dystrophy (LECD)**

Lisch epithelial corneal dystrophy (LECD) is an X-chromosomal recessive disease with mutation on the X chromosome, p.22.3. The onset of the disease is in childhood and is characterized by a slowly progressive feather-like opacification in the corneal epithelium, clinically presenting as band-like or whorl-like with microcysts in the epithelium. The disease is usually painless and there is a decrease in visual acuity but usually only in the older age.

- **Meesmann corneal dystrophy (MECD)**

Like most dystrophies, Meesmann corneal dystrophy (MECD) is inherited in an autosomal dominant manner. It is caused by a mutation in the *KRT3* gene on chromosome 12, q13.13 or *KRT12* gene on chromosome 17, q21.2. These genes are responsible for the coding of cytokeratin subunits.

The onset of MECD occurs in the first to second year of life. In most cases, both eyes are affected and multiple patchy opacities are found in the corneal epithelium: slit lamp microscopic examination reveals central superficial, fine and diffuse punctations in the corneal epithelium (compare Fig. 3.9). This frequently leads to a decrease

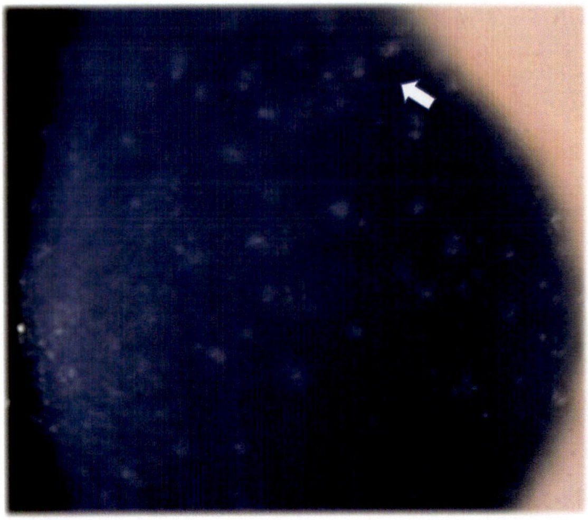

Fig. 3.9 Meesmann corneal dystrophy (MECD) in a child with microscopic central superficial, fine and diffuse punctations in the corneal epithelium

in visual acuity, which tends to be episodic. MECD favors the development of irregular astigmatism. Patients primarily show signs of photophobia. Corneal sensitivity is not reduced.

- **Epithelial-Stromal Dystrophies**

Clinically, there are five types: Granular corneal dystrophy (Classic) (GCD 1), Granular Corneal dystrophy type 2 (GCD 2), Reis–Buckler's corneal dystrophy (RBCD), Thiel-Behnke Corneal Dystrophy (TBCD) and Lattice corneal dystrophy type I (LCD 1). All five show progressive opacification of the cornea leading to severe visual handicap. All have been shown to have mutations in the gene encoding keratoepithelin, the TGFBI on chromosome 5q31.1.

- **Granular corneal dystrophy type I (GCD1)**

Granular corneal dystrophy type 1 is autosomal dominant.

The disease develops within the first 10 years of life and is associated with a slowly progressive visual reduction. Photophobia represents as an early sign. Patients with granular dystrophy often suffer from recurrent erosions. Slit lamp microscopic examination reveals small, white and irregularly shaped with sharply demarcated spots in the stroma that are embedded centrally in the cornea in clear corneal portions.

The periodic acid Schiff's (PAS) reagent and hematoxilin-eosin (HE) stains serve as an overview staining (compare Fig. 3.10a, b). Masson's trichrome stain serves as positive evidence of granular masses in granular corneal dystrophy, which stain bright red in the histologic section. (compare Fig. 3.11).

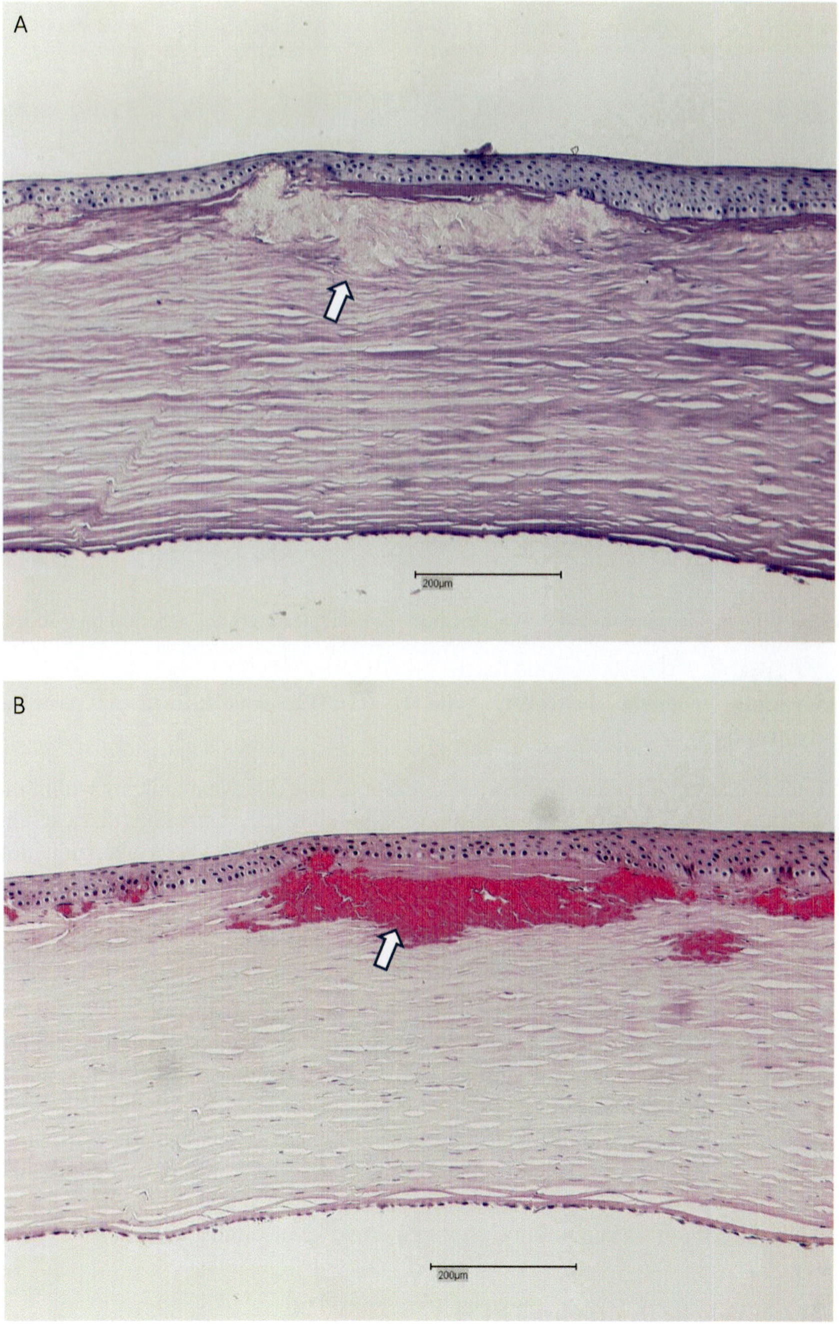

Fig. 3.10 Granular dystrophy in A) Hematoxilin-eosin coloring and B) periodic acid Schiff's reagent

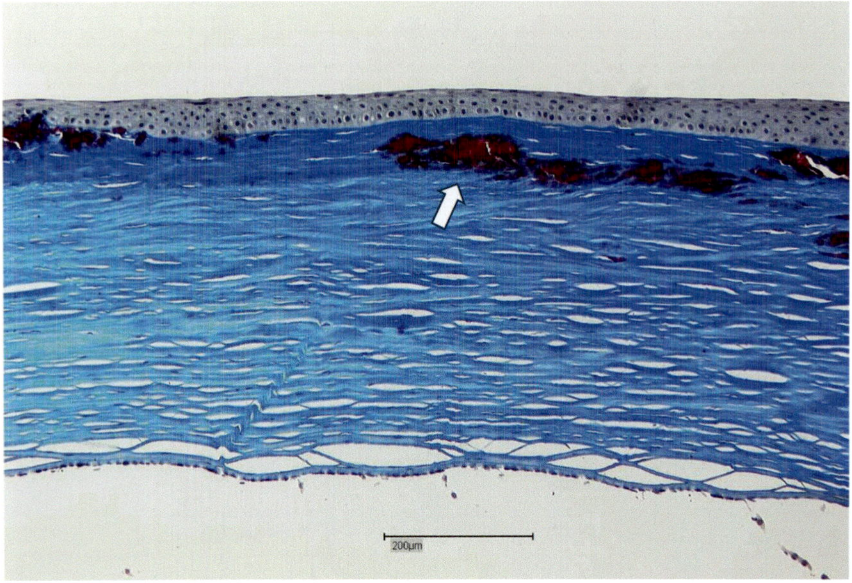

Fig. 3.11 Granular dystrophy in Masson's trichrome, which stain bright red in the histologic section

- **Granular corneal dystrophy type II (GCD2; was known as Avellino dystrophy)**

It is an autosomal dominantly inherited condition. The disease manifests within the first 10 years of life, with an earlier onset corresponding to homozygous disease. The disease shows a slow progression with a slow decrease in visual acuity. Examination shows linear or lattice-like deposits in the cornea, which are less numerous than in granular corneal dystrophy type I.

- **Rice-Bückler's corneal dystrophy (RBCD)**

Rice-Bückler's corneal dystrophy is inherited autosomal dominantly. It begins in early childhood and is characterized by recurrent erosions on both sides. Clinical findings are subepithelial opacities confined to Bowman's membrane with symmetrical, reticulate or ring-like inclusions.

Rice-Bückler's honeycomb dystrophy results in progressive visual loss with irregular astigmatism. There is often reduced corneal sensitivity. Remission is possible in early adulthood, as well as later recurrences.

Therapy comprises keratotomy, photorefractive keratectomy, or lamellar keratoplasty.

- **Thiele Behnke Dystrophy (TBCD)**

TBCD is caused by an autosomal dominant mutation in the *TGFBI* gene on chromosome 5, q31.1, and on the other gene locus on chromosome 10 (q23-q24). Clinically visible are honeycomb-shaped superficial corneal opacities, which are very difficult to distinguish from RBCD, especially in children, as they take a similar course.

- **Lattice Corneal Dystrophy (LCD I)**

There are three types of lattice dystrophy, but only type I has its onset in children. LCD1 is an uncommon dystrophy and is the result of abnormal deposition of amyloid within the cornea. The disease is bilateral, and changes can be seen in the first decade of life. The disease is autosomal dominant. Initially the lesions are small subepithelial dots or lines, originating in the central cornea. The lesions then progress and can become round, oval, speculated, or branching in nature. Although the intervening areas are initially clear, they progressively become opaque. Vision is diminished by the recurrent erosions and stromal haze.

3.5.1.2 Dystrophies of the Stroma

- **Macular corneal dystrophy**

Macular corneal dystrophy, also known as Groenouw II/Fehr syndrome, usually begins in the first decade of life and affects both eyes. Initially, macular dystrophy presents with a cloudy haze, and later parenchymatous patches and nodules (compare Figs. 3.12 and 3.13). With age, there is increasing visual loss, reduced corneal sensitivity, and recurrent erosions with pain, photophobia, and foreign body sensation.

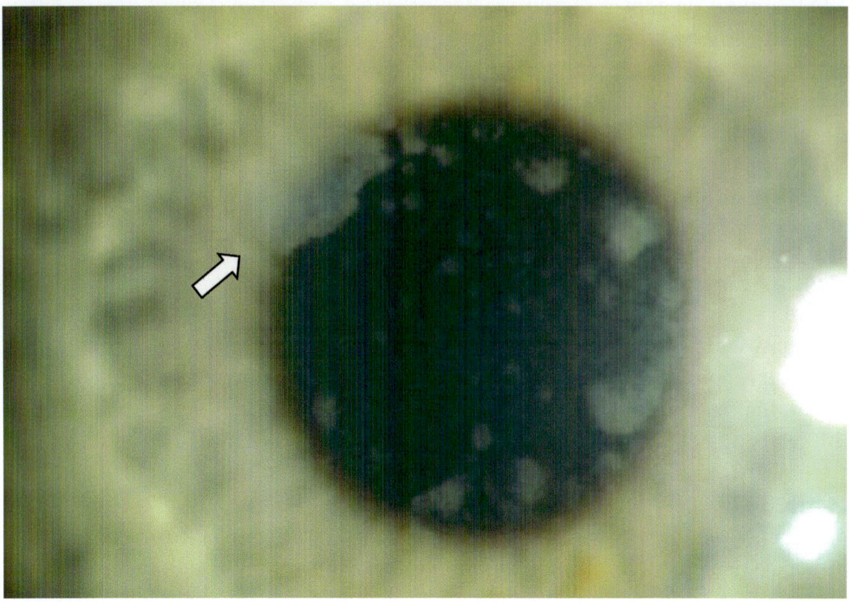

Fig. 3.12 Macular corneal dystrophy in an eight-year-old child with a cloudy haze and parenchymatous patches and nodules

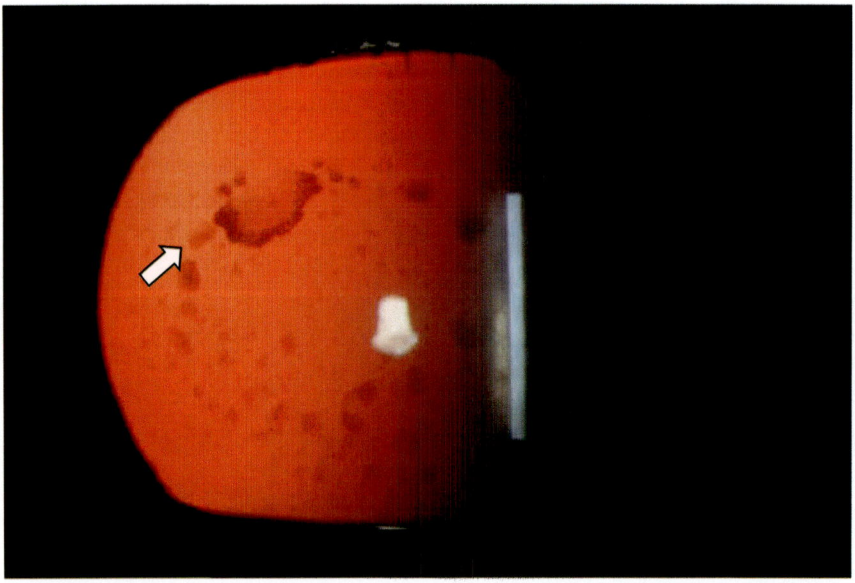

Fig. 3.13 Macular corneal dystrophy in an eight-year-old child: In regressed light, parenchymatous patches and nodules are also detectable

Differential diagnosis should include granular corneal dystrophy type I, lattice corneal dystrophy type I in early stages only; and corneal involvement in systemic mucupolysaccharidoses such as Hurler's disease, Scheie's disease but in these last two the clouding is diffuse and never nodular.

3.5.1.3 Endothelial Dystrophies in Childhood

- **Posterior polymorphous corneal dystrophy (PPCD)**

Posterior polymorphous corneal dystrophy (PPCD) is an endothelial corneal dystrophy, which often occurs asymmetrically. However, visual impairment at birth is rare but reported (see Fig. 3.14) and progression occurs slowly over many decades. The slit lamp shows retrocorneal geographical deposits of the Descemet membrane with partly vesicles and snail-like changes (compare Fig. 3.15) [51].

Corneal ectasias or peripheral irido-corneal adhesions and glaucoma have been described also described in some cases of PPCD speculatively due to abnormal corneal endothelial cells with epithelial characteristics affecting the trabecular meshwork and iris. Secondary complications are therefore common, e.g. corneal edema, glaucoma, iris adherence to the cornea, and corectopia. Patients may also have symptoms of pains, tearing, photophobia, foreign body sensation and blurred vision.

PPCD is a genetically heterogeneous condition with heterozygous mutations in the transcription factor encoding gene *ZEB1* (MIM: 189,909) (PPCD3 [MIM: 609141])

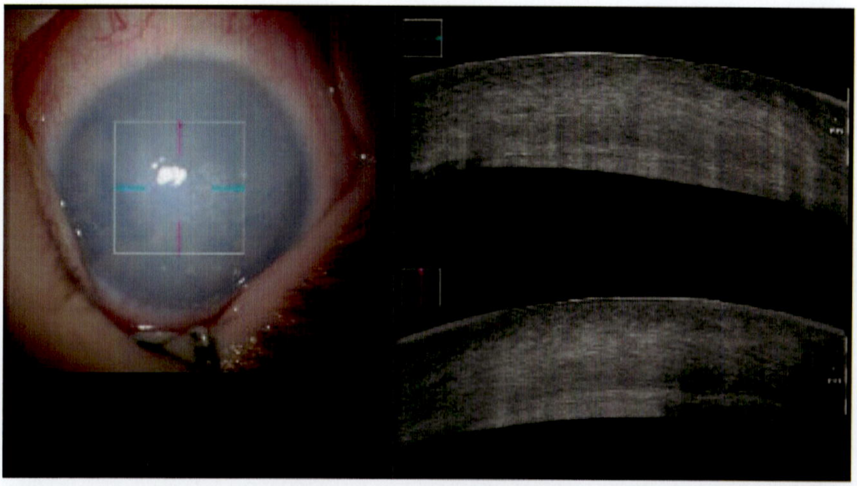

Fig. 3.14 22 months old with molecular confirmation of PPCD due to monoallelic mutation of ZEB1. The integrated OCT shows very thickened DM

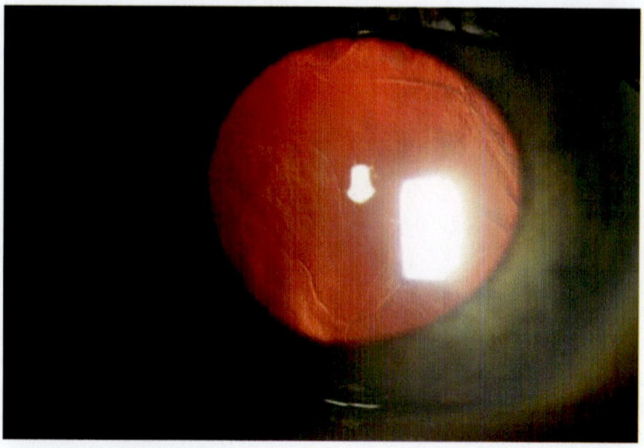

Fig. 3.15 Clinical picture of posterior polymorphic corneal dystrophy (PPCD) in a 14-year-old patient: Clearly visible endothelial cochlea-like changes, which can best be assessed in retroillumination. First publishe in "Die Ophthalmologie". https://doi.org/10.1007/s00347-022-01587-6

and it is established that heterozygous regulatory mutations in the 5´UTR promoter region c.-307T > C of the *OVOL2* gene (MIM: 616441) cause PPCD [46]. The function of *ZEB1* and *OVOL2* is to control the cell state, through regulation of epithelial-to-mesenchymal transition (EMT) and the converse process of mesenchymal-to-epithelial transition (MET), through a mutually inhibitory pathway. Central processes in the development are EMT and MET, and these finely tuned and reversible cell state transition pathways also support the maintenance of cellular function and identity. Aberrant regulation of MET and EMT underpins malignant transformation as well as tumor progression and are playing an important role in other disease conditions, e.g. inflammation, fibrosis and wound healing.

No *OVOL2* expression could be detected in human corneal endothelium, but multiple binding sites for transcription factors expressed in the corneal endothelium are located in the *OVOL2* promoter. The genetically heterogeneous clinical picture of PPCD can also be caused by mutations in the genes *COL8A2* and *GRHL2* in the long arm of chromosome 20q11 and is associated with the gene mutations on *VSX1* [4, 49, 50, 50, 51].

Histologically, the lesions of PPCD are located at the level of DM and the endothelium. The lesions have three different types: vesicle-type lesions, band lesions and diffuse opacities. The former two types are more common than the last one. The vesicles appear as blister or bleb-like under a slit lamp, with an optically clear center and a small halo of gray-white haze.

Previous studies have shown, that "epithelium-like" multilayered cells scattered in areas of normal endothelium and deposition of abnormal collagen material on DM, forming an abnormal posterior collagenous layer. The four types of cells shown on the posterior corneal surface in PPCD are normal ECs, attenuated or degenerating ECs, fibroblast-like cells, and epithelial-like cells. (compare Fig. 3.16).

- **Congenital hereditary endothelial dystrophy (CHED)**

The original classifications of congenital hereditary endothelial dystrophy (CHED) described two forms of CHED [3, 4]:

- **CHED1**: An autosomal dominant disease and presenting a progressive corneal clouding beginning within the first few years of life.
- **CHED2**: An autosomal recessive disease and presented with corneal clouding at birth or in the immediate newborn period.

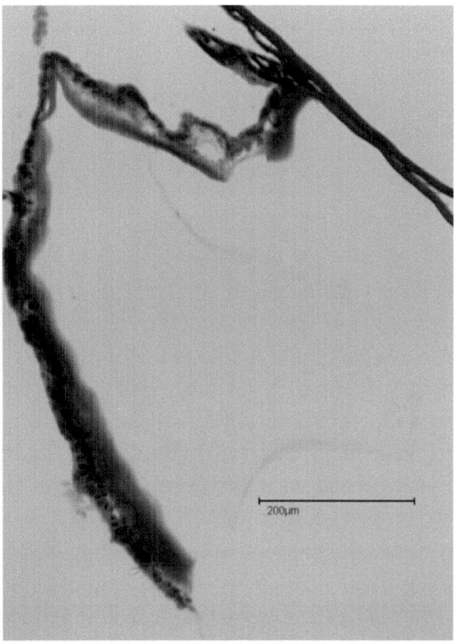

Fig. 3.16 Histological sample obtained intra-operatively in a patient with PPCD: Histologically, the lesions of PPCD are located at the level of DM and the endothelium

Genetic analyses and clinical findings confirmed that the previously termed autosomal dominant CHED (originally CHED1) is a form of PPCD with a severe and early corneal edema. Therefore it is no longer considered in the category of CHED, so that in consequence the entity of CHED1 is now classified with PPCD.

Based on the update to the International Classification of Corneal Dystrophies in 2015, the term "CHED" is now exclusively referred to the autosomal recessive CHED (originally CHED2).

CHED is a really rare disorder of the corneal endothelium with an early onset of corneal edema (central corneal thickness of up to 1000 μm and more) and it is characterized by non-progressive bilateral corneal edema and opacification combined with diffuse milky glass-like corneal opacity of varying severity at birth or shortly thereafter (compare Fig. 3.17).

Inflammation, epiphora or photophobia are not prominent features in CHED in contrast to PPCD in which Photophobia and epiphora are common.

Primary disease of the corneal endothelium is the culprit for edema in CHED. The normal hexagonal endothelial mosaic is altered or absent. The cells are attenuated and fibrotic, when endothelial cells are visualized by confocal microscopy.

The thickening of the endothelial basement membrane, Descemet's membrane, is visible by using slit lamp examination. These mice have progressive corneal swelling, doubling the thickness of the cornea, as well as thickening of Descemet's membrane.

This fact is usually the result of terminal mis-differentiation of the endothelial cells. As a result of this mis-differentiation, the development of stromal edema in CHED patients is favored, whereby the *SLC4A11* gene seems to play an essential role, as it encodes the bicarbonate transporter-related protein-1 (BTR1), which as a sodium-borate cotransporter physiologically pumps out excess water with the necessary nutrients for the cornea from the stroma [51, 51, 51].

In CHED, BTR-1 is often significantly limited in its function, which inevitably leads to clouding of the cornea.

In addition, the endothelial cells in CHED show a fibrotic remodeling, which additionally negatively affects the transparency of the cornea [46]. Also, the Descemet membrane as well as often the Bowman membrane is thickened in CHED and it

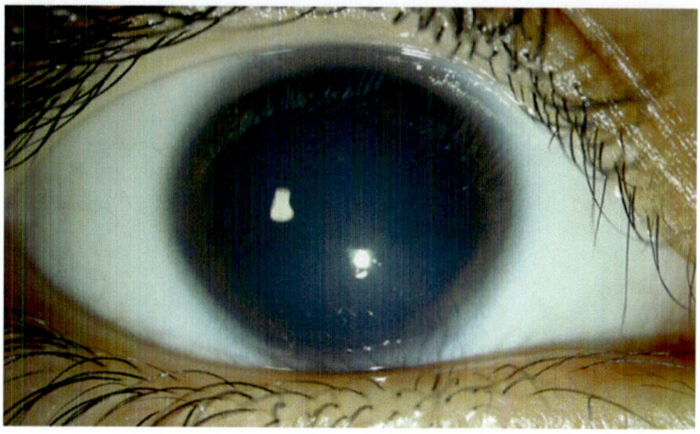

Fig. 3.17 Pre-operative findings after DSAEK in a 13-year-old child with congenital hereditary endothelial dystrophy (CHED): Pre-operative slit lamp photomicrograph showed marked diffuse milky opacity of the corneal and corneal edema

can also lead to vascularization and ligament keratopathy of the corneal surface. The resulting limited visual acuity can result in nystagmus and amblyopia.

As described above, homozygous or compound heterozygous mutations in *SLC4A11* gene 4 with autosomal recessive inheritance pattern provide genetic basis [4]. A present consanguinity thus increases the risk of the occurrence of CHED. PPCD and CHED have been mapped to chromosome 20 at two distinct loci: 20p11.2-q11.2 for PPCD and 20p13 for CHED. All cases of CHED should have a hearing test to exclude Harboyan syndrome.

- **Congenital hereditary stromal dystrophy (CHSD)**

CHSD is a very rare, at best slowly progressive congenital dystrophy of the corneal stroma. With a normal corneal surface, there is a diffuse opacity of the thickened corneal stroma with whitish deposits on both sides [55]. CHSD is caused by mutations in the decorin gene *DCN* and is autosomal dominantly segregated [4].

Five different heterozygous frameshift mutations have been described in the literature so far, which lead to a premature stop with C-terminal truncation of the protein and are all located in exon 8 of the *DCN* gene[26]. This suggests that exon 8 is a mutation hotspot and represents a functionally important area of the decorin protein.

Decorin is a leucine-rich proteoglycan, which binds as a component of the extracellular matrix to collagen type I and II, as well as to TGF-ß and fibronectin, regulates fibrillogenesis and fibril diameter and thus plays an important role in corneal transparency formation [56].

It has been shown that homozygous *DCN* mutations have no effect on corneal transparency, but heterozygous mutations lead to stromal corneal opacity [56]. It is assumed that the heterozygously mutated decorin cannot literally interact with the collagen fibrils and thus the corneal opacity occurs.

- **X-linked endothelial corneal dystrophy (XECD)**

XECD is very rare and was first described in 2006 [57]. Already at the birth there is a frosted glass-like opacity of the cornea with lunar crater-like changes in the corneal back surface. The changes can affect all corneal layers. By means of microsatellite analysis, the presumably disease-causing locus was mapped to the long arm of chromosome 23, q25 [4]. With X-linked dominant inheritance pattern, both men and women may be affected.

> **➢ Overview**
> **Important and amblyopia-relevant corneal dystrophies in children**
>
> - Posterior polymorphous corneal dystrophy (PPCD)
> - Congenital hereditary endothelial dystrophy (CHED)
> - Congenital hereditary stromal dystrophy (CHSD)
> - X-linked endothelial corneal dystrophy (XECD).

3.5.2 Corneal Structure Defects Due to Dermoids

A corneal dermoid is a congenital benign choristoma of mesodermal or ectodermal origin. Clinically there is a smooth whitish space requirement, which is often localized at the temporal lower limbus (compare Figs. 3.18 and 3.19a).

Dermoids can induce astigmatism or even obscure the optical axis. Histologically, hair-sebaceous gland complexes are usually found embedded in dense connective tissue [58]. Co-involvement of intraocular structures are rare.

Dermoids can also occur in the context of the Goldenhar syndrome, although the pathophysiology is not yet sufficiently clarified here. However, it has been shown that a mutation exists at the gene site 14q32, which are often spontaneous mutations [59]. In the literature, autosomal dominant as well as autosomal recessive inheritances are described. In addition to the corneal changes, changes to the retina, the optic nerve

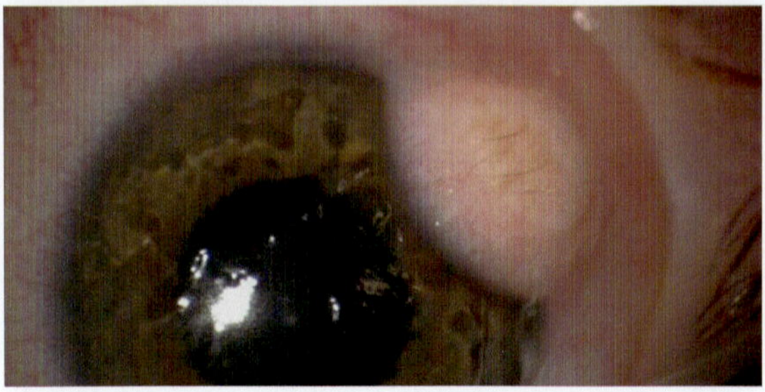

Fig. 3.18 Five-year-old patient with epibulbar dermoid and increasing astigmatism and surface inflammation: Microscopically a whitish, raised, limbus-crossing mass with hair growth temporally below could be seen. First published in "Die Ophthalmologie". https://doi.org/10.1007/s00347-022-01587-6

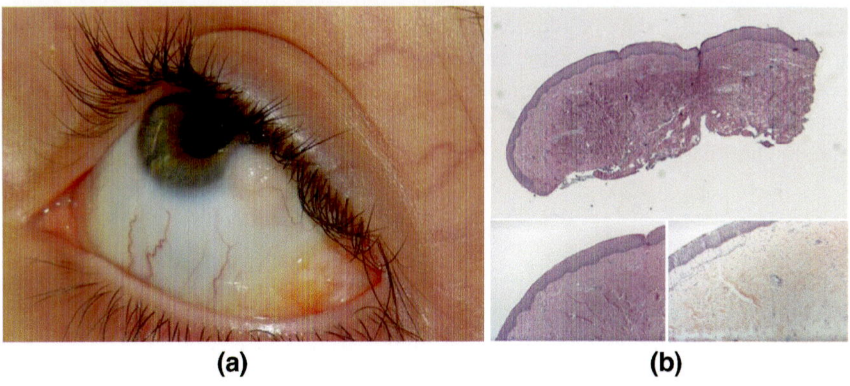

Fig. 3.19 a: Nine-year-old girl with a big temporal epibulbar dermoid and also surface inflammation. b: Correlating histological findings in the epibulbar dermoid of the nine-year-old girl in from Fig. 3.19a: Inconspicuous surface epithelium with stromal fibrosis

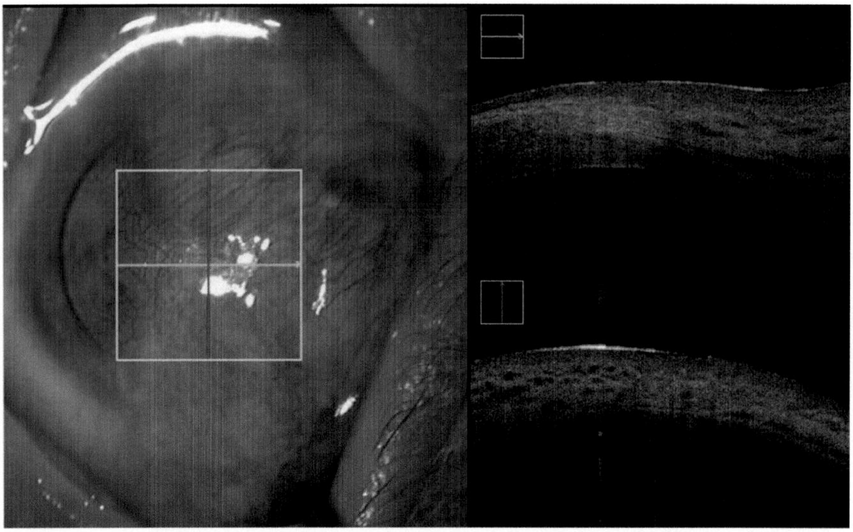

Fig. 3.20 Corneal dermoid in a case of Oculoectodermal syndrome due to mutation in KRAS; OCT shows that the dermoid is not full thickness

and the retinal vessels can also be observed [60]. Indications for surgical intervention are large limbal dermoid encroaching on the visual axis, large dermoid preventing lid closure or hairs growing from the dermoid and causing a keratopathy. Astigmatism is the cause of amblyopia: shaving excision or removal with lamellar keratoplasty does not improve the astigmatism but can allow the use of a contact lens to better correct the astigmatism.

More rarely, the lesion affects larger parts of the cornea or conjunctiva and sclera (Fig. 3.20). These are more typically associated with mosaic rasopathies. These dermoids often have fine vessels in what appears grossly to be clear cornea. Penetrating keratoplasty may be required in these cases. Mosaic rasopathies encompass three conditions which are on the spectrum: oculectodermal syndrome, linear sebaceous nevus syndrome and encephalo-cranio cutaneous lipomatosis. In these conditions lid notches maybe seen and a waxy alopecia (nevus psiloparus) of the scalp is often the hallmark of the condition.

3.5.3 CYP1B1 Cytopathy

Homozygous or compound heterozygous mutations in CYP1B1 occur in connection with primary congenital glaucoma (see below) and have also been associated with corneal opacity associated with the iris and lens not only by increased intraocular pressure and corneal adhesion [61]. The disease is inherited in an autosomal recessive manner.

3.5.4 Sclerocornea

This term is not helpful. It is typically a bilateral displacement of the limbus with a resulting small cornea (microcornea) or even a complete absence of the limbus and complete congenital corneal opacification. The peripheral cornea is often not distinguishable from the sclera, the center is sometimes slightly clearer than the periphery (compare Chap. 5, Fig. 3.7).

It is recommended to avoid the term sclerocornea because it is often just total corneal opacification due to a primary issue inside the eye; e.g. primary congenital aphakia due to biallelic mutations in FOXE3 results in bilateral opaque corneas.

The surface and stroma are often vascularized with altered, flattened epithelium and a missing Bowman lamella and disorganized collagen fibrils in the stroma, which explains the opacity of the cornea.

A planal sclerocornea is present in flat cornea and hyperopia and may be often associated with glaucoma, especially due to the flat anterior chamber [62].

Peripheral cornea is indeed a real entity and this may be associated with cornea plana; cornea plana may be inherited autosomal dominant (CNA1) or autosomal recessive (CNA2) [63]. A pedigree of peripheral sclerocornea was found to be due to mutations in *RAD21* are related to the development of sclerocornea [64].

3.6 Secondary Corneal Disease: Developmental Abnormalities of the Anterior Segment

The development of ocular anterior segment structures is a precisely coordinated process that is determined by both genetic and environmental factors. In humans, this process begins from week 6 of gestation, and it is characterized by the formation of the lens placode from overlying surface ectoderm. The cornea is derived after lens detachment, while several waves of tissue invade the primary mesenchyme that lies behind the surface ectoderm, ultimately giving rise to an anterior epithelium, and a posterior endothelium, with the corneal stroma laying between these layers. A number of genes that include transcription factors, nuclear proteins, structural proteins, and enzymes are known to be involved in this sophisticated process, and defects in these key genes may lead to severe congenital anterior segment dysgenesis (ASD) [67].

3.6.1 Irido-Corneal Dysgenesis

In the case of central and thus potentially surgical opacity due to dysgenesis, the opacity can affect the epithelium, stroma and endothelium separately or in combination. Dysgenesis of the corneal endothelium and, if necessary, of the stroma, in which the limbus is intact, but there is no microcornea and the peripheral cornea is often clear, are considered separately. These changes occur in conjunction with malformations of the chamber angle, iris and lens and are called **Peters anomaly** (compare Fig. 3.21) [68, 69].

Peters' anomaly (PA) is a rare form of ASD characterized by central corneal opacity, defects in Descemet's membrane and an abnormal structure of the stroma, accompanied by irido-corneal or lenticulo-corneal adhesions [70].

Peters anomaly is a sign and not a diagnosis. As such it is a homeotic gene disorder. Accompanying ocular signs may point to a molecular diagnosis. If aniridia is present, PAX 6 is likely while presence of Axenfeld–Rieger anomaly makes FOXC1 or PITX 2 more likely. CYP1B1 has also been implicated but so have many other genes. With the development of next-generation sequencing (NGS), the genetic spectrum of PA has been expanded to include *TFAP2A, HCCS, NDP, SLC4A11, FLNA, COL4A1* and *COL6A3* [71, 72]. However, all of these PA-causal genes identified can only explain a small proportion of the disease etiology, and most PA cases still lack a clear genetic diagnosis.

Peters plus syndrome (Peters anomaly, cleft lip and palate, brachydactyly and developmental delay) is due to bialleleic mutations in beta-1,3-galactosyltransferase-like gene (*B3GALTL*) [73, 74].

Heterozygous mutations in *FOXE3* also appear to play a role, although not all cases of failed lens-ectoderm separation are due to *FOXE3* mutations [75, 76]. A primary lens problem can lead to extralenticular changes such as corneal opacity with or without glaucoma.

A missing or insufficient differentiation of endothelial cells from mesenchymal cells and, accordingly, a lack of migration of endothelial cells between the stroma and lens vesicles causes the maldevelopment of the cornea and partly also of the lens.

As with all dysgenesis, the manifestations can be very different with a centrally emphasized absence of endothelium and partial iris system (Peter's anomaly type I) with correspondingly centrally emphasized opacity up to the complete attachment

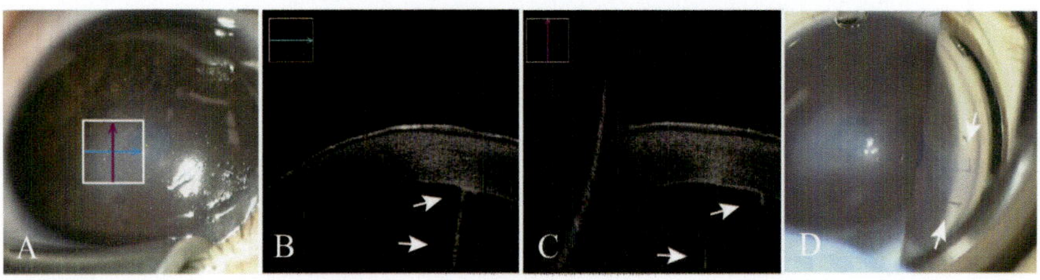

Fig. 3.21 Intraoperative optical coherence tomography (OCT) of a fourteen-week-old patient with Peters anomaly: Microscopically, a dense corneal opacity is seen within the optical axis. The superimposed cross shows the localization and direction of the OCT scan (A). Optical coherence tomography (OCT) shows anterior synechiae (arrows) in the horizontal (B) and vertical (C) sections. Gonioscopy also shows anterior synechiae (D). First published in "Die Ophthalmologie". https://doi.org/10.1007/s00347-016-0299-4

of the iris, a lens opacity with then often attachment of the lens to the corneal back surface (Peter's anomaly type II).

In type I of Peter's anomaly, there is also often a central, eccentric or rarely a total opacity of the cornea with simultaneous avascularity of the cornea. In contrast, in type II Peter's anomaly, there is always a central or even total clouding of the cornea with pronounced vascularization, which is probably due to a developmental failure of the separation of the invaginating lens vesicle from the surface ectoderm above it.

Clinically, in addition to the corneal opacity, a thinning of the cornea is shown simultaneously, combined with synechia (compare Fig. 3.22) of the iris in the chamber angle as well as an irido-lenticulo-corneal synechia and, if necessary, a lens displacement and/or cloudiness. With the help of the UBM and the anterior optical coherence tomography (A-OCT), the cataractous lens can be clinically detected, in which the anterior lens capsule is usually not recognizable at the attachment point. The prognosis of perforating keratoplasty in keratolenticular adhesion is in principle rather poor.

An indication that there is no failure of the separation of the lenses and cornea in the sense of Peters anomaly is the intact reflectivity of the anterior capsule of the lens visible in the A-OCT or UBM findings. Here, surgical removal of the lens instead of primary corneal transplantation is the most effective treatment, since removing the lens allows restoration of the intactness of the endothelium. This can be caused, for example, by persistent fetal vessels, whereby the retrolenticular membrane of the lens is pushed forward towards the cornea. This can also be observed in vitreoretinal dysplasia.

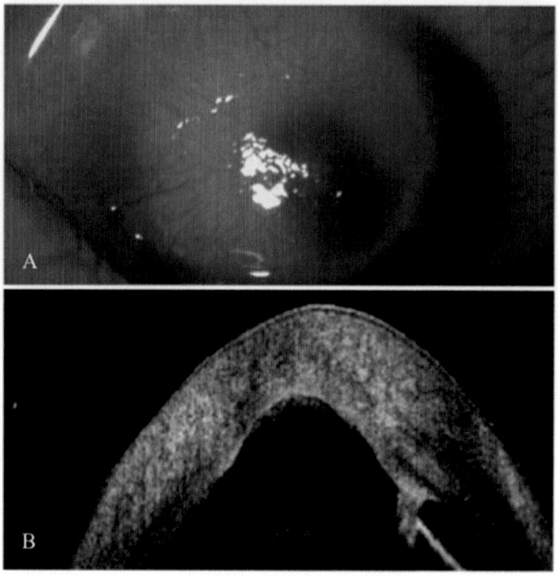

Fig. 3.22 Six-month-old patient with Peter's anomaly: microscopically, there is vascularized opacification of the midperipheral cornea (A). Optical coherence tomography (OCT) shows pervasive stromal hyperreflectivity with anterior synechiae of the iris (B)

➢ **Overview**

Possible manifestations of iridocorneal or keratolenticular adhesions (Peters Anomaly 1 or 2)

- Mutations in the beta-1,3-galactosyltransferase-like gene (B3GALTL).
- Mutations have also been described in PAX6, PITX2, FOXC1, FOXE3 and CYP1B1
- autosomal recessive or sporadic
- occurrence in siblings (kin connections)

➢ **Ophthalmological findings**

- dysgenesis: unilateral or bilateral
- corneal opacities with thinning of the cornea
- Synechiae iris in the chamber angle glaucoma
- Irido-lenticulo-corneal synechiae
- Lens displacement and/or opacities
- Unilateral or bilateral microphthalmia
- Nystagmus.

➢ **Overview: Peters-Plus-Syndrome**

- **Skeletal anomalies**
  - Short stature with comparatively short arms and legs
  - Brachydactyly and small feet, unusual joint mobility
  - Bending of the little finger towards the ring finger (clinodactyly)
  - Small head with an unusually large fontanelle after birth
- **Facial anomalies**
  - Round face, small ears, flat nasal bridge, narrow (upper) lip, pronounced philtrum, cleft palate
- **Cognitive and motor developmental delay**
- **Ear, nose and throat**
  - Conductive hearing loss, possible narrowing or occlusion of the auditory canal
- **Neurology**
  - Dilated brain ventricles

- **Multi-organ disease**
  - Disease of the kidneys, heart defects, common respiratory diseases
- **Gestation**
  - Clustered unusually large amount of amniotic fluid (polyhydramnios),
  - frequent miscarriage

Aniridia or **colobomas** can also lead to irido-corneal dysgenesis, as a very flat anterior chamber combined with the slightest kerato-lenticular touch or retrocorneal adhesion of the lens, leading also in consequence to a clouding of the cornea [77]. Similarly, a hypoxic environment can cause clouding of the cornea by the transcription factor HIV1aplha stimulating the production of VEGF and thus promoting angiogenesis and corneal vascularization [78].

Congenital aniridia (compare Figs. 3.23 and 3.27) is a rare genetic disorder disrupting normal development of the eye [79]. The incidence ranges from 1:40 000 to 1:100.000 [80].

Heterozygous mutations within the PAX6 gene (paired box gene 6) or associated regulatory regions are the most common cause of aniridia [81, 82].

These mutations reduce the expression of the PAX6 gene and lead to a shortage of functional PAX6 protein, which, among other effects, disrupts eye development [83]. This can lead to a spectrum of ocular anomalies, including incomplete development of the iris, fovea, and optic nerve; severely impaired vision; and nystagmus.

The progressive nature of aniridia frequently leads to secondary ocular complications such as cataract, glaucoma, and aniridia-associated keratopathy (AAK). The clinical phenotype is highly variable among individuals with different genotypes, as well as between individuals with the same genotype [84–86].

Typical ocular coloboma is caused by defective closure of the embryonal fissure. The occurrence of coloboma can be sporadic, hereditary (known or unknown gene defects) or associated with chromosomal abnormalities. Ocular colobomata are more often associated with systemic abnormalities when caused by chromosomal abnormalities. The ocular manifestations widely vary [87].

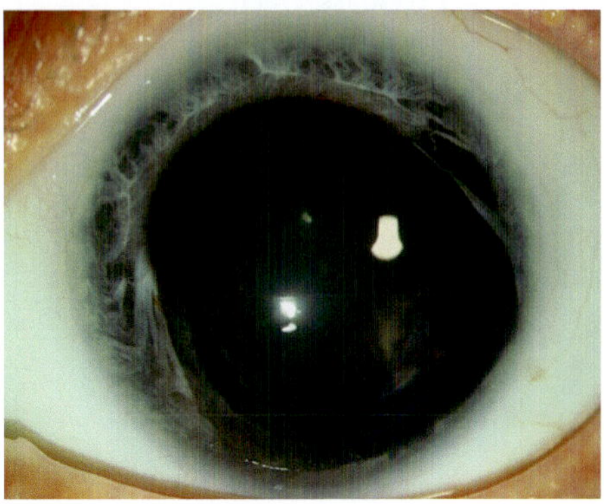

Fig. 3.23 Clinical picture of almost total congenital aniridia in a young patient. The anterior chamber is flattened. The patient complains of severe photophobia due to the missing iris

Inherited cases of coloboma and those associated with chromosomal defects can be associated with systemic anomalies in addition to the ocular coloboma (compare Table 3.2) [87].

Another form of Kerato-irido-corneal dysgenesis is described in which the lens separates from the corneal back surface but does not further form.

In most cases, this results in a total corneal opacity with vascularization, which can only be diagnosed by UBM or OCT of the anterior segment of the eye. Since there is usually only one lens residue, an accompanying vitrectomy for corneal transplantation is often required, which significantly reduces the success rate of the transplant.

Table 3.2 Systemic anomalies in ocular coloboma

Type of aberration	Syndrome/location of chromosomal aberration	Coloboma	Systemic and other ocular associations
Triploldy	69; XXY chromosomes	Iris	Persistent hyperplastic primary vitreous, retinal dysplasia, cebocephaly, single mldllne nostril, syndactyly
Trisomy	Patau syndrome (Trisomy 13)	Iris	Microphthalmos, short survival, holoprosencephaly, cardiac and urogenital anomalies
	Trisomy 22	Chorioretinal	Craniofacial anomalies
Deletions	16q syndrome (16q23.1-16q24.2 del)	Iris	Broad prominent forehead, large nose and mouth, short stature
	Cranlosynostosls (2q24.3 and 2q31 del)	Iris; chorio retinal; optic disc	Cranlosynostosls, mental retardation, syndactyly, campodactyly, small mandible, hypertelorism, proptosls
	Wolf-Hlrschhom syndrome (4pl6.3 del)	Iris	Microcephaly, seizures, characteristic fades: high forehead, frontal bossing, hypertelorism, low set ears
	4q26 deletion syndrome (4q23-q27del)	Iris, chorioretinal	Microphthalmos, prominent forehead, eplcanthus, broad nose
	7q deletion syndrome (7q34-ter.del)	Chorioretinal	Psychomotor retardation, dysmorphlsm
	Charge syndrome with micro deletion 8ql2.1	Iris; chorio retinal; optic disc	Cardiac defects, choanal atresia, growth retardation, genital hypoplasia, cleft palate, facial nerve palsy, deafness

(continued)

Table 3.2 (continued)

Type of aberration	Syndrome/location of chromosomal aberration	Coloboma	Systemic and other ocular associations
	Jacobsen syndrome (Uq23-q25 del)	Iris; chorlo-retlnal	Growth retardation, telecanthus, CNS abnormalities, endocardial cushion defect, trigonocephaly, facial dysmorphlsm, heart defects
	13q deletion syndrome (13-ql3.2 ter del; 13ql2-q32 del; 13ql4-13q32 del)	Iris; chorlo-retlnal	Microphthalmos, holoprosencephaly, absent corpus callosum, skeletal anomalies, retinoblastoma described
	DIGeorge syndrome (22.11.2 del)	Iris; chorlo-retlnal	Microphthalmos, thalamic aplasia, heart defects, chronic Infections, skeletal and renal anomalies, dysmorphlsm, hypotonia
Inversion	Baraltser-Wlnter syndrome (2pl2-ql4 Inv)	Iris; chorlo-retlnal	Mental retardation, pachygyria and cortical atrophy
Translocation	Hypomelanosts of Ito (Xp 11.2 Mosaicism)	Iris; chorlo-retlnal	Incontinentia plgmentl achromlans, hypomelanosts of Ito, developmental delay, dental anomalies
	Coloboma with agenesis of corpus callosum (2p24 and 9q32)	Iris; chorlo retinal	Agenesis of corpus callosum, periventricular nodular heterotopia
Duplication	Cat eye syndrome (22qll)	Iris; chorlo-retlnal	Hypertelorism, pne-aurlcular skin tags or pits, anal anomalies, heart defects, down slanting palpebral fissure, micrognathia, renal, genital and skeletal anomalies, developmental delay/mental retardation

This is different from the cataracts of the membranous type that can be observed in Hallermann-Streiff syndrome [88, 89].

> **Overview**
> **Important irido-corneal dysgenesis**
>
> - Peters Anomaly
> - Aniridia
> - Coloboma.

A rare form in this context is the **primary congenital aphakia**, in which the lens also does not develop and shape. Clinically, this dysgenesis manifests itself as a silver-gray cornea, which despite this is still translucent. The eyes can be microphthalmic and associated with congenital glaucoma. Often there is a homozygous or compound heterozygous mutation in *FOXE3* [90–92].

Irido-corneal endothelial syndrome (ICE syndrome) must be distinguished from this. ICE syndrome is a group of very rare diseases of the cornea with progressive proliferation of the endothelium and includes Chandler syndrome, Cogan-Reese syndrome and essential iris atrophy. The clinical pictures differ in each case by the extent of atrophy of the iris and changes in the cornea. Viral infections such as herpes simplex viruses or Epstein-Barr viruses are discussed as the cause. The finding is usually one-sided and clinical manifestations are colobomas and atrophy of the iris, corneal opacity, synechia and deformed pupils. Ice syndrome is usually associated with secondary glaucoma and neuropathy of the optic nerve and nodule formation of the iris [93, 94].

3.6.2 Irido-Trabecular Dysgenesis

Dysgenesis in the irido-trabecular area often leads to the clinical picture of primary congenital glaucoma. Most often, this is caused by mutations in the *CYP1B1* gene. Mutations in *LTBP2* [106] are also associated with this disease [95–97].

The **Axenfeld-Rieger anomaly/syndrome (ARA/ARS)** is also a rare ASD and is often, but not regularly, combined with a stromal corneal opacity.

This condition was originally described by Axenfeld in 1920 as a bilateral, white line on the posterior aspect of the cornea with strands from the peripheral iris to this line [98].

In 1934, Rieger described the same changes but with the addition of changes in the iris structure such as pulling of the iris towards part of the angle (corectopia), thinning of the iris and, if this is severe, hole formation in the iris, sometime mimicking multiple pupils (compare Table 3.3) [99, 100].

Due to the combined occurrence of iris dysplasia, in the form of colobomas or synechia, and possible additional iris atrophy as well as displaced Schwalbe line, which can lead to secondary glaucoma, the corneal transparency of the cornea could also be affected. Moreover, a limbus-spreading, corneal vascularization can lead to a corneal clouding (compare Fig. 3.24).

Histologically, ARA is characterized by a distinct irregular arrangement of collagen fibrils and increased stromal H_2O retention (compare Fig. 3.25).

It has been noted that the severity of both anomalies can vary quite considerably, with a severe Axenfeld little different from a mild Rieger and for this reason the spectrum of abnormalities is often called Axenfeld-Rieger anomaly (ARA) [100]. For the moment, it may still be useful to attempt to separate classical Axenfeld-type changes (i.e. only peripheral iris involvement) from classical Rieger type changes, as it may be that they represent different mutations of the same gene [101].

Table 3.3 Overview diagnostic table for ASD

	Cornea				Iris		Pupil	Angle	Lens	Systematic Associations	Disc	Genotyp/ Locus
	Post. Embryotoxon	Corneal Diam > 13 mm & normal IOD	Corneal Opacity & normal IOD	Corneal Opacity with Iris/lens Adherence	Featureless/ Hypoplastic Iris	Absent Iris Collarette	Corectopia/ Polycoria	PAS or abnormal angel	abnormal		cupped	
Megalo-cornea		■								■		Xq21-q26
ARA	■						■	■			±	PITX2 FOXC1 13q14
ARS	■						■	■		■	±	PITX2 FOXC1 13q14
CHED			■								±	20p13
Peters			■	■			■	■		■	±	PAX6 PITX2
Iris-hypoplasia					■	■		■		■	±	PITX2 FOXC1

■ Sign present — Sign absent — ± Sign can be present

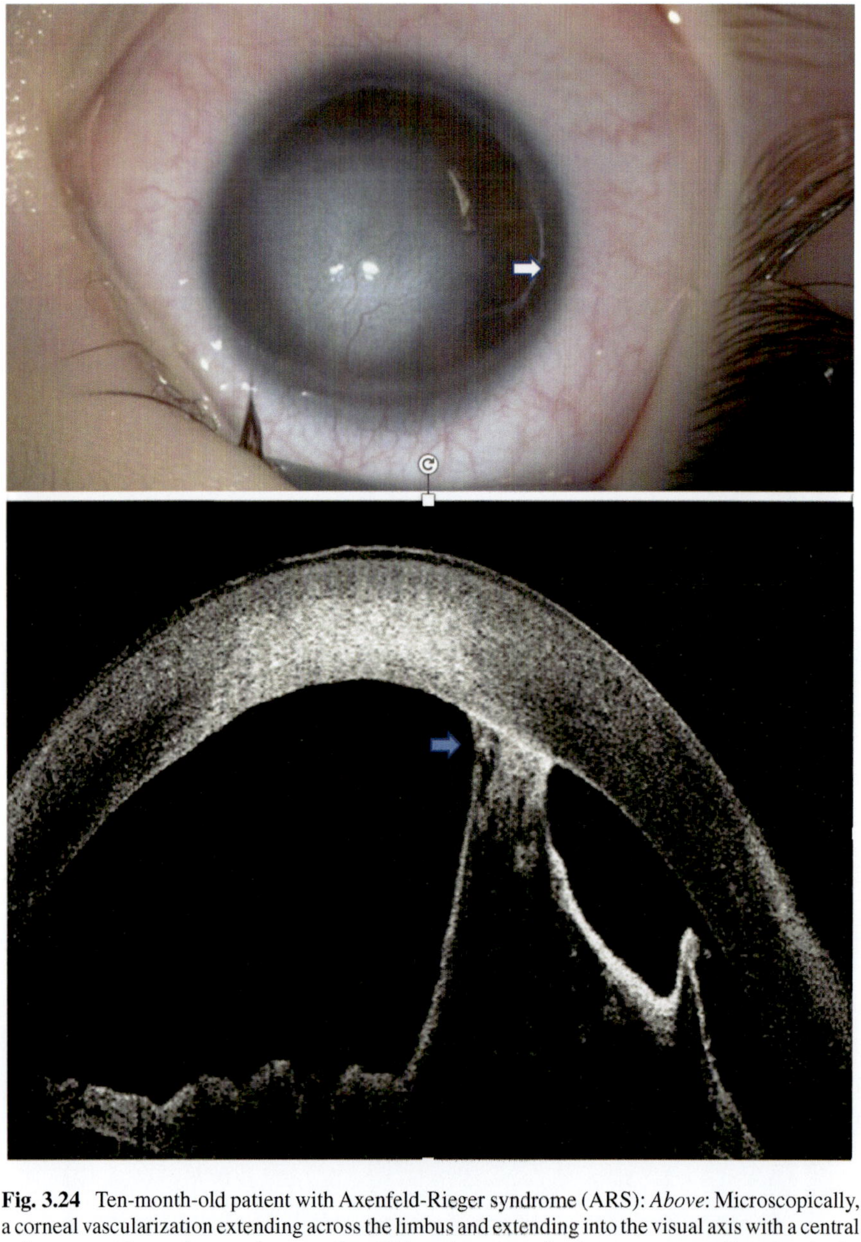

Fig. 3.24 Ten-month-old patient with Axenfeld-Rieger syndrome (ARS): *Above*: Microscopically, a corneal vascularization extending across the limbus and extending into the visual axis with a central stricter stromal scarring can be seen. In addition, there is a clearly upstream swallow line in the middle periphery of the cornea in the sense of an ARS (white arrow). *Below*: Intraoperative optical coherence tomography (iOCT) shows thorough stromal hyperreflectivity with clearly pronounced irido-corneal synechiation with thickening of the Descemet membrane in the area of adhesion (blue arrow). At the periphery, the cornea appears clearer with reduced hyperreflectivity in the iOCT

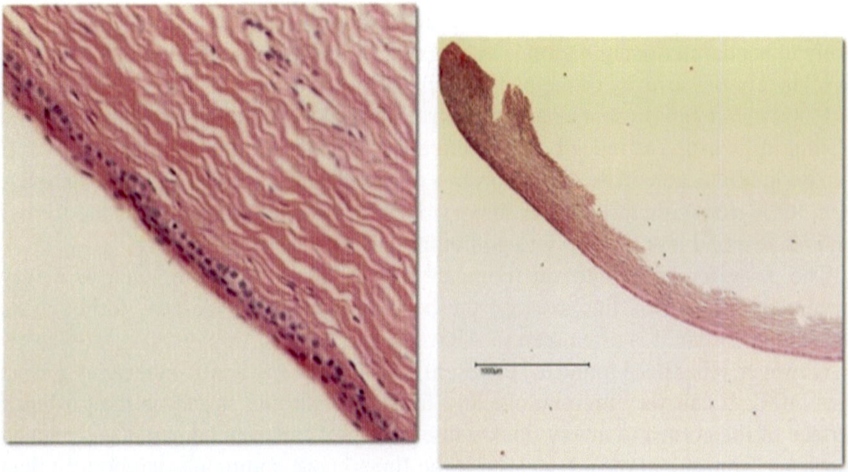

Fig. 3.25 Histological cross-section of the cornea with hematoxilin-eosin (HE) staining under light microscopy in a child with ARS: Right: section of the specimen showing marked irregular arrangement of collagen fibrils and increased stromal H_2O retention. Left: Overview slice preparation of the performed DALK. in a ten-month-old patient with Axenfeld-Rieger syndrome

Often there is an autosomal dominant inheritance with mutations in the gene *FOXC1 (6p25)* and *PITX2* (4q25) [102–104]. The inheritance pattern is autosomal dominant.

There is fluctuating expression, so that sometimes a generation seems to have been skipped. Often an increase in expression can be observed, although sporadic cases are also possible. When they are associated with systemic anomalies, they are given the suffix-syndrome, namely Axenfeld-Rieger syndrome (ARS).

➢ Notes

Axenfeld-Rieger-Syndrom (ARS): Axenfeld-Rieger-Syndrom (ARS)

- **Clinical ophthalmologic picture**
  - Iris dysplasia: colobomas or synechiae.
  - Iris atrophy with anteriorly displaced Schwalbe line
  - Secondary glaucoma.
- **Systemic**
  - middle ear hearing loss
  - cerebral retardation
  - dental, maxillofacial malformation (microdontia or hypodontia)
  - increased incidence of umbilical hernias
  - generalized bone forming disorders.

Around 50% of those with ARA develop glaucoma, and a rise in IOP is most likely to occur later in childhood. The risk of developing glaucoma does not seem to be related to the severity of the phenotype [105, 106].

However, it can present at any time from birth to adulthood, and patients need lifelong follow-up (as indeed do all patients with anterior segment dysgeneses). If the rise in IOP occurs in the first two years of life it is important to differentiate ARA from ICG (from either the family history or, if possible, examination) as the former tends to respond less favorably to goniotomy [107].

The posterior **embryotoxon** (compare Fig. 3.26) is the name given to a very prominent Schwalbe's line seen on the peripheral posterior Cornea. Although its origin is uncertain it is often seen in ARA/ARS.

However, it has been found to be present in 8–15% of apparently otherwise normal eyes [108]. It can vary morphologically from a subtle thin strand on the posterior surface of the cornea to a very thick white band and can even be partially detached and hang from the cornea. It is seen three times more commonly temporally than nasally and is often not seen superiorly and inferiorly as the sclera extends further forward here. In the presence of other anterior segment anomalies, the presence of a posterior embryotoxon indicates that the diagnosis is ARA.

> **Notes: Axenfeld-Rieger-Syndrome (ARS)**

- extremely rare disease
- autosomal dominant disease: often *FOXC1* on 6p25 and *PITX 2* on 4q25
- fluctuating expressivity sometimes skipping one generation
- often increase in expressivity
- sporadic cases are possible
- embryotoxon posterior
- **corneal opacity**.

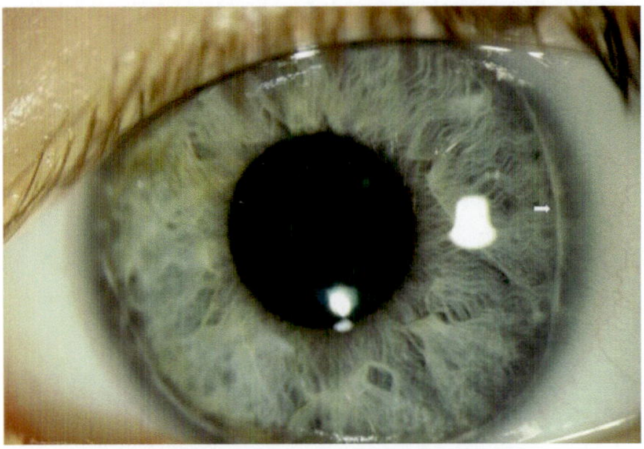

Fig. 3.26 Young adult with a posterior embrytoxon with prominent swallow line with known ARA

In children with bilateral corneal opacity, without posterior embryotoxon, but with extraocular features for ARS (maxillofacial hypoplasia, abnormal dentition, paraumbilical hernia and generalized bone formation disorders in the skeletal system), testing for *PITX2* and *FOXC1* should be considered. Magnetic resonance imaging should also be performed to rule out problems of the pituitary axis, as this is also affected by *PITX2* mutations. The constellation of findings sometimes complicates the differentiation of ARS to Peters Plus anomaly, so that pediatric and genetic clarification in interdisciplinary cooperation is very useful.

> **Overview**
>
> **Important irido-trabecular dysgenesis, to be distinguished from irido-corneal dysgenesis**
>
> - Axenfeld-Rieger syndrome (ARS)
> - Posterior Embryotoxon
> - Aniridia.

In the maximum variant of irido-trabecular dysgenesis, the **aniridia**, there is partial or complete hypoplasia (compare Fig. 3.27) of the iris. This can result in the attachment of the lens to the corneal back surface with subsequent corneal opacity. Corneal opacity can also be caused by associated limbal stem cell insufficiency.

In addition to cataract and glaucoma, the development of a pannus, a nystagmus, as well as foveal and opticus hypoplasia are also possible ocular side effects [80]. There is usually a mutation in *PAX6* [109–113].

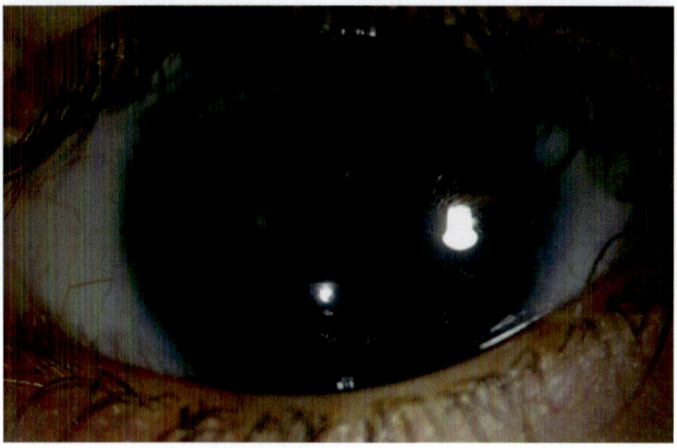

Fig. 3.27 Clinical picture of a nine-year-old child with congenital aniridia and buphthalmos: There is marked hypoplasia of the iris and an enlarged corneal radius

In the case of sporadic mutations, a deletion is often the cause, so that in these patients the presence of a Wilms tumor must also be excluded, since the gene for the Wilms tumor (*WT1*) is located near *PAX6* on chromosome 11p13 [80].

As described above, comorbidities are often present in the diseases mentioned, such as ASD, optic nerve damage, cataract, or retinopathy, which increase the complexity of surgical interventions. Not infrequently, in addition to corneal opacity, limbal stem cell insufficiency is also present, which leads to a pathological sprouting of vessels into the cornea.

This neovascularization, possibly combined with a conjunctivalization of the cornea, produces a significant reduction in transparency of the cornea, which makes surgery unavoidable. Secondary corneal cloudiness in buphthalmos, for example, in congenital glaucoma also plays an important role and is often an indication for pediatric corneal surgery. The secondary corneal opacity will be discussed in further detail below.

3.6.3 Ectasia of the Anterior Segment

In **keratoconus**, there is a progressive thinning and cone-shaped deformation of the cornea of the eye. The disease is always bilateral, but can be weaker in one eye or not symptomatic at all (form frustration keratoconus).

The disease is therefore characterized by two characteristics, which leads first to a progressive thinning and sharping of the cornea (compare Fig. 3.28) and secondary

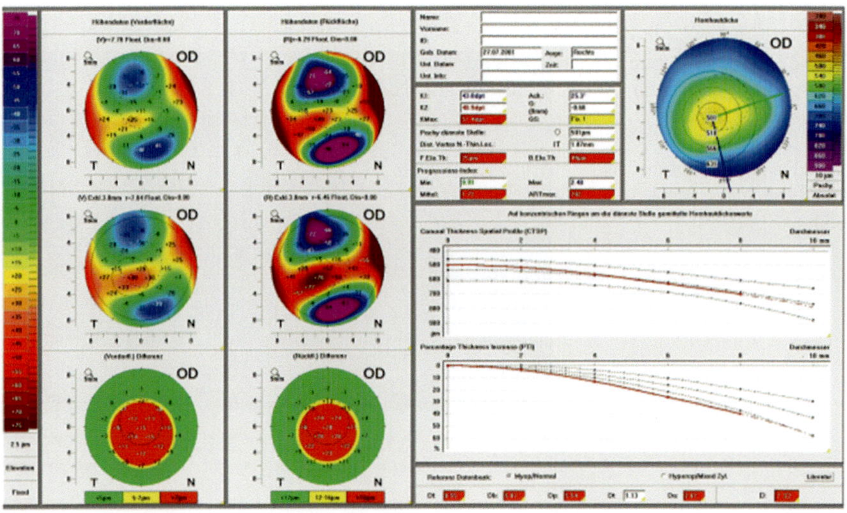

Fig. 3.28 Measurement of corneal topography using Oculus Pentacam: Typical for keratoconus are the progressive thinning and sharpening of the cornea

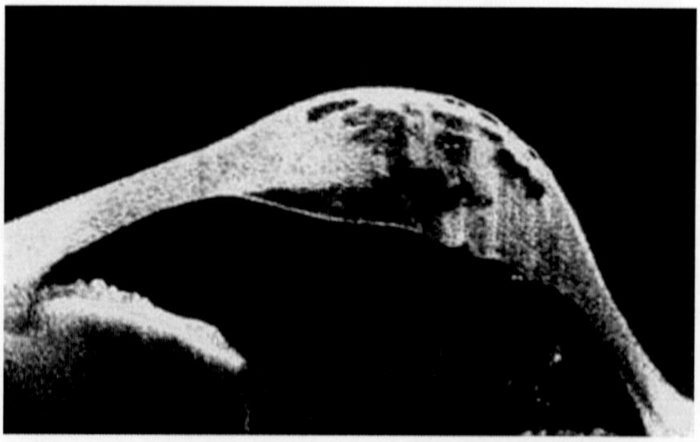

Fig. 3.29 Acute hydrops in a 15 years -old boy with trisomy 21 and keratoconus. The Descemet's tear and the resulting bullous stromal and epithelial edema can be detected in the anterior OCT scan

to a decreasing visual acuity due to the irregular deformation of the cornea. However, this myopia cannot be completely corrected with a visual aid, as the cone-shaped corneal protrusion causes irregular astigmatism.

Clinical features of keratoconus may be a hemosiderin ring (Fleischer's rings), known as keratoconus lines. Here, a yellow–brown to green–brown coloration occurs, which moves the base of the cone as a half or closed circle, visible in good lighting.

During the further course, superficial, irregular scars and opacities as well as tears in the Descemet membrane may become visible and Vogt's lines may occur. When corneal edema occurs, there is acute keratoconus. This can heal after three to four months if scarring.

There may rarely be cracks in the posterior cornea, so that fluid from the anterior chamber of the eye penetrates into the cornea, coming to a hydrops or acute keratoconus. This also manifests itself in an acute, strong clouding of the cornea, due to the stromal- and epithelial bullous edema (compare Fig. 3.29). The hydrops generally regresses on its own. Surgical care using Murrain sutures or a mini DMEK is also possible but rarely practiced in children, as hydrops are observed less often here [114].

Childhood keratoconus is often seen mainly in the context of genetically induced syndromic diseases, such as trisomy 21, monosomy X syndrome, Ehlers-Danlos syndrome, Marfan syndrome, Alport syndrome, Silver-Russell syndrome, Noonan syndrome, Mulvihill-Smith syndrome, as well as Urrets-Zavalia syndrome and floppy eyelid syndrome [115–121].

3.6.4 Keratoglobus

Keratoglobus is a rare disorder of the cornea, which is noninflammatory and is characterized by generalized thinning and globular protrusion of the cornea. It was first described as a separate clinical entity by Verrey in 1947 [122].

The congenital and as well as the acquired form of keratoglobus have been shown to occur, and may be associated with various other ocular and systemic syndromes including the connective tissue disorders, such as collagen disorders and Osteogenis imperfecta [123].

Osteogenesis imperfecta is caused by various disorders in the biosynthesis of collagen, a very important component of the bone matrix. In 95% of cases, genes that are important for the synthesis of collagen type I are affected (*COL1A1* and *COL1A2*). If there is a loss of one *COL1A1* allele, only a reduced synthesis of collagen type I is possible.

However, the collagen is intact, so that the expression of the disease is mild. However, if mutations occur in the *COL1A1* or *COL1A2* gene (e.g. by point mutation, or alternative splicing), predominantly defective and only slightly intact type I collagen is produced. In most cases, this occurs by substitution of the major amino acid glycine in the triple helix of collagen with another amino acid. In addition, the twisting of the collagen triple helix is often disturbed, resulting in reduced stability. These facts leads to the ophthalmological clinical fining of blue sclera and kertoglobus. However, the exact genetics and pathogenesis remain unknown [123].

Similarities have been also found with other noninflammatory thinning disorders like keratoconus.

The clinical findings in keratoglobus is characterized by a progressive diminution resulting from irregular corneal topography with increased corneal fragility due to extreme thinning (compare Fig. 3.30a). It usually occurs on both sides and varies in severity [124].

Unlike keratoconus, in which only the central area of the cornea is affected, in keratoglobus peripheral areas of the cornea are also damaged. The cornea is too large (megalocornea Ø > 13 mm up to 18 mm). Myopia and irregular astigmatism cause a worsening of visual acuity.

Acute keratoglobus can occur when the cornea is injured at the endothelium and Descemet's membrane. Like acute keratoconus, acute keratoglobus can heal spontaneously (compare Fig. 3.30b).

Conservative and surgical management for visual rehabilitation and improved tectonic stability have been described but remains challenging.

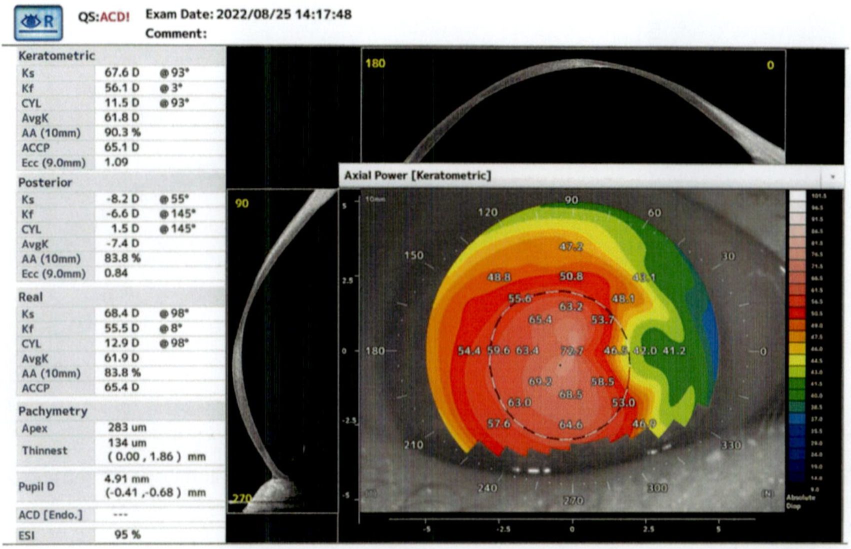

(a)

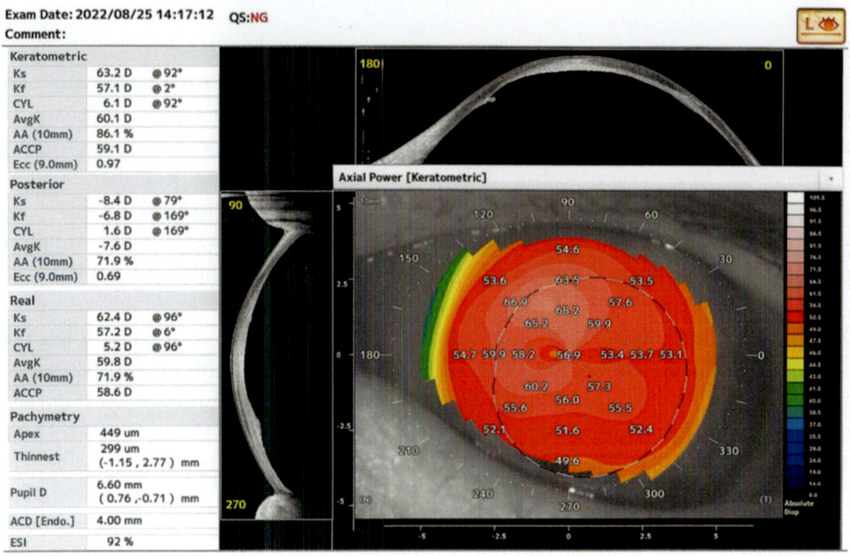

(b)

Fig. 3.30 a: Thinning of the cornea up to 283 μm centrally with an irregular astigmatism in a child with keratoglobus with osteogeneis imperfecta. Clinical the sclera also thin, which occurs blue. The anterior chamber is also very deppen. b: Stromal and endothelial scaring after an acute hydrops with spontaneous healing with a simultaneous thinning of to cornea in a child with Osteogenesis imperfecta and keratglobus

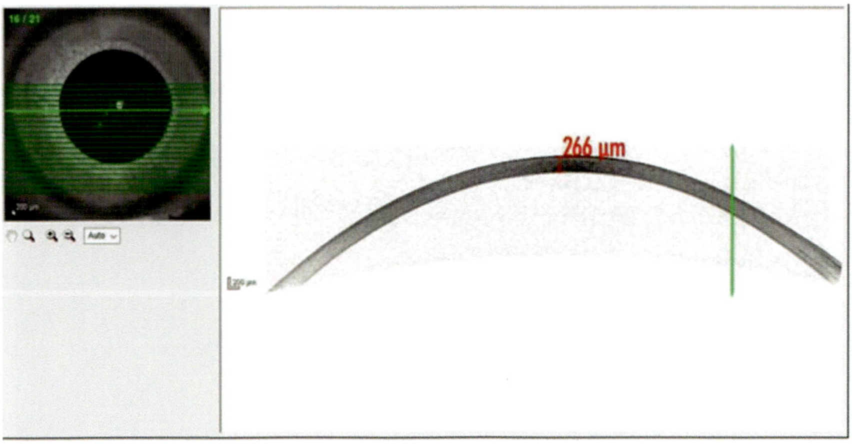

Fig. 3.31 Massively thinned cornea of a 13 year old patient to 266 µm at the apex of the cornea with BCS

3.6.5 *Brittle Cornea Syndrome (BCS)*

BCS is a genetic disease involving the connective tissue in the eyes, ears, joints, and skin. The symptoms of BCS typically involve thinning of the cornea in the form of keratoconus or keratoglobus, which may lead to tearing or rupture after minor injury. This may occur as early as two years of age. The corneal thinning usually worsens over time (compare Fig. 3.31). Scarring of the cornea may be found in areas where rupture has occurred. Other eye symptoms may include a blue tint to the sclera of the eye, myopia and retinal detachment [125]. Other systemic symptoms may include hearing loss, People with BCS may also experience musculoskeletal symptoms, including hip dysplasia and abnormal curvature of the spine (scoliosis). Other symptoms may include low muscle tone (hypotonia) in infancy, long and slender fingers and toes (arachnodactyly) and above-average joint flexibility. People with BCS may also experience a tightening and shortening of muscles around the joints (contractures), particularly involving the pinky (small, fifth finger) [126]. There are two types of BCS. BCS type 1 is caused by mutations in the *ZNF469* gene and BCS type 2 is caused by changes in the *PRDM5* gene [126–128]. BCS is inherited in an autosomal recessive manner. The diagnosis of BCS is made based on symptoms and may be confirmed through genetic testing.

3.6.6 *Microcornea as a Form of Anterior Section Anomaly*

In **microcornea**, the corneal diameter is less than 8 mm in the newborn. Microcornea is often found in microphthalmia. Microphthalmia is based on a disorder of morphogenesis of eye development. It is often accompanied by a coloboma. In microphthalmia, there is an association with fetal alcohol syndrome, mother's vitamin A deficiency, radiation exposure and infections during pregnancy such as rubella in pregnancy, herpes simplex and cytomegaly [134]. Thalidomide (Contergan®) can also induce this developmental disorder.

Microphthalmia is usually genetic (e.g. in connection with trisomy 13, trisomy 8, triploidy or Peters Plus syndrome) and can occur together with other inhibition malformations, e.g. in Delleman syndrome or Wolf-Hirschhorn syndrome [130–133].

Microcornea by itself is also associated with myopia with a need of correction. Often only one eye is affected. The microcornea itself can be used in the context of retinopathy of prematurity and other syndromes such as Lenz syndrome, micro syndrome or geroderma osteodysplastica and is a leading symptom in the following syndromes, for example the Juvenile cataract—microcornea—renal glucosuria, underlying mutations in the SLC16A12 gene at location 10q23.31, the CCMCO syndrome (cataract, congenital—microcornea—corneal opacity), the Cataract-microcornea syndrome as well as the MRCS syndrome (microcornea—cone-rod dystrophy—cataract—posterior staphylom), autosomal dominant inheritance, mutations in the *PXDN* gene at location 2p25.3 [131, 134–137].

3.6.7 Primary Congenital Glaucoma

Primary congenital glaucoma manifests itself clinically within the first six months with increased intraocular pressure and resulting in corneal opacity, buphthalmos with Haab's striae (compare Fig. 3.32) and increased optic disc cupping [138, 139]. Disease-causing mutations have been described in *CYP1B1 and LTBP2*, and four gene locations with the disease have been identified: *GLC3A* (2p22-p21), *GLC3B* (1p36.2–36.1), *GLC3C* (14q24.3), and *GLC3D* (14q24.2–24.3) [95, 140, 141].

Primary congenital glaucoma is mostly caused by mutations in CYP1B1 with autosomal recessive inheritance. In addition, mutations in *LTBP2* have been described [95].

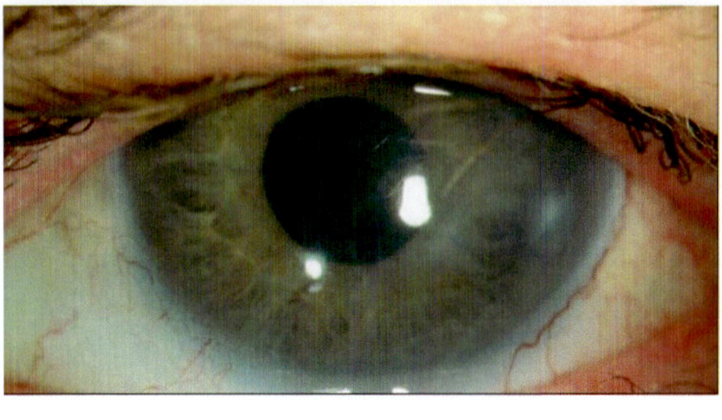

Fig. 3.32 Haab's Striae in an adolescent with congenital glaucoma: In the area of Haab's Striae a slight stromal opacity is detectable

3.6.8 Intracorneal Cyst

Intracoreal cysts in children are not common in everyday clinical practice, but a large number of individual case descriptions can be found in the literature. The intracorneal cysts as well as the cysts at the limboscleral junction are an abnormal proliferation of the epi- and/or endothelial cells, combined with fluid retention, which can be optimally diagnosed using slit lamp microscopy and OCT of the anterior segment of the eye (compare Fig. 3.33a, b).

This shows a corneal liquid gap, usually together with a decrease in the density of the affected area. Patients show signs of photophobia and often redness of the eyes. In the anamnesis, in most cases, no previous trauma and no previous operation on the affected eye is associable. The cysts can enlarge over time and lead to sequestration of the affected tissue area, which consequently makes surgical care unavoidable.

Surgical care is also indicated if the optical axis is affected by the cyst and amblyopia, especially due to the resulting irregular astigmatism, threatens [142–145]. Differential diagnosis in these cases should also be thought of terrien-marginal-degeneration [146].

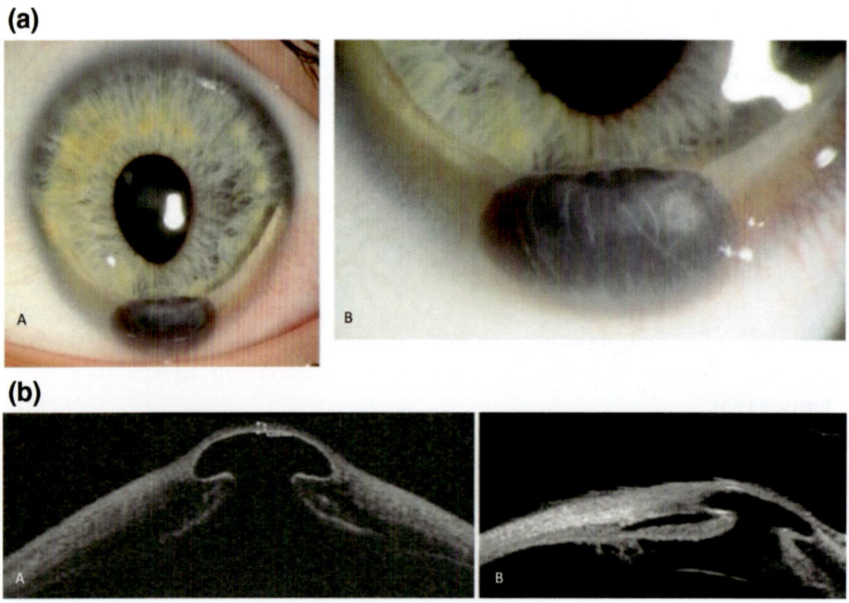

Fig. 3.33 a: Limbosceral pigmented intracorneal cysts in a child in slit lamp examination with an abnormal proliferation of the epi- and endothelial cells. b: Corresponding intracorneal cysts detected in optical coherence tomography with obvious with fluid retention

3.7 Secondary Corneal Disease: Acquired Corneal Disease

Acquired, secondary corneal diseases associated with corneal opacity in newborns can essentially be divided into metabolic diseases, trauma and infectious keratitis.

3.7.1 Metabolic Disease

Metabolic diseases that lead to an accumulation of various substances in tissues, including the cornea, are to be distinguished from dysgenesis due to enzyme defects. However, these are rarely already severely clouded at the time of birth, as accumulation increases over time. In mucolipidosis and mucopolysaccharidoses, enzyme defects cause the accumulation of mucopolysaccharides and mucolipids in the tissue [147]. Inheritance is usually autosomal recessive (exception: Hunter syndrome). The clouding of the cornea usually appears only in the months/years after birth. Clouding of the cornea may be seen at birth in Mucolipidosis II and IV.

The clinical picture is variable and dependent on the affected enzyme and the severity of its disorder. Important ocular characteristics include corneal opacity, cataract, abnormalities of the retina and retinal pigment epithelium, and glaucoma and optic atrophy [148]. If suspected, systemic involvement should be thoroughly clarified via a pediatrician. The very rare mucolipidose IV alone presents itself early within a few weeks after birth. It is associated with a severe psychomotor developmental delay [148, 149]. In rare autosomal recessively inherited cystinosis, increased intracellular levels of free cystine lead to deposits in numerous gives, including the cornea, which usually manifest themselves in the first year of life [150]. Other possible systemic metabolic diseases in this context include, for example, LCAT deficiency, tyrosinemia type 2, X-linked ichthyosis, as well as liposomal storage diseases and Fabry's disease [148, 150]. In the following, the most important systemic diseases will be briefly discussed in further detail.

- **LCAT deficiency**

Clinically, two forms of LCAT deficiency can be distinguished: Familial form, synonymous is Complete LCAT deficiency, with corneal opacities, anemia, and renal insufficiency.

In the second variant, Fish Eye Syndrome, Partial LCAT deficiency is present, also associated with corneal opacities and sometimes arteriosclerosis.

Underlying both forms are mutations in the LCAT gene in chromosome 16 at gene locus q22.1, which encodes the LCAT enzyme involved in the conversion of cholesterol esters to lipoproteins.

Clinical signs of LCAT deficiency are corneal opacities with small gray dots on the cornea starting in early childhood, renal insufficiency as well as renal hypertension, arteriosclerosis and xanthelasma. In rare cases, hepatomegaly, splenomegaly, and/or lymphadenopathy may be present,

In fisheye syndrome, the corneal opacities are much more pronounced and therefore also lead to early impairment of visual acuity.

- **Cystinosis**

Three forms of the disease are distinguished, with infantile or nephropathic cystinosis being the most common form. This is caused by a defect in the *CTNS* gene on chromosome 17, which codes for the lysosomal membrane protein cystinosin. The disease is inherited in an autosomal recessive manner. Cystinosin is responsible for the transport of cystine from the lysosome.

After the first symptom-free months of life, the disease initially begins with non-specific general symptoms such as fever, nausea, vomiting, loss of appetite, chronic constipation, weight loss, vitamin D-refractory rickets and dystrophy, polydipsia, polyuria. Due to the damaged kidneys there is hypokalemia and acidosis. Especially in the course of infections, this can lead to severe metabolic derailments in infants and young children. Mental retardation is usually not present in the mostly light-blond and light-shy patients.

Slit lamp examination can reveal multiple light-scattering cystine crystals in the cornea and conjunctiva.

- **Tyrosinemia type 2**

Tyrosinemia type 2 is a congenital defect in the metabolism of tyrosine and is inherited in an autosomal recessive manner. It is caused by mutations in the *TAT* gene (16q22.1), which encodes tyrosine aminotransferase (TAT). As a consequence of TAT deficiency and the resulting elevated tyrosine level, formation of tyrosine crystals is favored, triggering an inflammatory oculo-cutaneous reaction and the ocular symptoms.

These skin lesions are present in 80% of cases, and the eyes are involved in 75% of cases. 60% of patients show neurological symptoms as well as intellectual deficit.

The onset of the disease is variable and usually becomes apparent within the first year of life. Ocular findings include corneal opacification with bilateral dendritiform corneal lesions (pseudodendritic keratitis), vascularization, and corneal ulceration with scarring. Patients present symptoms of ocular redness, photophobia, epiphora, and pain, as well as reduced visual acuity. Skin symptoms usually begin after the first year of life, but may occur together with ocular symptoms.

Treatment is aimed at limiting phenylalanine and tyrosine. Oral retinoids can be used to treat the skin lesions. Under controlled diet, plasma tyrosine levels decrease and the eye and skin symptoms regress.

- **Fabry Disease**

Fabry disease is a lysosomal storage disease caused by a defect in alpha-galactosidase A, which leads to intracellular storage of the ceramide trihexoside globotriaosylceramide (Gb3), a sphingolipid.

The disease is inherited in an X-chromosomal recessive manner and usually causes first symptoms in late childhood, such as pain attacks and paresthesias in hands and feet and angiokeratomas of the skin.

In the course of the disease, nephropathies, cardiomyopathy, sensorineural hearing loss and visually limiting corneal opacities may occur.

Myocardial infarction, renal infarction, and stroke are possible due to Gb3 storage in vessels. The autonomic nervous system may also be affected in the form of hypohydrosis and disturbed temperature regulation.

Diagnosis is made by sequencing the GLA gene. Onion-skin-like intracellular Gb3 accumulations can be found in biopsies in semithin sections or by electron microscopy.

The disease is treated by enzyme replacement therapy with alpha-galactosidase. For some missense mutations, it is also possible to stabilize the defective enzyme using the pharmacological chaperone migalastat.

Currently (2023), Fabry disease is not yet part of the basic newborn screening. Life expectancy is limited.

3.7.2 Ichthyosis, X-linked Recessive

X-linked recessive ichthyosis (RXLI) is a genodermatosis. and affects almost exclusively the male sex.

X-linked ichthyosis is an abnormality of epidermal lipid metabolism based on inactivating mutations or deletions in the *steroid sulfatase gene* (STS; Xp22.3). Steroid sulfatase (STS) is a lipid hydrolase of the stratum corneum, and is involved in the regulation of the permeability barrier and desquamation of the skin as well as cornea via hydrolysis of steroid sulfates. STS deficiency results in increased concentrations of CSO4, inhibiting epidermal serine proteases, with consequent reduced desquamation of corneocytes and retention hyperkeratosis.

Symptoms often appear in the first days of life. Non-erythematous, polygonal, loosely adherent and later gray and painful adherent scales may form, appearing predominantly on the trunk, extensor and flexor sides of the extremities and neck.

Attention deficit hyperactivity disorder is also frequently present. Other extracutaneous manifestations include maldescensus testis and hypogonadism. Corneal opacities are frequently found in RXLI, but do not usually affect vision severely.

3.7.3 Trauma

Likewise, traumatic events such as a forceps birth can lead to corneal opacity, which usually occurs clinically linear and usually one-sided. This shows a mostly vertical Descemet tear, which can initially lead to focal corneal edema and later to corneal curvature (cave: horizontal Descemet membrane tears in the buphthalmos/Haab striae).

In the rare amniocentesis injury, a one-sided angular or linear opacity according to a needle perforation can be observed.

If an amniocentesis injury is suspected, cataracts, iris or pupil abnormalities and eyelid damage should always be excluded [151].

3.7.4 Infectious Keratitis

Infections can also lead to secondary corneal opacity. Viral and bacterial infections are the most common, but infections by fungi and protozoa are also possible [152–155].

The most common viral infection in newborns is the herpes simplex virus, which usually occurs in the birth canal or postnatally and manifests itself clinically within the first two weeks of life (compare Fig. 3.34). Clinically, conjunctivitis and corneal opacity are often present with a large geographical/dendritic epitheloid infection and eyelid swelling with vesicles [155].

A systemic pediatric examination is essential to rule out concomitant and potentially life-threatening pneumonitis, hepatitis and/or encephalitis at an early stage.

Among the most common bacterial pathogens that lead to serious infectious keratitis are the gonococci and chlamydia. Compared to herpes infection, a bacterial infection with gonococci usually manifests itself within the first days of life and infection with chlamydia within the first week of life.

Gonococcal infection first shows conjunctivitis with eyelid swelling and chemosis, and finally mucopurulent pseudomembranes of the conjunctiva and keratitis [156]. Chlamydia infection also results in massive conjunctivitis [157]. However, ulcerative keratitis is less common.

The correct diagnosis is relevant here given that many changes also allow layer-by-layer ablation, for example by means of a keratectomy or a lamellar kreatoplasty as a therapy, which is accompanied by a significantly better prognosis of the medium- to long-term results than with a complete perforating keratoplasty, for example [158].

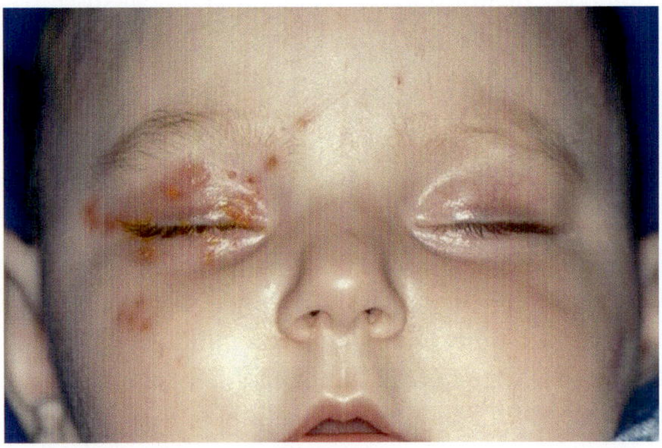

Fig. 3.34 Herpes simplex infection in a newborn: First published in "Lautenschlager, S. (2018). Humane Herpesviren. In: Plewig, G., Ruzicka, T., Kaufmann, R., Hertl, M. (eds) Braun-Falco's Dermatologie, Venerologie und Allergologie. Springer Reference Medizin. Springer, Berlin, Heidelberg". https://doi.org/10.1007/978-3-662-49544-5-9

3.7.5 *Vernal Conjunctivitis*

Vernal conjunctivitis and atopic keratoconjunctivitis can rarely lead to acquired infantile corneal opacity in infancy. It is a chronic recurrent disease with inflammation of the conjunctiva and cornea.

The disease often begins between the 4th and 7th year of life and occurs mainly in the months of January/February to September/October. A palpebral form is distinguished from a bulbar/limbal form, which is clinically manifested by papillae of the bulbar conjunctiva and Horner Tranta spots (eosinophilic cells and degenerated epithelium). The resulting puncate epitheliopathy and possible corneal neovascularization with lipid exudations cause pseudogerontoxon and corneal opacification, which may increase the risk of amblyopia. Possible complications of vernal keratoconjunctivitis may include keratoconus due to frequent eye rubbing. Likewise, a shield ulcer and pannus may develop.If a shield ulcer forms with a plaque, the plaque must be removed.

In most cases, the inflammation heals on its own during and after puberty. Risk factors for vernal conjunctivitis include chronic exposure to dust and smoke, UV light, allergies and asthma.

3.8 Surgical Procedures for Congenital Corneal Opacity

Surgical intervention should be reserved for clinically significant corneal opacities. Among the corneal dystrophies CHED is often the most common to need intervention. In the case of CHED endothelial keratoplasty may be considered but the age of the child will determine if this can be done; the depth of the anterior chamber may be too shallow to allow a safe endothelial keratoplasty and instead a penetrating keratoplasty may be needed.

In the case of a significant central corneal opacity due to anterior segment developmental anomaly the opacity can affect either the epithelium, or stroma, or endothelium or any combination of the three.

In total corneal opacification with disruption of corneal stromal lamellae, the surface and stroma are often vascularized with altered, flattened epithelium, missing Bowman layer and disorganized collagen fibrils in the stroma, which explains the whitish opacity of the cornea. At the same time, this opacity is accompanied by dysgenesis of the iris and drainage angle.

Thus far, no surgical interventions are recommended for such eyes, as a significantly reduced survival rate of the graft with a mean survival time of 36.4 months is described in studies [159]. However in bilateral cases at least one eye could be considered as long as VEP and ERG confirm visual potential.

Corneal surgery in early childhood due to Haab Striae is rare, as during this time the focus of treatment is on pressure-lowering measures and the effects of endothelial damage on corneal clarity can only be estimated after normalization of intraocular pressure.

The correct diagnosis holds strong relevance, as many changes also allow layer-by-layer ablation, for example by means of a keratectomy or a lamellar keratoplasty as a therapy, which is accompanied by a significantly better prognosis of medium to long-term results than, for example, with a complete perforating keratoplasty. The correct diagnosis thus helps to better assess the extent to which the cornea needs surgery.

> **Note**
>
> - The ophthalmologic workup of patients with congenital corneal opacities includes a thorough history with subsequent clinical examination, often performed under general anesthesia and supported by new imaging modalities such as optical coherence tomography.
> - The structured classification of congenital corneal opacities provides the basis for targeted therapy and should be focused on the limited to the affected layers/areas if possible.

3.8.1 Special Features of Corneal Surgery and Post-operative Examination

Cornea and sclera have a low intrinsic stiffness in children, which is why corneal incisions are always leaking and must be sutured closed.

Due to the small dimensions, a high vitreous body pressure, which leads to protrusion of the iris-lens diaphragam with an open eye, as well as a thick lens in relation to the anterior chamber depth, there is an increased risk of intraoperative lens injuries in perforating keratoplasty and transplantation of the corneal endothelium and increased trauma to the graft during suturing.

Children are prone to an increased fibrin reaction, partly also due to leaks of sutures and the resulting hypotension, whereby secondary increase in intraocular pressure can occur more often postoperatively. Wound healing is significantly accelerated compared to adults, which is why the corneal sutures are removed by 6 weeks post-surgery in infants under the age of 6 months; for every year in addition of age, 4 weeks are added to removal of sutures: e.g. an 18 month old post PKP would have sutures removed at 10 weeks while 3 yr old would have sutures removed at (6 + 4 + 4 =) 14–16 weeks.

The sutures also often loosen prematurely due to the described reduced rigidity of the cornea, making a suture repositioning necessary, which should be best achieved by means of interrupted single sutures [158, 160, 161]. Depending on age, suture checks and removals usually have to be carried out under anesthesia. Experience has shown that in children from the age of 6–7 years, depending on their willingness to cooperate, it is worthwhile to first try to remove individual sutures under local anesthesia. In this way, the already increased burden of general anesthesia can be reduced under certain circumstances.

In order for the children to cooperate in the examination, unpleasant procedures for the child, such as dressing removal or the dripping of local anesthetic, should be carried out in a timely manner before the examination and not by the ophthalmologists. This prevents the automatic association of negative experiences with the examination and the examiner. The examination itself should be well prepared. Hand slit lamp, iCare and objects to distract the child (colorful pictures, smartphone videos, pacifiers, ...) should be ready to make good use of short intervals of cooperation.

Once the decision for a child's corneal surgery has been made, the optimal time for surgery should be determined. Although a corneal transplant shows a significantly better prognosis, the older the child is, the indication of surgical therapy should be made earlier to reduce the risk of deprivation amblyopia.

In principle, earlier interventions for amblyopia reduction are to be preferred. In the case of superficial scars or scars in the anterior stromal area, which are only treated by a phototherapeutic keratectomy or anterior lamellar keratoplasty, surgery should be carried out accordingly quickly. In the case of perforating keratoplasties or endothelial transplants, the smaller dimension of the eye with the above limitations during transplantation must be weighed against the extent and anatomical location of the opacity.

Opacity of the cornea in the first months of life can still change and it can come to the receding of the findings, so that the situation for vision can improve. For this reason, and in view of the very high intraoperative vitreous pressure, it makes sense in many situations to avoid transplantation in the first 3–4 months of life and wait for the development of findings.

The risk of amblyopia must be weighed against the risks of pediatric anesthesia and a possible increased risk of graft failure during early surgical intervention.

> **Overview**
>
> **Special aspects of paediatric corneal surgery**
>
> - Sclera with low inherent stiffness, therefore corneal incisions are often leaky
> - High vitreous pressure
> - With open globe: risk of protrusion of the iris-lens diaphragm
> - Very thick lens in relation to the anterior chamber depth
> - Increased fibrin reactions post-operatively
> - Frequent suture leakage with necessity of suture repositioning suture repositioning/suture repositioning
> - Bulbar hypotony
> - Post-operative often secondary increase of intraocular pressure
> - Suture control and removal usually have to be performed under anesthesia.

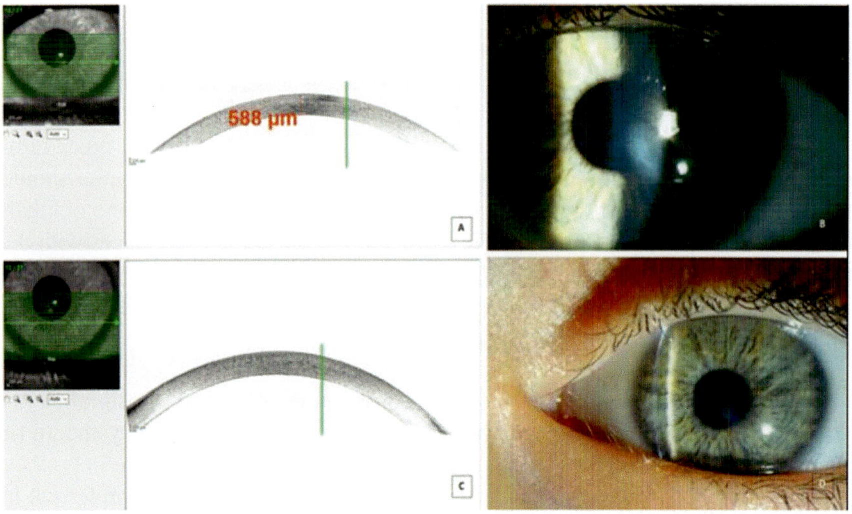

Fig. 3.35 Phototherapeutic keratectomy in children: A: Image of the left eye of an eight-year-old child with a unilateral paracentral hypertrophic corneal scar before manual keratectomy and phototherapeutic excimer laser keratectomy in anterior segment OCT. B shows the correlate in slit lamp microscopic findings. C and D show the immediate post-operative result with cleared findings after removal of the hypertrophic scar

3.8.2 The Child's Phototherapeutic Keratectomy (PTK)

PTK in children is analogous to treatment in adults with the difference that the procedure is performed under general anesthesia. With patience and a little effort, even without anesthesia, the indication and the depth of ablation can often be determined in infants by new very fast OCT devices for the anterior segment of the eye (compare Fig. 3.35) [162–164].

PTK shows a good prognosis for superficial corneal opacities, provided there is no further deeper or intraocular structural damage of the eye. If irregularities persist after PTK, further refractive correction can be performed with a dimensionally stable contact lens.

3.8.3 Crosslinking for Keratoconus

In children, keratoconus is usually more pronounced and progressive than in adults and is often already advanced by diagnosis [162, 165, 166]. As a rule, the disease is only noticeable from puberty but younger children have been reported with it too.

Risk factors for early onset and progressive progression include Down syndrome, frequent eye rubbing, Asian or Arab ethnicity, and connective tissue diseases such as Ehler-Danlos syndrome and Marfan syndrome [116–118, 162, 167].

An early onset can be more easily overlooked, as children under the age of 8 year old might not notice or do not notice the often-one-sided reduction in visual acuity. A childhood keratoconus (children under 15 years of age) thus has a seven-fold increased risk of needing keratoplasty in life. In children, progression occurs in up to 88% of cases [168]. Crosslinking should be carried out early due to the often rapid progression. In order to determine the progression even at the first presentation, a comparison with if necessary. older refraction values determined elsewhere.

Crosslinking is usually carried out in accordance with the Dresden Protocol [169]: After topical anesthesia of the affected eye, the epithelium is manually removed centrally with a diameter of approx. 9 mm ("Epi-off"). Subsequently, a solution of 0.1% riboflavin in 20% dextran is dropped into the eye every 2–3 min for 30 min, followed by UV-A irradiation (365–370 nm) at 3 mW/cm^2 for 30 min (total energy 5.4 J/cm^2).

A therapeutic contact lens and antibiotic local therapy is applied. Only patients with a corneal thickness of at least 400 μm after corneal epithelium removal are eligible.

In young children, this procedure must be performed under anesthesia. Even in children aged 14 and over, larger studies show good effects of crosslinking on the stabilization of the disease, a significant reduction in K_{max} and partial visual acuity improvements [170, 171].

In a study with 47 patients between 8 and 18 years of age, 80% of the progression could be stopped in the follow-up period of 10 years [171]. In case of recurrence, the procedure can be repeated if necessary.

> **Overview: Dresden Protocol for Crosslinking**
>
> - Topical anesthesia of the affected eye
> - Removal of the central epithelium ("Epi-off")
> - Administration of 0.1% riboflavin in 20% dextran every 2–3 min for 30 min into the affected eye
> - Treatment with UV-A irradiation (365–370 nm) at 3 mW/cm2 for 30 min
> - Postoperative insertion of a therapeutic contact lens combined with antibiotic with antibiotic local therapy.

3.8.4 Sectoral Iridectomy

The optical sectoral iridectomy can be useful in children in whom pronounced central opacity of the cornea with clear corneal parts in the lower area occurs. If an iridectomy is created in projection to this area, an optical window can be opened.

This procedure is suitable for children with severe corneal opacity, in whom e.g. vascularization and/or malformations of the chamber angle or iris increase the risk of perforating keratoplasty and in whom lamellar surgical therapy is not possible [172].

3.8.5 Selective Endothelialectomy or Removal (SER)

The principle here is that for central significant opacities due to iridocorneal adhesions, after lysis of the iridocorneal adhesions, using a low vacuum, the endothelium in the area of the opacity is very gently vacuumed off the DM; DM must not be damaged. By doing this the surrounding healthy endothelial cells can migrate into the area of the abnormal endothelial cells which have been removed. This causes the cornea to clear faster [173].

3.8.6 Pediatric Penetrating Keratoplasty (PKP)

At present, there is no consensus among studies on the optimal timing of perforating keratoplasty, although there tends to be better survival rates in older children. Infants have worse graft survival than children aged 5–12 years [174]. However, regarding the depth of amblyopia, the earliest possible operations are advantageous.

However, childhood cataract surgery is known to increase the risk of developing aphakia glaucoma in the first few months of life. In principle, the indication for bilateral surgery should be weighed well in view of the high risk of complications of the operation (intraoperative lens damage, post-operative increase in intraocular pressure, high astigmatism, wound dehiscences and thread loosening with the need for anesthesia, primary graft failure). Transplants on the second eye at short intervals theoretically have the charm of reducing the risk of amblyopia. However, an advantage for vision on the already operated eye should be able to be safely derived before the second eye is operated.

There is also no uniform recommendation for donor age. Corneas from very young donors are limited in availability and too elastic to be used for perforating keratoplasty. For this reason, tissue from adult donors who are as young as possible is usually used. The oversizing of donor tissues by 0.5–1 mm results in easier wound closure and provides a deeper anterior chamber and also increases the morphological success of corneal transplantation in pediatric eyes, thereby reducing the incidence of keratoplasty-associated glaucoma [175].

After the operation, prophylactic local antibiotic therapy with fluoroquinolones, in children preferably with moxifloxacin, should be carried out until the complete removal of the sutures, as well as regular checks of intraocular pressure. Corneal sutures are removed by 6 weeks post-surgery in infants under the age of 6 months; for every year in addition of age, 4 weeks are added to removal of sutures: e.g. an 18 month old post PKP would have sutures removed at 10 weeks while 3 yr old would have sutures removed at $(6 + 4 + 4 =)$ 14–16 weeks.

Superficial neovascularization in the area of loose sutures can favor graft rejection. Any loose or broken suture should be therefore removed as soon as possible, as they also pose an increased risk of infection [176, 177].

Transplant survival rates depend enormously on the underlying diagnosis. In principle, the rate of rejection in children is higher than in adults. The probability of transplant rejection is 50% in the first four years of life and 27% by the age of 12. At the age of 13th to 19th year, the rejection rate is reduced to about 10% [178]. In most studies, congenital corneal opacity shows worse results than acquired corneal opacity. The average graft survival is 45.2 ± 5.8 months [179].

Complications of pediatric keratoplasty primarily include an increased risk of rejection, the development of infectious keratitis, suture loosening, the development of glaucoma, as well as the development of phthisis. These complications are usually more common and severe than in adults and can be difficult to diagnose and manage in children who have limited communication [180]. Recognizable symptoms of complications can be photophobia and epiphora.

No intervention by means of PKP is recommended in acute keratoconus (very rare in children) or in the rare disease of "brittle cornea," in which there is an extremely high fragility of the tissue, which can even lead to spontaneous perforations. In the acute process, in these cases, a pure suture supply of the findings should be carried out. After the healing process and the scarring reconstruction, a keratoplasty can then be considered.

Since a number of alternative surgical therapy methods are now available, the need for PKP (compare Fig. 3.36) in children is reducing.

➢ Overview

Possible complications of PKP in children

- intraoperative lens damage
- postoperative increase in intraocular pressure
- high astigmatism
- wound dehiscences
- thread loosening with the need for anesthesia
- primary graft failure
- risk of rejection
- the development of infectious keratitis
- development of glaucoma
- development of phthisis.

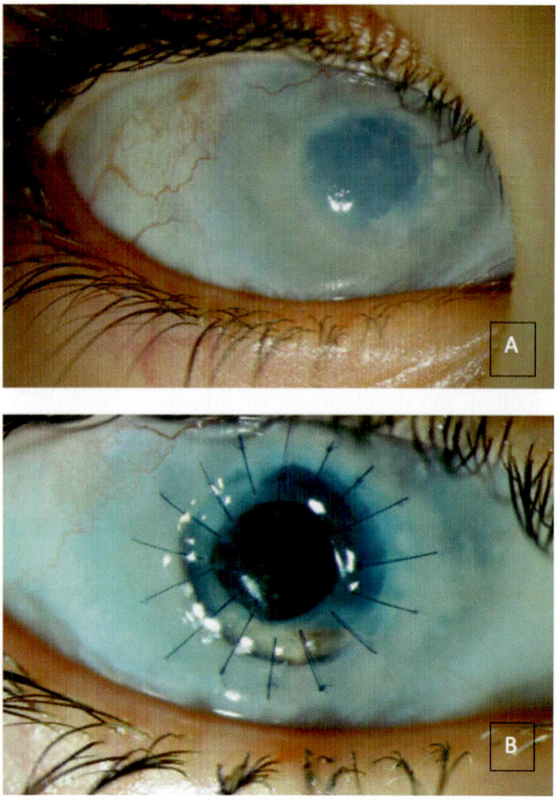

Fig. 3.36 Performed PKP (B) in condition after multiple amotio surgery with use of oil and resulting secondary corneal decompensation with stromal fibrosis and scarring (A) in an 11-year-old boy

3.8.7 Sandwich Technique of PKP in Infants

In this technique to try and maintain a closed chamber, as the host tissue is trephined a single 8/0 nylon suture is used to secure the cut edge of the host button to the host peripheral cornea. Four 8/o nylon sutures are placed securing the cut host button. The donor tissue has copious amounts of Healon GV placed on its endothelial side; the graft is placed on top of the diseased cornea. Now 10/0 nylon is used to secure the donor cornea to the host in three cardinal suture positions. Before placing the fourth, the 8/0 nylon sutures securing the host button to the host peripheral cornea are cut and the host button slipped out from under the donor cornea. The final cardinal suture is placed. The remaining 12 interrupted 10/0 nylon sutures are then placed to secure host to donor (compare Fig. 3.37). This technique reduces the chances of extrusion of ocular contents.

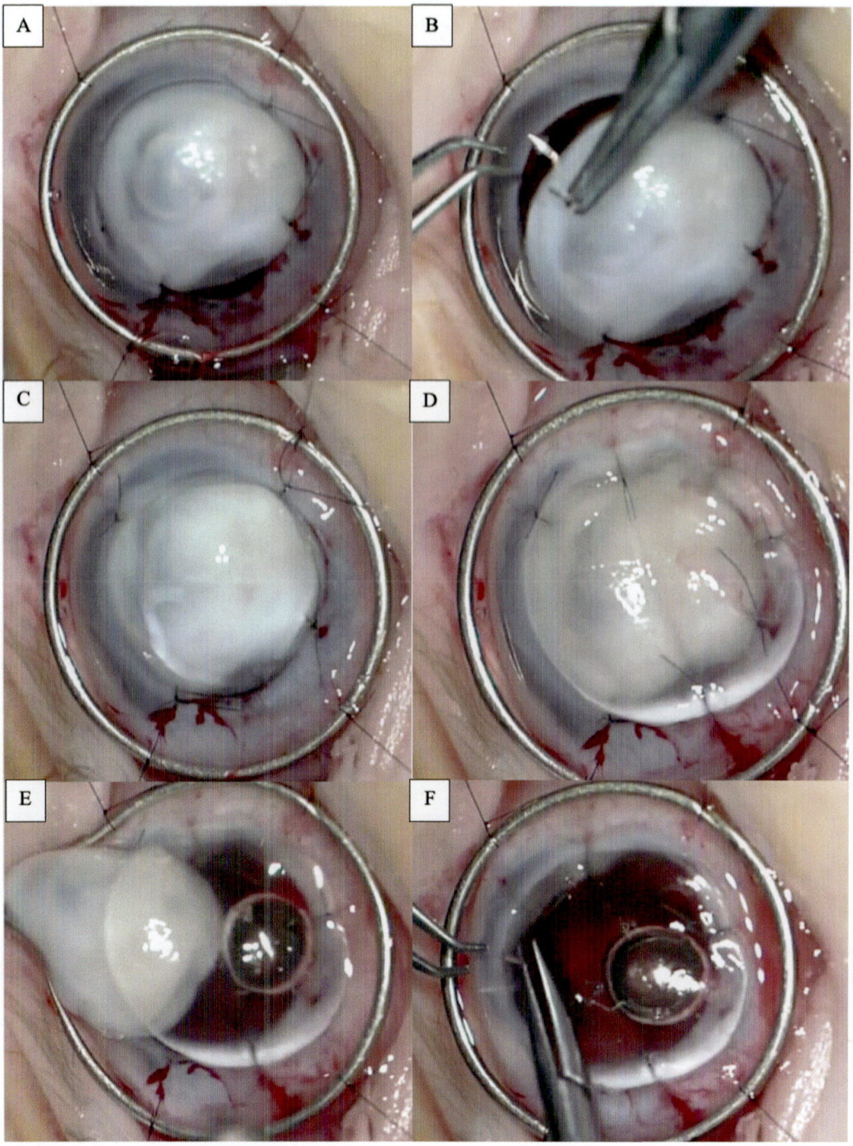

Fig. 3.37 Figures showing a PKP by using the Sandwich technique; in (A) and (B) there has been a partial trephination of the host tissue followed by quadrant by quadrant penetration; after each quadrant is opened a 8/0 nylon suture is placed to secure the host tissue in place. (C) Viscoelastic is placed on the host tissue and the donor button (D) is secured with three cardinal 10/0 nylon sutures. The 8/0 nylon sutures securing the host tissue are cut (E) and the host tissue removed. A final 10/0 nylon is used to secure the donor button (F). In this way an open sky situation is avoided

3.8.8 Pediatric Deep Anterior Lamellar Keratoplasty (DALK)

Deep anterior lamellar keratoplasty (DALK) is performed in the case of corneal opacity limited to the stroma and in which a proper endothelial function is present, for example in the case of scarring of the stroma e.g. after inflammation, in childhood keratoconus or in the cases of stromal clouding in the context of systemic diseases, such as mucopolysaccharidosis (compare Figs. 3.38 and 3.39) [162, 181].

The DALK can thus represent a good compromise if a perforating keratoplasty is considered too risky. In addition to the reduced risk of transplant rejection in lamellar keratoplasty, preference is given to a non-eye-opening procedure, which reduces the risk of intraoperative complications, such as expulsive suprachoroidal bleeding. The risk of secondary glaucoma is also reduced due to the reduced immune response in lamellar keratoplasty.

Due to the reduced fibrin reaction, the risk of synechiation of the chamber angles is reduced, so that a secondary increase in intraocular pressure occurs less frequently. A worsening of any existing glaucoma can also be avoided in this way. However, post-operative dehiscence with fluid accumulation in the interface may result, which may require a gas/air injection (rebubbling) into the anterior chamber, associated with renewed anesthesia in small children.

In severe cases, where limbal stem cell insufficiency is present with clinically significant cross-limbal corneal neovascularization, combined surgery with limbal stem cell transplantation may be an operative option.

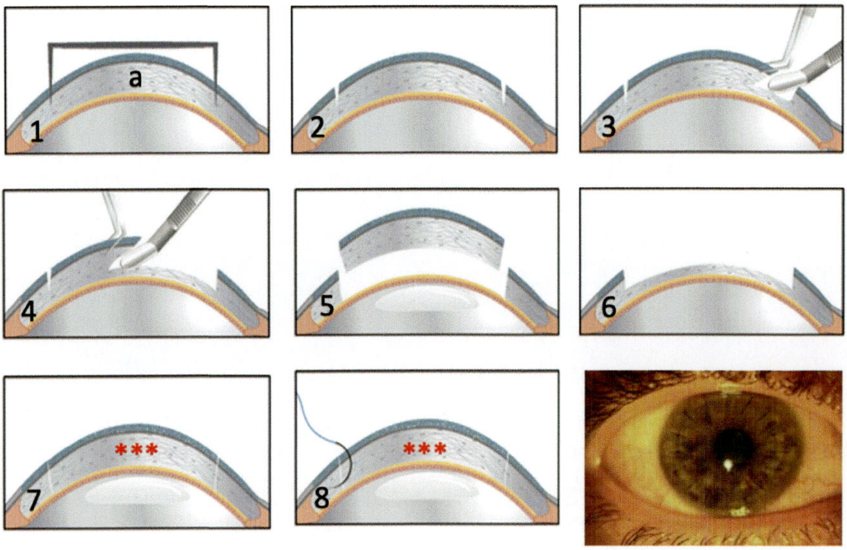

Fig. 3.38 Schematic overview of deep anterior lamellar keratoplasty (DALK) with "a" the defect anterior stroma of the patient and the postoperative donor tissue as replacement, marked with 'red ***'

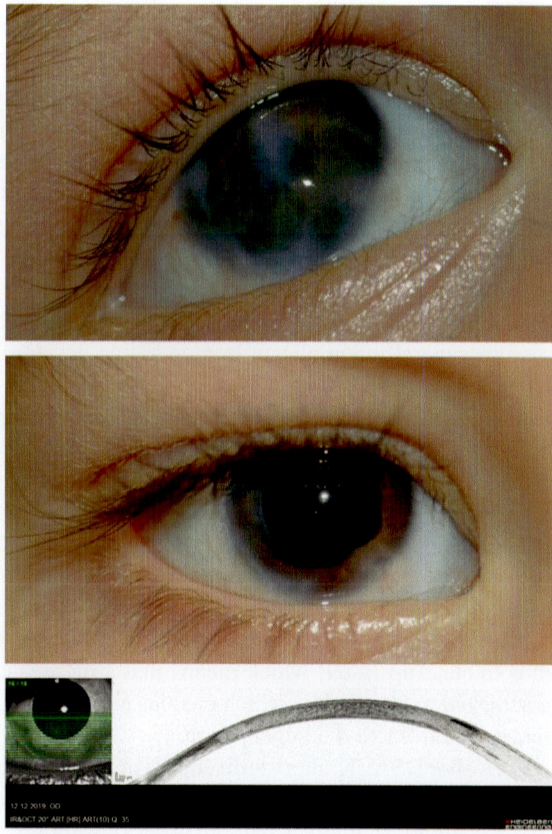

Fig. 3.39 Five-year-old child with condition after perilimbal dermoid cyst and persistent corneal scar up to the optical axis. Initially a lamellar keratectomy and a PTK was performed. Because of too thin corneal residual thickness, a DALK was performed. Below is the clinical picture after DALK and the corresponding anterior segment OCT, which shows the DALK lamella still well 2 years postoperatively

However, rejection of the transplanted limbal stem cells happens very often, which is why the indication for such interventions must be made depending on the extent of the pre-existing opacity.

➢ Overview

Advantages of deep anterior lamellar keratoplasty (DALK)

- Reduced risk of transplant rejection due to a non-eye-opening procedure
- Reduced risk of expulsive suprachoroidal bleeding
- Reduced risk of secondary glaucoma
- Reduced immune response due to the reduced fibrin reaction, so that the risk of synechiation of the chamber angles is also reduced
- A secondary increase in intraocular pressure occurs is less frequent.

3.8.9 Pediatric Endothelial Transplantation

The lamellar endothelial keratoplasties are currently performed as Descemet's stripping (automated) endothelial keratoplasty (DS(A)EK) or Descemet membrane endothelial keratoplasty (DMEK) for isolated endothelial dysfunction. DSAEK, in which the graft has a thin stromal lamella in addition to the endothelium/Descemet complex, has the disadvantage of a higher rejection rate and a slightly worse visual acuity result compared to DMEK with transplantation of exclusively the Descemet membrane and corneal endothelium in adults.

In children, the narrow anterior chamber conditions and the high vitreous body pressure generally complicate intraoperative development. In addition, there is an increased risk of lens injury, as in children the lens is further anterior compared to the adult eye. In addition, the diseased endothelium in small children is very difficult and may not be removed, which significantly reduces the adhesion of the endothelial grafts.

The DSAEK lamella has been shown to show improved adherence after transplantation in adults, which manifests itself in a reduced rate of rebubblings. This aspect of better graft adherence and reduced rebubbling rate is beneficial in young children, as rebubbling is always associated with anesthesia in an infant [182].

In addition, in posterior lamellar keratoplasty in the form of a DSAEK, the cornea tends to clear up faster, which means that a more stable refraction in children can be achieved more quickly, which enables early amblyopia treatment with occlusion therapy and refraction compensation.

Even after DSAEK, short-term checks under anesthesia with possibly renewed gas input into the anterior chamber may be necessary for graft dehiscences. Dehiscences have been more common in children in various studies, as consistent back positioning in infants is difficult to impossible during the phase, in which the anterior chamber is filled with gas/air, which can lead to graft dislocation or dehiscence.

Here, the advantage of DSAEK over DMEK outweighs the possibility of suture fixation of the DSAEK graft. This can significantly reduce the risk of graft dehiscence/dislocation.

For this reason, DSAEK is currently still preferred for small children (compare Figs. 3.40 and 3.42).

For older children, a DMEK can certainly be considered, although the published data remain small, since so far only a case-by-case description of a 12-year-old child is available [183]. An increased use of early pediatric DMEK will essentially depend on fixation possibilities of the graft to reduce the rebubbling rate in the future, and a possibility to fix the DSAEK grafts with the suture already exists (compare Fig. 3.41).

The endothelium is difficult or not to remove in CHED patients, as already described above. In a first publication on the attempt of endothelial transplantation in a patient with CHED, the DSAEK procedure was therefore discontinued and intra-operatively switched to a PKP because the endothelium was too firmly attached [184]. Meanwhile, endothelial transplantation is performed in such situations without stripping.

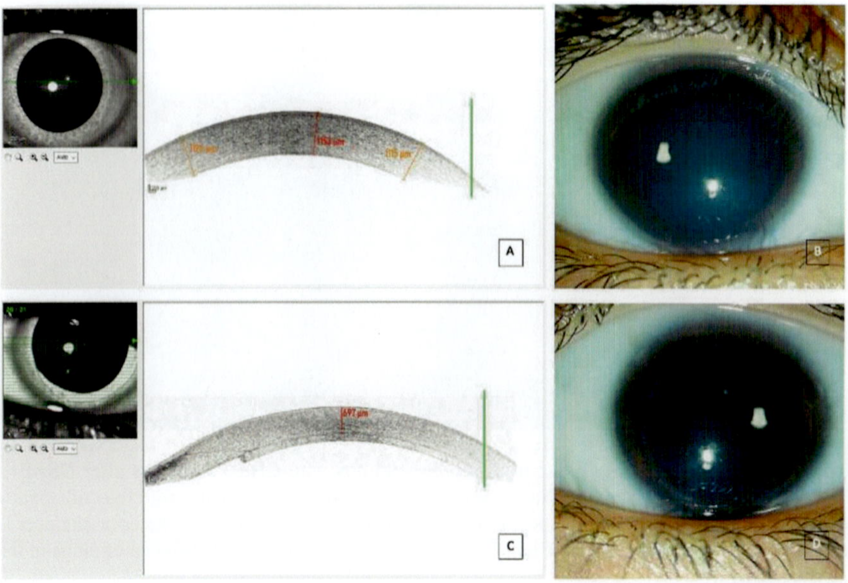

Fig. 3.40 Pre- and post-operative findings after DSAEK in a 13-year-old child with congenital hereditary endothelial dystrophy (CHED): Pre-operative slit lamp photomicrograph showed marked diffuse milky opacity of the corneal stroma (B) with thickening of the cornea to over 1153 μm on the performed anterior segmental OCT. The cornea appeared clearer as early as 2 weeks after DSAEK (D). The central corneal thickness reduced postoperatively to 697 μm (C) with nicely adherent DSAEK flap (C)

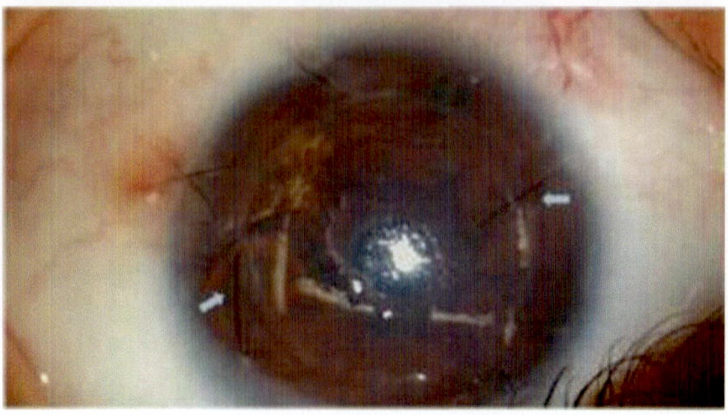

Fig. 3.41 DSAEK in a four year old child with CHED: The transplant was fixed by single sutures (see arrows at 2 and 7 o'clock) to avoid dislocation of the transplant and thus reduce the risk of rebubbling under anesthesia for the child

It is known from adult patients that after DMEK and DSAEK a significantly faster clearing of the cornea is achieved compared to the PKP, the post-operative astigmatism is significantly lower and the rejection rate is significantly lower due to the rarer immune reaction. The extent to which these benefits apply to children is not well documented.

A larger series (30 eyes of 16 children) according to DSAEK at CHED suggests that the earliest possible grafts in infancy lead to better visual acuity results after an

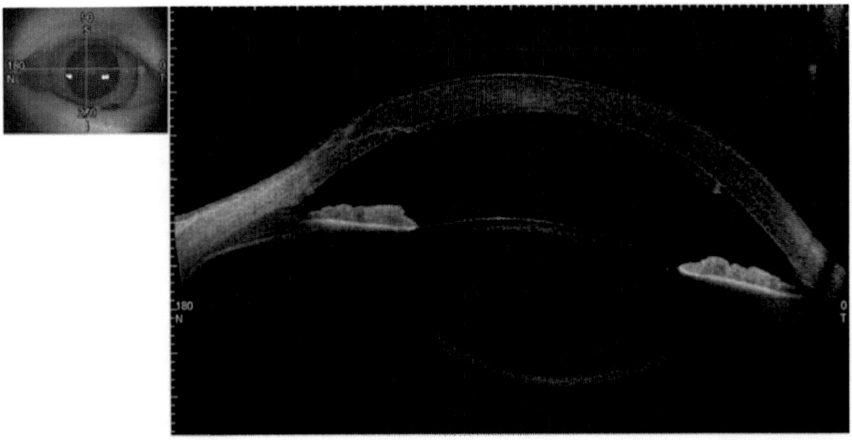

Fig. 3.42 Examination with Casia2 in a five-year-old boy with CHED 9 months after DSAEK: The cornea is clear without any scaring. The transplant is in place without any graft rejection or any dehiscens. The central cornea thickness is almost normally up to 606 μm. The anterior chamber is deep without any synechiation. The lens is also clear and without any pathological findings in the anterior segment

average of 4 years than transplants in older childhood [184]. Patients who received their first keratoplasty before age 6 tend to show a better post-operative visual outcome than those who underwent surgery after age 6 [180].

> **Note**
> **Advantages of DSAEK in children**
>
> - Improved adherence of the transplantat
> - Reduced rate of rebubblings: beneficial in young children, as rebubbling is always associated with anesthesia in an infant
> - DSAEK tends to clear up faster
> - More stable and quicker rehabilitation of refraction in children: advantage in amblyopia treatment in combination with occlusion therapy.

3.8.9.1 Pediatric Autorotational Keratoplasty

Autorotational keratoplasty can occur on corneas with central sweeping scars, where the peripheral cornea is clear. The principle comprises a peripherally shifted trepanation with the inclusion of the central opacity and rotation of the trephinnated cornea, so that the opacity is shifted to the periphery (compare Figs. 3.43 and 3.44).

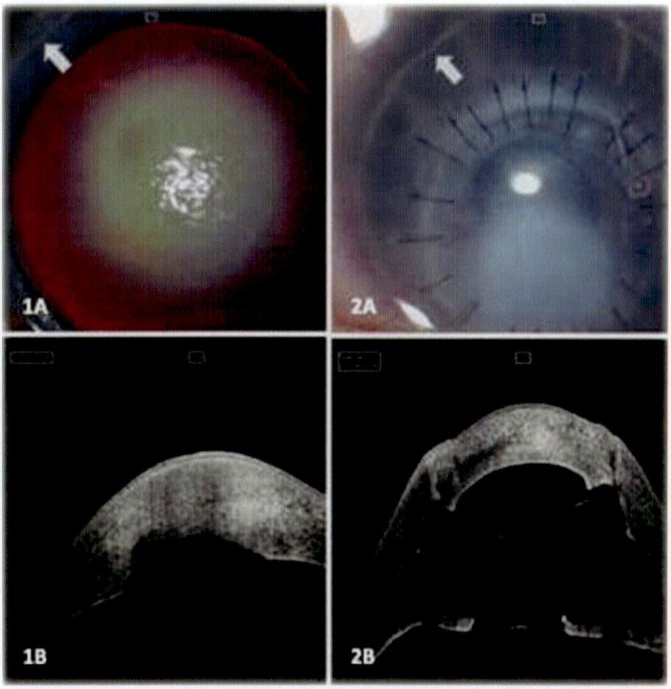

Fig. 3.43 Pediatric autorotation keratoplasty in a three- year old child: 1A: Pre-operatively, there is a dense central corneal opacity within the central optical axis and an advanced Schwalbe line (see white arrows). Before the operation, the pupil was therapeutically dilated far a better vision development of the child. 1B: Intraoperative microscopic picture: iOCT with hyperreflectivity of the entire stroma in the opacity area and a missing endothelium in the opacity zone. If there is no endothelium, a decision should be made against a DALK and for an autorotation keratoplasty with an upwardly decentered trepanation under the entire opacity zone. 2A: Postoperatively, the pupil can be seen centrally and the central optical axis is largely exposed. 2B: In the post-operative iOCT, the central cornea was thinner with an intact endothelial layer and improved reflectivity

> **Note**
> The advantages of the lack of rejection should be compared with the disadvantages of a higher irregularity and possibly only incomplete central clarity if a decision has to be made between an autorotation and an allogeneic keratoplasty.

In auto-keratoplasty, a distinction is made between ipsilateral and contralateral autokeratoplasty [186–190].

This procedure offers a longer, better prognosis in children than the allogeneic PKP, but the refractive result is worse due to the decentered trephination through partially different corneal tissue and due to the lack of oversizing of the transplant. For a good cosmetic result, the persistent corneal opacity should be rotated under the upper eyelid.

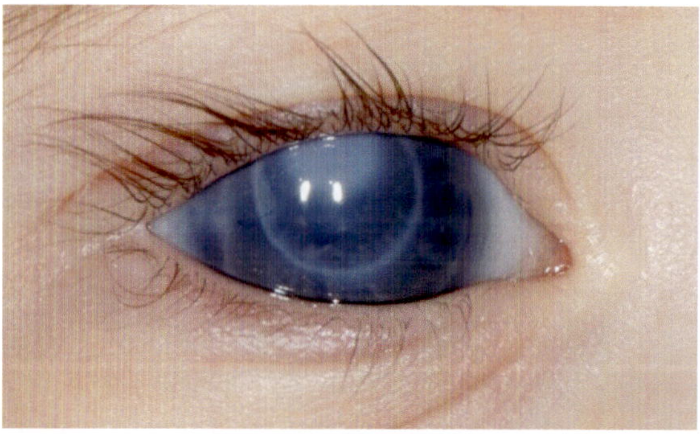

Fig. 3.44 Pediatric autorotation keratoplasty in a three- year old child: Post-operative findings after autorotation keratoplasty in a child with chamber angle dysgenesis and anteriorly displaced Schwalbe line as well as central corneal opacity in the sense of a Peters anomaly in a one-year-old child. The opacity was rotated out of the optic axis under the upper eyelid. A deep stromal suture remnant in the interface is still present. First published in "Die Ophthalmologie" https://doi.org/10.1007/s00347-022-01612-8

Advantages of these procedures are the lack of rejection reactions, the only short-term need for steroids, and the long retention of the endothelium compared to allogeneic transplantation (15% endothelial cell loss after one year with autorotation keratoplasty vs. 40% with PKP after one year) [186–190].

Disadvantages are the induction of astigmatism, which in some cases can even be higher than with an allogeneic PKP, due to the suture of the pathological tissue in the interface with increased suture tension and the eccentric trepanation [186–190].

Further disadvantages are the persistent residual opacities on the transplant, which are left on the periphery, and that overall only a few patients are eligible for this procedure and therefore no larger studies are available.

> **Note**
> **Autokeratoplasty is divided into ipsilateral and contralateral autokeratoplasty**
>
> - The contralateral autokeratoplasty is performed when an eye with a clear cornea has a low prognosis of vision due to a e.g. retinal disease, and the partner eye has a good retinal function, while the cornea is cloudy. During this procedure a perforating keratoplasty (PKP) is performed on both sides and the corneas change the sides.
> - For ipsilateral auto-rotation keratoplasty, patients are eligible whose cornea still has transparent areas that can be rotated centrally. These corneas are trephined mostly eccentrically and rotated in a position that the center is clear postoperatively in consequence. The target size for this clear area is a free optical axis of 4-5 mm.

> **Note**
> If a decision has to be made between an autorotation and an allogeneic keratoplasty, the advantage of the lack of rejection should be compared with the disadvantage of a higher irregularity and possibly only incomplete central clarity.

3.8.9.2 Pediatric Keratoprosthesis

The keratoprosthesis is an artificial cornea with a central optics, made of clear inerated material that allows the transmission of images through an otherwise cloudy natural cornea (compare Fig. 3.45).

The most commonly used keratoprosthesis in children was Boston keratoprosthesis type I (B-KPro I, compare Fig. 3.46).

The back wall of B-KPro I was available for pediatric patients with a smaller diameter (7.0 mm diameter). In most cases, aphacization was also carried out intraoperatively in children, as a cataract often develops in the process.

With the B-KPro I, there are models for aphak and pseudophake eyes [191, 192].

Since the complication rate B-KPro I is already very high in adults and in children it is even more frequently and poorly controllable, absolute glaucoma and endophthalmitis can develop, B-KPro I is no longer used in children.

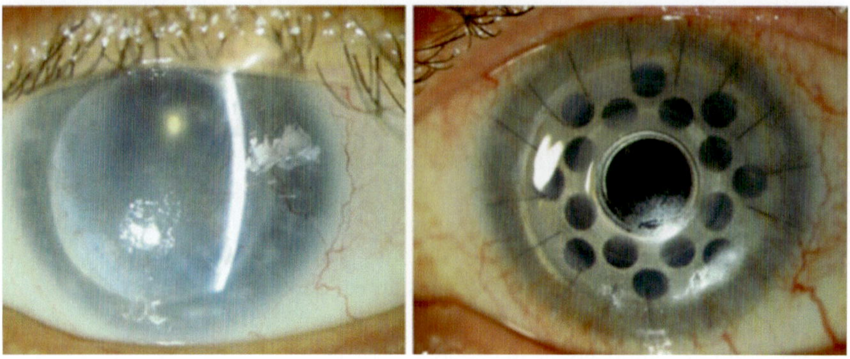

Fig. 3.45 Slit lamp biomicroscopic findings of limbal stem cell insufficiency in congenital aniridia and graft failure in a young adult. (preoperative visual acuity: 1/25 m visual acuity, MV; postoperative visual acuity after 2 months: 0.2 decimal) [192]. First published in “Die Ophthalmologie”. https://doi.org/10.1007/s00347-017-0581-0

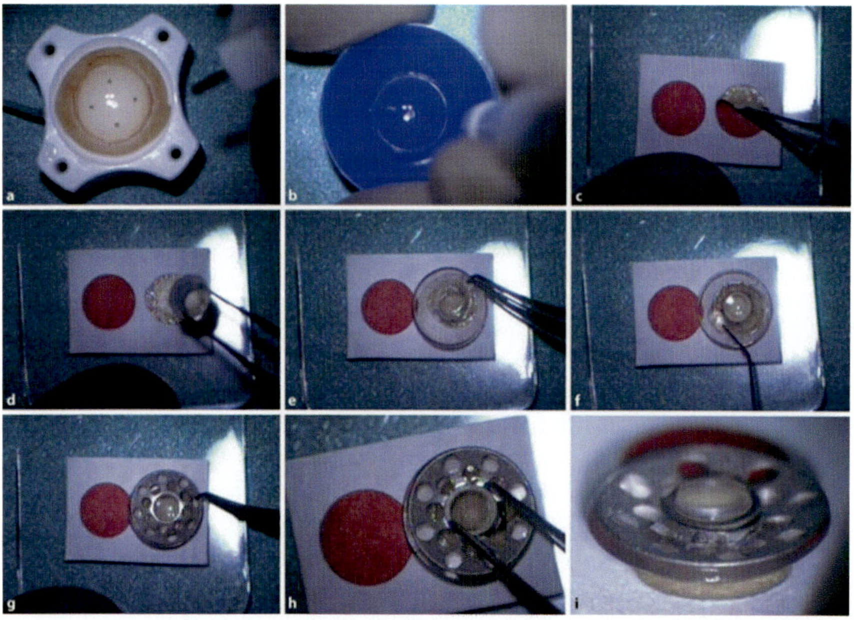

Fig. 3.46 Preparation of the Boston type 1 keratoprosthesis(B-KPro): **a)** Trephination of the donor cornea as a whole with Barron trephine. **b)** Repeated central trephination of the donor cornea with 3 mm Trepan. **c)** Apply the fixation points to the microscope slide. **d)** Fixation of the B-KPro optic. Subsequently, layer-by-layer application of **e)** donor cornea, **f)** viscoelastic, **g)** titanium backplate and blocking with h titanium compression ring **i)** Fully assembled B-KPro [192]. First published in "Die Ophthalmologie" https://doi.org/10.1007/s00347-018-0806-x

3.9 Conclusion

The causes and the clinic of congenital corneal opacity are diverse. An early and correct diagnosis holds central importance to counteract the impending development of amblyopia in a targeted manner. New diagnostic modalities such as OCT offer important assistance in this regard.

In children with congenital corneal opacity, there are many unique challenges in surgical care that must always be considered. Improved examination options and new lamellar treatment options help to avoid perforating keratoplasty with its high spectrum of complications in children to enable these young patients to see as satisfactorily as possible in the long term.

Acknowledgement of Sarah Barbara Zwingelberg: With everlasting love for my beloved mother and my protective brother.

I am deeply grateful for the unwavering, educational, and patient guidance of Prof. Dr. Claus Cursiefen, MD, and Prof. Björn Bachmann, MD—you instilled in me a love and passion for the cornea.

Thank you for everything.

References

1. Vanathi M, Panda A, Vengayil S, Chaudhuri Z, Dada T. Pediatric keratoplasty. Surv Ophthalmol. 2009;54(2):245–71.
2. Bermejo E, Martinez-Frias ML. Congenital eye malformations: clinical-epidemiological analysis of 1,124,654 consecutive births in Spain. Am J Med Genet. 1998;75(5):497–504.
3. Weiss JS, Rapuano CJ, Seitz B, Busin M, Kivelä TT, Bouheraoua N, Bredrup C, Nischal KK, Chawla H, Borderie V, Kenyon KR, Kim EK, Møller HU, Munier FL, Berger T, Lisch W. IC3D classification of corneal dystrophies-edition 3. Cornea. 2024. https://doi.org/10.1097/ICO.0000000000003420.
4. Weiss JS, Møller HU, Lisch W, et al. IC3D classification of corneal dystrophies–edition 2. Cornea. 2015;34(2):117–59.
5. Schröder S, Eppig T, Langenbucher A. A Concept for the analysis of repeatability and precision of corneal shape measurements. Z Med Phys. 2016;26(2):150–8.
6. Augustin AJ. York SBHN, editor. Augenheilkunde; 2007. p. 229.
7. Sridhar MS. Anatomy of cornea and ocular surface. Indian J Ophthalmol. 2018;66(2):190–4.
8. Meek KM, Knupp C. Corneal structure and transparency. Prog Retin Eye Res. 2015;49:1–16.
9. Lang GK, Oskar Gareis JE, Lang GE, Lang SJ, Spraul CW, Wagner P. In: Lang GK, editor. Augenheilkunde. Georg Thieme Verlag KG; 2019. p. 105–107.
10. Sachsenweger M. In: Bob AuK, editor. Duale Reihe Augenheilkunde. Deutschland: Georg Thieme Verlag; 2003. p. 100, 101.
11. Burk RB, Checkliste Augenheilkunde. In: Überarbeitete und erweiterte Auflage, vol. 4. Stuttgart: Georg Thieme Verlag; 2005. p. 192–195.
12. Price MO, Mehta JS, Jurkunas UV, Price FW. Corneal endothelial dysfunction: Evolving understanding and treatment options. Prog Retin Eye Res. 2021;82:100904.
13. Siebelmann S, Scholz P, Sonnenschein S, Bachmann B, Matthaei M, Cursiefen C, Heindl LM. Anterior segment optical coherence tomography for the diagnosis of corneal dystrophies according to the IC3D classification. Surv Ophthalmol. 2018;63(3):365–80.
14. Nicolay N, Güler I. Bradytroph [Webpage] 2019 [cited 2019 20.08.2019]; Available from: https://flexikon.doccheck.com/de/Bradytroph.
15. Hos D, Matthaei M, Bock F, Maruyama K, Notara M, Clahsen T, Hou Y, Le VNH, Salabarria A-C, Horstmann J, Bachmann BO, Cursiefen C. Immune reactions after modern lamellar (DALK, DSAEK, DMEK) versus conventional penetrating corneal transplantation. Prog Retin Eye Res. 2019;73:100768.
16. Kitazawa K, Hikichi T, Nakamura T, Nakamura M, Sotozono C, Masui S, Kinoshita S. Direct reprogramming into corneal epithelial cells using a transcriptional network comprising PAX6, OVOL2, and KLF4. Cornea; 2019.
17. Di Girolamo N. Stem cells of the human cornea. Br Med Bull. 2011;100(1):191–207.
18. Ma J, Wang Y, Wei P, Jhanji V. Biomechanics and structure of the cornea: implications and association with corneal disorders. Surv Ophthalmol. 2018;63(6):851–61.
19. Lüllmann-Rauch R, Taschenlehrbuch Histologie, vol 3. Auflage: Georg Thieme Verlag; 2009. p. 25, 26, 27.
20. Pricopie S, Istrate S, Voinea L, Leasu C, Paun V, Radu C. Pseudophakic bullous keratopathy. Rom J Ophthalmol. 2017;61(2):90–4.
21. Tan DTH, Dart JKG, Holland EJ, Kinoshita S. Corneal transplantation. The Lancet. 2012;379(9827):1749–61.
22. Grehn F. In: Medizin S, editor. Augenheilkunde, vol. 31. Auflage. Springer Science+Business Media; 2012, p. 111.
23. Komai Y, Ushiki T. The three-dimensional organization of collagen fibrils in the human cornea and sclera. Invest Ophthalmol Vis Sci. 1991;32(8):2244–58.
24. Costagliola C, Romano V, Forbice E, Angi M, Pascotto A, Boccia T, Semeraro F. Corneal oedema and its medical treatment. Clin Exp Optom. 2013;96(6):529–35.
25. https://www.upi.com/Science_News/2013/06/11/Scientists-discover-new-layer-of-human-cornea/3121370965203/?ur3=1

26. Augustin AJ. Augenheilkunde, vol. 3. In: Marion Philipp H, editor. Komplett überarbeitete und erweiterte Auflage. Berlin: Springer; 1997, 2001, 2007.
27. Matthaei M, Hribek A, Clahsen T, Bachmann B, Cursiefen C, Jun AS. Fuchs endothelial corneal dystrophy: clinical, genetic, pathophysiologic, and therapeutic aspects. Ann Rev Vis Sci. 2019;5(1):151–75.
28. Elhalis H, Azizi B, Jurkunas UV. Fuchs endothelial corneal dystrophy. Ocul Surf. 2010;8(4):173–84.
29. Lang GK, Gareis O, Lang GE, Lang SJ, Spraul CW, Wagner P. In: Lang GK, editor. Augenheilkunde. Georg Thieme Verlag KG; 2019. p. 2.
30. Fan T-J, Wu S-X, Jiang G-J. Apoptotic effects of norfloxacin on corneal endothelial cells. Naunyn-Schmiedeberg's Arch Pharmacol. 2019.
31. Wacker K, Reinhard T, Maier P. Pathogenese, Diagnose und Klinik der Fuchs-Endotheldystrophie. Ophthalmologe. 2019;116(3):221–7.
32. Fautsch MP, Wieben ED, Baratz KH, Bhattacharyya N, Sadan AN, Hafford-Tear NJ, Tuft SJ, Davidson AE. TCF4-mediated Fuchs endothelial corneal dystrophy: Insights into a common trinucleotide repeat-associated disease. Prog Retin Eye Res. 2021;81:100883–100883.
33. Augustin AJ. In: York SBHN, editor. Augenheilkunde; 2007. p. 955.
34. Feizi S. Corneal endothelial cell dysfunction: etiologies and management. Therap Adv Ophthalmol. 2018;10:2515841418815802–2515841418815802.
35. Joyce NC. Proliferative capacity of corneal endothelial cells. Exp Eye Res. 2012;95(1):16–23.
36. Rembold M, Loosli F, Adams RJ, Wittbrodt J. Individual cell migration serves as the driving force for optic vesicle evagination. Science. 2006;313(5790):1130–1134.
37. White D, Rabago-Smith M. Genotype–phenotype associations and human eye color. J Hum Genet. 2011;56:5–7.
38. Ein wanderndes Auge. Das Biotechnologie und Life Sciences Portal Baden-Württemberg; 2006.
39. Grainger RM. Embryonic lens induction: shedding light on vertebrate tissue determination. Transgen. 1992;8:349–355.
40. Schnorr B, Kressin M. Embryologie der Haustiere. 6. Auflage. Enke.
41. Zuber ME, Gestri G, Viczian AS, Barsacchi G, Harris WA. Specification of the vertebrate eye by a network of eye field transcription factors. Development. 2003;130:5155–5167.
42. Lane N. Leben – Verblüffende Erfindungen der Evolution. Kap. 7: Sehen. Primus Verlag; 2013.
43. Faszination Lebenswissenschaften. Wiley-VCH; 2002.
44. Lüllmann-Rauch R., Paulsen F.: Taschenbuch der Histologie. 4. Auflage. Thieme, Stuttgart.
45. Eguchi G, et al. Regenerative capacity in newts is not altered by repeated regeneration and ageing. Nat Commun. 2011;384.
46. Kumar P, Hammersmith KM, Eagle Jr. RC. In: Congenital corneal opacities: diagnosis and management. Mannis M, Holland E, editors. Cornea. 5 ed.: Elsevier; 2021. p.185–203.
47. Weiss JS, Møller HU, Lisch W, et al. The IC3D classification of the corneal dystrophies. Cornea. 2008;27:1–83.
48. Dana MR, Moyes AL, Gomes JA, et al. The indications for and outcome in pediatric keratoplasty: a multicenter study. Ophthalmology. 1995;102(8):1129–38.
49. Frueh BE, Brown SI. Transplantation of congenitally opaque corneas. Br J Ophthalmol. 1997;81(12):1064–9.
50. Stulting RD, Sumers KD, Cavanagh HD, Waring GO 3rd, Gammon JA. Penetrating keratoplasty in children. Ophthalmology. 1984;91(10):1222–30.
51. Zaidman GW. Pediatric corneal transplant surgery. In: CopelandAfshari RA, editor. Principles and practice of cornea. Jaypee Brothers Medical Publishers; 2013. p. 1072–8.
52. Nischal KK Keratoplasty P. In: Cornea. 5 ed. Mannis M, Holland E, editors. Elsevier; 2021. p. 1277.
53. Nischal KK. Genetics of congenital corneal opacification-impact on diagnosis and treatment. Cornea. 2015;34(Suppl 10):S24-34.

54. Nischal KK. A new approach to the classification of neonatal corneal opacities. Curr Opin Ophthalmol. 2012;23(5):344–54.
55. Fayed MA, Chen TC. Pediatric intraocular pressure measurements: Tonometers, central corneal thickness, and anesthesia. Surv Ophthalmol. 2019;64(6):810–25.
56. Majander AS, Lindahl PM, Vasara LK, Krootila K. Anterior segment optical coherence tomography in congenital corneal opacities. Ophthalmology. 2012;119(12):2450–7.
57. Siebelmann S, Bachmann B, Lappas A, Dietlein T, Steven P, Cursiefen C. Intraoperative optical coherence tomography for examination of newborns and infants under general anesthesia. Ophthalmologe. 2016;113(8):651–5.
58. Siebelmann S, Bachmann B, Matthaei M, et al. Microscope-integrated intraoperative optical coherence tomography in examination of pediatric patients under anesthesia. Ophthalmologe. 2018;115(9):785–92.
59. Siebelmann S, Hermann M, Dietlein T, Bachmann B, Steven P, Cursiefen C. Intraoperative optical coherence tomography in children with anterior segment anomalies. Ophthalmology. 2015;122(12):2582–4.
60. Siebelmann S, Matthaei M, Heindl LM, Bachmann BO, Cursiefen C. Intraoperative Optical Coherence Tomography (MI-OCT) for the treatment of corneal dystrophies. Klin Monbl Augenheilkd. 2018;235(6):714–20.
61. Northup JK, Matalon D, Hawkins JC, Matalon R, Velagaleti GVN. Pericentric inversion, inv(14)(p11.2q22.3), in a 9-month old with features of Goldenhar syndrome. Clin Dysmorphol. 2010;19(4):185–189.
62. Lisch W, Weiss JS. Clinical and genetic update of corneal dystrophies. Exp Eye Res. 2019;186:107715.
63. Kelberman D, Islam L, Jacques TS, Russell-Eggitt I, Bitner-Glindzicz M, Khaw PT, Nischal KK, Sowden JC. CYP1B1-related anterior segment developmental anomalies novel mutations for infantile glaucoma and von Hippel's ulcer revisited. Ophthalmology. 2011;118(9):1865–73.
64. Rajagopal R, Giridhar D, Biswas J. Overview of sclerocornea. Taiwan J Ophthalmol. 2023;13(4):461–466. https://doi.org/10.4103/tjo.TJO-D-23-00070. PMID: 38249514; PMCID: PMC10798383. Tahvanainen E, Forsius H, Kolehmainen J, Damsten M, Fellman J, de la Chapelle A. The genetics of cornea plana congenita. J Med Genet. 1996;33(2):116–9. https://doi.org/10.1136/jmg.33.2.116.
65. Zhang BN, Chan TCY, Tam POS, Liu Y, Pang CP, Jhanji V, Chen LJ, Chu WK. A Cohesin Subunit Variant Identified from a Peripheral Sclerocornea Pedigree. Dis Markers. 2019;12(2019):8781524.
66. Zhang BN, Wong TCB, Yip YWY, Liu Z, Wang C, Wong JSC, He JN, Chan TCY, Jhanji V, Pang CP, Zhao H, Chu WK. A sclerocornea-associated RAD21 variant induces corneal stroma disorganization. Exp Eye Res. 2019;185:107687. https://doi.org/10.1016/j.exer.2019.06.001.
67. Harissi-Dagher M, Colby K. Anterior segment dysgenesis: Peters anomaly and sclerocornea. Int Ophthalmol Clin. 2008;48(2):35–42. https://doi.org/10.1097/IIO.0b013e318169526c.
68. Bhandari R, Ferri S, Whittaker B, Liu M, Lazzaro DR. Peters anomaly: review of the literature. Cornea. 2011;30(8):939–44. https://doi.org/10.1097/ICO.0b013e31820156a9.
69. Zhang Z, Syed NA, Alward WLM. Peters anomaly. Ophthalmol Glaucoma. 2019;2(4):266. https://doi.org/10.1016/j.ogla.2019.03.005. PMID: 32672549.
70. Khasnavis A, Fernandes M. Peters anomaly: an overview. Taiwan J Ophthalmol. 2023;13(4):434–42. https://doi.org/10.4103/tjo.TJO-D-23-00065.
71. Faber H, Puk O, Holz A, Biskup S, Voykov B. Identification of a new genetic mutation associated with peters anomaly. Cornea. 2021;40(3):373–6. https://doi.org/10.1097/ICO.0000000000002611.
72. Weh E, Reis LM, Happ HC, Levin AV, Wheeler PG, David KL, Carney E, Angle B, Hauser N, Semina EV. Whole exome sequence analysis of Peters anomaly. Hum Genet. 2014;133(12):1497–511. https://doi.org/10.1007/s00439-014-1481-x.

73. Lesnik Oberstein SAJ, Ruivenkamp CAL, Hennekam RC. Peters plus syndrome. [updated 2017 Aug 24]. In: Adam MP, Feldman J, Mirzaa GM, Pagon RA, Wallace SE, Bean LJH, Gripp KW, Amemiya A, editors. GeneReviews® [Internet]. Seattle (WA): University of Washington, Seattle; 2007. p. 1993–2024.
74. Zhang A, Venkat A, Taujale R, Mull JL, Ito A, Kannan N, Haltiwanger RS. Peters plus syndrome mutations affect the function and stability of human β1,3-glucosyltransferase. J Biol Chem. 2021;297(1):100843. https://doi.org/10.1016/j.jbc.2021.100843. Epub 2021 May 28.
75. Ormestad M, Blixt A, Churchill A, Martinsson T, Enerbäck S, Carlsson P. Foxe3 haploinsufficiency in mice: a model for Peters' anomaly. Invest Ophthalmol Vis Sci. 2002;43(5):1350–7.
76. Nischal KK. Genetics of congenital corneal opacification-impact on diagnosis and treatment. Cornea. 2015;34(Suppl 10):S24-34. https://doi.org/10.1097/ICO.0000000000000552.
77. Hingorani M, Hanson I, van Heyningen V. Aniridia. Eur J Hum Genet. 2012;20(10):1011–7. https://doi.org/10.1038/ejhg.2012.100. Epub 2012 Jun 13.
78. Safvati A, Cole N, Hume E, Willcox M. Mediators of neovascularization and the hypoxic cornea. Curr Eye Res. 2009;34(6):501–14. https://doi.org/10.1080/02713680902919557.
79. Calvão-Pires P, Santos-Silva R, Falcão-Reis F, Rocha-Sousa A. Congenital Aniridia: clinic, genetics, therapeutics, and prognosis. Int Sch Res Notices. 2014;29(2014):305350. https://doi.org/10.1155/2014/305350.
80. https://eyewiki.org/Aniridia#Molecular_and_Genetic_Basis_of_Aniridia
81. Moosajee M, Hingorani M, Moore AT. PAX6-Related Aniridia. 2003 May 20 [updated 2018 Oct 18]. In: Adam MP, Feldman J, Mirzaa GM, Pagon RA, Wallace SE, Bean LJH, Gripp KW, Amemiya A, editors. GeneReviews® [Internet]. Seattle (WA): University of Washington, Seattle; p. 1993–2024. PMID: 20301534.
82. Käsmann-Kellner B, Seitz B. Kongenitale Aniridie oder PAX6-Syndrom? [Congenital aniridia or PAX6 syndrome]. Ophthalmologe. 2014;111(12):1144. German. https://doi.org/10.1007/s00347-014-3058-4.
83. Pedersen HR, Baraas RC, Landsend ECS, Utheim ØA, Utheim TP, Gilson SJ, Neitz M. PAX6 genotypic and retinal phenotypic characterization in congenital aniridia. Invest Ophthalmol Vis Sci. 2020;61(5):14. https://doi.org/10.1167/iovs.61.5.14.
84. Landsend ECS, Lagali N, Utheim TP. Congenital aniridia—a comprehensive review of clinical features and therapeutic approaches. Surv Ophthalmol. 2021;66(6):1031–50. https://doi.org/10.1016/j.survophthal.2021.02.011. Epub 2021 Mar 4.
85. Lee HK, Kim MK, Oh JY. Corneal abnormalities in congenital aniridia: congenital central corneal opacity versus aniridia-associated keratopathy. Am J Ophthalmol. 2018;185:75–80. https://doi.org/10.1016/j.ajo.2017.10.017. Epub 2017 Oct 31.
86. Bremond-Gignac D. Aniridie congénitale de l'enfant [Congenital aniridia in children]. Rev Prat. 2019;69(1):67–70.
87. Lingam G, Sen AC, Lingam V, Bhende M, Padhi TR, Xinyi S. Ocular coloboma-a comprehensive review for the clinician. Eye (Lond). 2021;35(8):2086–2109. https://doi.org/10.1038/s41433-021-01501-5. Epub 2021 Mar 21.
88. Caspersen I, Warburg M. Hallermann-Streiff syndrome. Acta Ophthalmol (Copenh). 1968;46(3):385–90. https://doi.org/10.1111/j.1755-3768.1968.tb02820.x.
89. Ide CH, Webb RW. Hallermann-Streiff syndrome. Am J Ophthalmol. 1969;67(1):151–3. https://doi.org/10.1016/0002-9394(69)90023-3.
90. Ernst J, Medsinge A, Scanga HL, Hiasat J, Moore W, Ali A, Levin AV, Stahl ED, Nischal KK. Congenital primary aphakia. J AAPOS. 2022;26(1):4.e1-4.e5. https://doi.org/10.1016/j.jaapos.2021.09.008. Epub 2022 Jan 17.
91. Valleix S, Niel F, Nedelec B, Algros MP, Schwartz C, Delbosc B, Delpech M, Kantelip B. Homozygous nonsense mutation in the FOXE3 gene as a cause of congenital primary aphakia in humans. Am J Hum Genet. 2006;79(2):358–64. https://doi.org/10.1086/505654. Epub 2006 Jun 8 PMID: 16826526.
92. Deml B, Reis LM, Lemyre E, Clark RD, Kariminejad A, Semina EV. Novel mutations in PAX6, OTX2 and NDP in anophthalmia, microphthalmia and coloboma. Eur J Hum Genet. 2016;24(4):535–41. https://doi.org/10.1038/ejhg.2015.155. Epub 2015 Jul 1.

93. Herde J. Iridocorneo-endotheliales Syndrom (ICE-S): Klassifikation, Klinik und Diagnostik [Iridocorneal endothelial syndrome (ICE-S): classification, clinical picture, diagnosis]. Klin Monbl Augenheilkd. 2005;222(10):797–801. https://doi.org/10.1055/s-2005-858119.
94. Denis P. Le glaucome du syndrome irido-cornéo-endothélial [Iridocorneal endothelial syndrome and glaucoma]. J Fr Ophtalmol. 2007;30(2):189–95. https://doi.org/10.1016/s0181-5512(07)89575-1.
95. Abu-Amero KK, Edward DP. Primary Congenital Glaucoma. 2004 Sep 30 [updated 2017 Aug 17]. In: Adam MP, Feldman J, Mirzaa GM, Pagon RA, Wallace SE, Bean LJH, Gripp KW, Amemiya A, editors. GeneReviews® [Internet]. Seattle (WA): University of Washington, Seattle; p. 1993–2024.
96. Lewis CJ, Hedberg-Buenz A, DeLuca AP, Stone EM, Alward WLM, Fingert JH. Primary congenital and developmental glaucomas. Hum Mol Genet. 2017;26(R1):R28–36. https://doi.org/10.1093/hmg/ddx205.
97. Lim SH, Tran-Viet KN, Yanovitch TL, Freedman SF, Klemm T, Call W, Powell C, Ravichandran A, Metlapally R, Nading EB, Rozen S, Young TL. CYP1B1, MYOC, and LTBP2 mutations in primary congenital glaucoma patients in the United States. Am J Ophthalmol. 2013;155(3):508-517.e5. https://doi.org/10.1016/j.ajo.2012.09.012. Epub 2012 Dec 4.
98. https://eyewiki.org/Axenfeld_Rieger_Syndrome
99. Zamora EA, Salini B. Axenfeld-Rieger Syndrome. 2022 Oct 24. In: StatPearls [Internet]. Treasure Island (FL): StatPearls Publishing; 2024.
100. Michels K, Bohnsack BL. Ophthalmological manifestations of axenfeld-rieger syndrome: current perspectives. Clin Ophthalmol. 2023;10(17):819–28. https://doi.org/10.2147/OPTH.S379853.
101. Alward WL. Axenfeld-Rieger syndrome in the age of molecular genetics. Am J Ophthalmol. 2000;130(1):107–15. https://doi.org/10.1016/s0002-9394(00)00525-0.
102. Chang TC, Summers CG, Schimmenti LA, Grajewski AL. Axenfeld-Rieger syndrome: new perspectives. Br J Ophthalmol. 2012;96(3):318–22. https://doi.org/10.1136/bjophthalmol-2011-300801. Epub 2011 Dec 23.
103. Strungaru MH, Dinu I, Walter MA. Genotype-phenotype correlations in Axenfeld-Rieger malformation and glaucoma patients with FOXC1 and PITX2 mutations. Invest Ophthalmol Vis Sci. 2007;48(1):228–37. https://doi.org/10.1167/iovs.06-0472.
104. Weisschuh N, Dressler P, Schuettauf F, Wolf C, Wissinger B, Gramer E. Novel mutations of FOXC1 and PITX2 in patients with Axenfeld-Rieger malformations. Invest Ophthalmol Vis Sci. 2006;47(9):3846–52. https://doi.org/10.1167/iovs.06-0343.Erratum.In:InvestOphthalmolVisSci.2006;47(12):5162.
105. Shields MB. Axenfeld-Rieger syndrome: a theory of mechanism and distinctions from the Iridocorneal Endothelial Syndrome. Trans Am Ophthalmol Soc. 1983;81:736–84.
106. Shields MB, Buckley E, Klintworth GK, Thresher R: Axenfeld-Rieger syndrome. A spectrum of developmental disorders. Surv Ophthalmol. 1985;29:387–409
107. McPherson SD Jr, Berry DP. Goniotomy versus external trabeculectomy for developmental glaucoma. Am J Ophthalmol. 1983;95:427–31.
108. Ho DK, Levin AV, Anninger WV, Piccoli DA, Eagle RC Jr. Anterior chamber pathology in Alagille syndrome. Ocul Oncol Pathol. 2016;2(4):270–5. https://doi.org/10.1159/000446804.
109. Ton CC, Hirvonen H, Miwa H, et al. Positional cloning and characterization of a paired box- and homeobox-containing gene from the aniridia region. Cell. 1991;67:1059–74.
110. Dahl E, Koseki H, Balling R. Pax genes and organogenesis. BioEssays. 1997;19(9):755–65.
111. Prosser J, van Heyningen V. PAX6 mutations reviewed. Hum Mutat. 1998;11:93–108.
112. Sérgio Rodrigues Gonçalves, Correlações Genótipo-Fenótipo numa população de doentes com aniridia, Trabalho final do 6º ano com vista à atribuição do grau de mestre no âmbito do ciclo de estudos de mestrado integrado em medicina, Faculdade de Medicina da Universidade de Coimbra, Março 2009. https://eyewiki.aao.org/Aniridia#cite_ref-goncalves15_13-0
113. Glaser T, Jepeal L, Edwards JG, et al. PAX6 gene dosage effect in a family with congenital cataracts, aniridia, anophthalmia and central nervous system defects. Nat Genet. 1994;7:463–71.

114. Bachmann BO, Matthaei M, Schlereth S, Cursiefen C. Corneal hydrops—aetiology and advanced therapeutic strategies. Klin Monbl Augenheilkd. 2023;240(6):795–802. English, German. https://doi.org/10.1055/a-2048-6703. Epub 2023 May 5.
115. Mukhtar S, Ambati BK. Pediatric keratoconus: a review of the literature. Int Ophthalmol. 2018;38(5):2257–66. https://doi.org/10.1007/s10792-017-0699-8. Epub 2017 Aug 29.
116. Unni P, Lee HJ. Systemic associations with keratoconus. Life (Basel). 2023Jun 10;13(6):1363. https://doi.org/10.3390/life13061363. PMID: 37374145.
117. Maumenee IH. The eye in the Marfan syndrome. Trans Am Ophthalmol Soc. 1981;79:684–733 PMID: 7043871.
118. Robertson I. Keratoconus and the Ehlers-Danlos syndrome: a new aspect of keratoconus. Med J Aust. 1975;1(18):571–3. https://doi.org/10.5694/j.1326-5377.1975.tb111590.x.
119. Moshirfar M, Skanchy DF, Gomez AT, Ronquillo YC, Buckner B, Hoopes PC. Keratoconus in a patient with Alport syndrome: a case report. World J Clin Cases. 2019;7(19):3012–7. https://doi.org/10.12998/wjcc.v7.i19.3012.
120. Ascaso FJ, Del Buey MA, Huerva V, Latre B, Palomar A. Noonan's syndrome with keratoconus and optic disc coloboma. Eur J Ophthalmol. 1993;3(2):101–3. https://doi.org/10.1177/112067219300300210.
121. Rau S, Duncker GI. Keratokonus bei Mulvihill-Smith-Syndrom [Keratoconus in Mulvihill-Smith syndrome]. Klin Monbl Augenheilkd. 1994;205(1):44–6. https://doi.org/10.1055/s-2008-1045490
122. Wallang BS, Das S. Keratoglobus. Eye (Lond). 2013;27(9):1004–12. https://doi.org/10.1038/eye.2013.130. Epub 2013 Jun 28.
123. Marom R, Rabenhorst BM, Morello R. Osteogenesis imperfecta: an update on clinical features and therapies. Eur J Endocrinol. 2020;183(4):R95–106. https://doi.org/10.1530/EJE-20-0299.
124. Ong APC, Zhang J, Vincent AL, McGhee CNJ. Megalocornea, anterior megalophthalmos, keratoglobus and associated anterior segment disorders: a review. Clin Exp Ophthalmol. 2021;49(5):477–97. https://doi.org/10.1111/ceo.13958. Epub 2021 Jun 27.
125. Dhooge T, Van Damme T, Syx D, Mosquera LM, Nampoothiri S, Radhakrishnan A, Simsek-Kiper PO, Utine GE, Bonduelle M, Migeotte I, Essawi O, Ceylaner S, Al Kindy A, Tinkle B, Symoens S, Malfait F. More than meets the eye: Expanding and reviewing the clinical and mutational spectrum of brittle cornea syndrome. Hum Mutat. 2021;42(6):711–30. https://doi.org/10.1002/humu.24199.
126. Porter LF, Gallego-Pinazo R, Keeling CL, Kamieniorz M, Zoppi N, Colombi M, Giunta C, Bonshek R, Manson FD, Black GC. Bruch's membrane abnormalities in PRDM5-related brittle cornea syndrome. Orphanet J Rare Dis. 2015;11(10):145. https://doi.org/10.1186/s13023-015-0360-4.
127. Stanton CM, Findlay AS, Drake C, Mustafa MZ, Gautier P, McKie L, Jackson IJ, Vitart V. A mouse model of brittle cornea syndrome caused by mutation in Zfp469. Dis Model Mech. 2021;14(9):dmm049175. https://doi.org/10.1242/dmm.049175. Epub 2021 Sep 22.
128. Abu A, Frydman M, Marek D, Pras E, Nir U, Reznik-Wolf H, Pras E. Deleterious mutations in the Zinc-Finger 469 gene cause brittle cornea syndrome. Am J Hum Genet. 2008;82(5):1217–22. https://doi.org/10.1016/j.ajhg.2008.04.001.
129. Verma AS, Fitzpatrick DR. Anophthalmia and microphthalmia. Orphanet J Rare Dis. 2007;26(2):47. https://doi.org/10.1186/1750-1172-2-47.
130. Sanderson B, Leach C, Zein M, Islam O, MacLean G, Strube YNJ, Guerin A. Bilateral severe microphthalmia in a neonate with trisomy 8 mosaicism: A new finding. Am J Med Genet A. 2021;185(2):534–8. https://doi.org/10.1002/ajmg.a.61955.
131. Jamjoom H, Osman M, AlMoallem B, Osman EA. Oculocerebrocutaneous syndrome (Delleman Oorthuys syndrome) associated with congenital glaucoma: a case report. Eur J Ophthalmol. 2020;4:1120672120964696. https://doi.org/10.1177/1120672120964696.
132. Dickmann A, Parrilla R, Salerni A, Savino G, Vasta I, Zollino M, Petroni S, Zampino G. Ocular manifestations in Wolf-Hirschhorn syndrome. J AAPOS. 2009;13(3):264–7. https://doi.org/10.1016/j.jaapos.2009.02.011.

133. Sohajda Z, Holló D, Berta A, Módis L. Microcornea associated with myopia. In: Graefe's archive for clinical and experimental ophthalmology = Albrecht von Graefes Archiv für klinische und experimentelle Ophthalmologie. 2006;244(9):1211–1213. https://doi.org/10.1007/s00417-006-0264-z
134. Kelly SP, Fielder AR. Microcornea associated with retinopathy of prematurity. Br J Ophthalmol. 1987;**71**(3):201–203.
135. Kloeckener-Gruissem B, Vandekerckhove K, Nürnberg G, Neidhardt J, Zeitz C, Nürnberg P, Schipper I, Berger W. Mutation of solute carrier SLC16A12 associates with a syndrome combining juvenile cataract with microcornea and renal glucosuria. Am J Hum Genet. 2008;82(3):772–9. https://doi.org/10.1016/j.ajhg.2007.12.013.
136. Khan K, Al-Maskari A, McKibbin M, Carr IM, Booth A, Mohamed M, Siddiqui S, Poulter JA, Parry DA, Logan CV, Hashmi A, Sahi T, Jafri H, Raashid Y, Johnson CA, Markham AF, Toomes C, Rice A, Sheridan E, Inglehearn CF, Ali M. Genetic heterogeneity for recessively inherited congenital cataract microcornea with corneal opacity. Invest Ophthalmol Vis Sci. 2011;52(7):4294–9. https://doi.org/10.1167/iovs.10-6776.
137. Cai XB, Wu KC, Zhang X, Lv JN, Jin GH, Xiang L, Chen J, Huang XF, Pan D, Lu B, Lu F, Qu J, Jin ZB. Whole-exome sequencing identified ARL2 as a novel candidate gene for MRCS (microcornea, rod-cone dystrophy, cataract, and posterior staphyloma) syndrome. Clin Genet. 2019;96(1):61–71. https://doi.org/10.1111/cge.13541.
138. Weisschuh N, Wolf C, Wissinger B, et al. A clinical and molecular genetic study of German patients with primary congenital glaucoma. Am J Ophthalmol. 2009;147:744–53.
139. Kaur K, Gurnani B. Primary congenital glaucoma. In: StatPearls [Internet]. Treasure Island (FL): StatPearls Publishing; 2021.
140. Faiq M, Mohanty K, Dada R, Dada T. Molecular diagnostics and genetic counseling in primary congenital glaucoma. J Curr Glaucoma Pract. 2013;7(1):25–35. https://doi.org/10.5005/jp-journals-10008-1133.
141. Ava S, Demirtaş AA, Karahan M, Erdem S, Oral D, Keklikçi U. Genetic analysis of patients with primary congenital glaucoma. Int Ophthalmol. 2021;41(7):2565–74. https://doi.org/10.1007/s10792-021-01815-z.
142. AlQahtani E, Godoy F, Lyons C. Enlarging corneoscleral cyst in a 2-year-old girl. J AAPOS. 2015;19(4):389–91.
143. Park MS, Yoon CH, Kim YW, Lee HJ, Yu YS, Oh JY. Progressive intrascleral epithelial cyst with intracorneal extension. J Pediatr Ophthalmol Strabismus. 2019;25(56):e20–3.
144. Mahmood MA, Awad A. Congenital sclerocorneal epithelial cyst. Am J Ophthalmol. 1998;126(5):740–1.
145. Kalamkar C, Mukherjee A. Primary corneoscleral cyst in a pediatric patient. Case Rep Ophthalmol. 2017;8(2):425–8.
146. Lee TL, Lee HY, Tan JCH. Terrien marginal degeneration complicated by a corneoscleral cyst. Cornea. 2018;37(5):658–66.
147. Sornalingam K, Javed A, Aslam T, Sergouniotis P, Jones S, Ghosh A, Ashworth J. Variability in the ocular phenotype in mucopolysaccharidosis. Br J Ophthalmol. 2019;103(4):504–10. https://doi.org/10.1136/bjophthalmol-2017-311749.
148. Lisch W, Pitz S, Geerling G. Therapy for systemic metabolic disorders based on the detection of basic corneal landmarks in childhood. Klin Monbl Augenheilkd. 2013;230(6):575–81. https://doi.org/10.1055/s-0032-1328524.
149. Reich M, Reinhard T, Lagrèze WA. Corneal changes in infancy and childhood as an expression of systemic metabolic diseases. Klin Monbl Augenheilkd. 2020;237(6):761–771. https://doi.org/10.1055/a-1114-1887.
150. Naik MP, Sethi HS, Dabas S. Ocular cystinosis: rarity redefined. Indian J Ophthalmol. 2019;67(7):1158–9. https://doi.org/10.4103/ijo.IJO_1467_18.
151. Rohrbach JM, Szurman P, Bartz-Schmidt KU. Eye trauma in childhood and youth. Klin Monbl Augenheilkd. 2004;221(8):636–45. https://doi.org/10.1055/s-2004-812903. PMID: 15343447.

152. Whitcher JP, Srinivasan M, Upadhyay MP. Corneal blindness: a global perspective. Bull World Health Organ. 2001;79(3):214–21.
153. Di Zazzo A, Antonini M, Fernandes M, Varacalli G, Sgrulletta R, Coassin M. A global perspective of pediatric non-viral keratitis: literature review. Int Ophthalmol. 2020;40(10):2771–88. https://doi.org/10.1007/s10792-020-01451-z.
154. Kunimoto DY, Sharma S, Reddy MK, Gopinathan U, Jyothi J, Miller D, Rao GN. Microbial keratitis in children. Ophthalmology. 1998;105(2):252–7. https://doi.org/10.1016/s0161-6420(98)92899-8. PMID: 9479283.
155. Gallardo MJ, Johnson DA, Gaviria J, et al. Isolated herpes simplex keratoconjunctivitis in a neonate born by cesarean delivery. J AAPOS. 2005;9:285–7.
156. Ullman S, Roussel TJ, Culbertson WW, Forster RK, Alfonso E, Mendelsohn AD, Heidemann DG, Holland SP. Neisseria gonorrhoeae keratoconjunctivitis. Ophthalmology. 1987;94(5):525–31. https://doi.org/10.1016/s0161-6420(87)33415-3.
157. Coppens I, Abu el-Asrar AM, Maudgal PC, Missotten L. Incidence and clinical presentation of chlamydial keratoconjunctivitis: a preliminary study. Int Ophthalmol. 1988;12(4):201–5. https://doi.org/10.1007/BF00133933.
158. Bachmann B, Avgitidou G, Siebelmann S, Cursiefen C. Pediatric corneal surgery and corneal transplantation. Ophthalmologe. 2015;112(2):110–7.
159. Kim YW, Choi HJ, Kim MK, et al. Clinical outcome of penetrating keratoplasty in patients 5 years or younger: peters anomaly versus sclerocornea. Cornea. 2013;32:1432–6.
160. Di Zazzo A, Bonini S, Crugliano S, Fortunato M. The challenging management of pediatric corneal transplantation: an overview of surgical and clinical experiences. Jpn J Ophthalmol. 2017;61(3):207–17. https://doi.org/10.1007/s10384-017-0510-4.
161. Vanathi M, Panda A, Vengayil S, Chaudhuri Z, Dada T. Pediatric keratoplasty. Surv Ophthalmol. 2009;54(2):245–71. https://doi.org/10.1016/j.survophthal.2008.12.011.
162. Schlereth SL, Gietzelt C, Zwingelberg Cursiefen C, et al. Surgical treatment options for congenital/infantile corneal opacities and anterior segment dysgenesis. Ophthalmologe. 2022;119(5):453–461. https://doi.org/10.1007/s00347-022-01612-8 Epub 2022 Apr 4.
163. Kollias AN, Spitzlberger GM, Thurau S, Grüterich M, Lackerbauer CA. Phototherapeutic keratectomy in children. J Refract Surg. 2007;23(7):703–8.
164. Autrata R, Rehurek J, Vodicková K. Phototherapeutic keratectomy in children: 5-year results. J Cataract Refract Surg. 2004;30(9):1909–16. https://doi.org/10.1016/j.jcrs.2004.02.047.
165. Padmanabhan P, Rachapalle Reddi S, Rajagopal R, et al. Corneal collagen cross-linking for Keratoconus in pediatric patients-long-term results. Cornea. 2017;36:138–43.
166. Mukhtar S, Ambati BK. Pediatric keratoconus: a review of the literature. Int Ophthalmol. 2018;38:2257–66.
167. Torres Netto EA, Al-Otaibi WM, Hafezi NL, et al. Prevalence of keratoconus in paediatric patients in Riyadh, Saudi Arabia. Br J Ophthalmol. 2018;102:1436–41.
168. Chatzis N, Hafezi F. Progression of keratoconus and efficacy of pediatric [corrected] corneal collagen cross-linking in children and adolescents. J Refract Surg. 2012;28:753–8.
169. Wollensak G, Spoerl E, Seiler T. Riboflavin/ultraviolet-a-induced collagen crosslinking for the treatment of keratoconus. Am J Ophthalmol. 2003;135:620–7.
170. Li J, Ji P, Lin X. Efficacy of corneal collagen cross-linking for treatment of keratoconus: a meta-analysis of randomized controlled trials. PLoS ONE. 2015;10:e0127079.
171. Mazzotta C, Traversi C, Baiocchi S, et al. Corneal collagen cross-linking with riboflavin and ultraviolet a light for pediatric keratoconus: ten-year results. Cornea. 2018;37:560–6.
172. Junemann A, Gusek GC, Naumann GO. Optical sector iridectomy: an alternative to perforating keratoplasty in Peters' anomaly. Klin Monbl Augenheilkd. 1996;209:117–24.
173. Ramappa M, Chaurasia S, Mohamed A, Ramya Achanta DS, Mandal AK, Edward DP, Gokhale N, Swarup R, Nischal KK. Selective endothelialectomy in peters anomaly: a novel surgical technique and its clinical outcomes in children. Cornea. 2022;41(12):1477–86.
174. Alldredge OC, Krachmer JH. Clinical types of corneal transplantat rejection. Their manifestations, frequency, preoperative correlates and treatment. Arch Opthalmol. 1981;99:599.

175. Trief D, Marquezan MC, Rapuano CJ, Prescott CR. Pediatric corneal transplants. Curr Opin Ophthalmol. 2017;28(5):477–84.
176. Karadag R, Chan TC, Azari AA, Nagra PK, Hammersmith KM, Rapuano CJ. Survival of primary penetrating keratoplasty in children. Am J Ophthalmol. 2016;171:95–100.
177. Hos D, Matthaei M, Bachmann BO, Cursiefen C, et al. Immune reactions after modern lamellar (DALK, DSAEK, DMEK) versus conventional penetrating corneal transplantation. Prog Retin Eye Res. 2019;73:100768.
178. Williams KA, Lowe MT, Keane MC et al. The Australian corneal graft registry 2012 report. SnapPrinting Adelaide. 2012;235–242
179. Xavier Dos Santos Araújo ME, Santos NC, Souza LB, Sato EH, de Freitas D. Primary Pediatric keratoplasty: etiology, graft survival, and visual outcome. Am J Ophthalmol. 2020;212:162–168.
180. Seitz B, Naumann G, Seitz B, et al. Keratoplasty in children. Klin Monbl Augenheilkd. 2013;230(6):587–94.
181. Harding SA, Nischal KK, Upponi-Patil A, Fowler DJ. Indications and outcomes of deep anterior lamellar keratoplasty in children. Ophthalmology. 2010;117(11):2191–5. https://doi.org/10.1016/j.ophtha.2010.03.025. Epub 2010 Jul 21 PMID: 20663562.
182. Anwar HM, El-Danasoury A. Endothelial keratoplasty in children. Curr Opin Ophthalmol. 2014;25(4):340–6.
183. Gonnermann J, Klamann MK, Maier AK, et al. Descemet membrane endothelial keratoplasty in a child with corneal endothelial dysfunction in kearns-sayre syndrom. Cornea. 33:1232–1234.
184. Yang F, Hong J, Xiao G, Feng Y, Peng R, Wang M, Qu H. Descemet Stripping Endothelial Keratoplasty in pediatric patients with congenital hereditary endothelial dystrophy. Am J Ophthalmol. 2020;209:132–40.
185. Price FW Jr, Hanna SI. Bilateral penetrating autokeratoplasty. J Refract Surg. 1995;11:494–6.
186. Bourne WM, Brubaker RF. A method for ipsilateral rotational autokeratoplasty. Ophthalmology. 1978;85:1312–6.
187. Arnalich-Montiel F, Dart JK. Ipsilateral rotational autokeratoplasty: a review. Eye (Lond). 2009;23:1931–8.
188. Bertelmann E, Hartmann C, Scherer M, et al. Outcome of rotational keratoplasty: comparison of endothelial cell loss in autografts vs allografts. Arch Ophthalmol. 2004;122:1437–40.
189. Jonas JB, Rank RM, Budde WM. Autologous ipsilateral rotating penetrating keratoplasty. Am J Ophthalmol. 2001;131:427–30.
190. Aquavella JV, Gearinger MD, Akpek EK, McCormick GJ. Pediatric keratoprosthesis. Ophthalmology. 2007;114(5):989–94.
191. Matthaei M, Bachmann B, Cursiefen C, et al. Boston type I keratoprosthesis implantation technique: video article. Ophthalmologe. 2019;116(1):67–72. https://doi.org/10.1007/s00347-018-0806-x.
192. Schaub F, Cursiefen C, et al. Boston keratoprosthesis: 73 eyes from Germany: an overview of experiences from two centers. Ophthalmologe. 2018;115(9):744–753. https://doi.org/10.1007/s00347-017-0581-0.

Chapter 4
Congenital Cataract

Ken K. Nischal and Sarah Zwingelberg

Abstract Congenital cataract is a hereditary opacification of the lens that has been present since birth. Congenital cataracts often occur sporadically or are inherited in an autosomal recessive, dominant or X-linked manner. Furthermore, syndrome-related congenital cataracts are common. They are often combined with other eye malformations, for example with microphthalmos and coloboma of the uvea in trisomy 13 or 15. Alport syndrome and Hallermann-Streiff syndrome also manifest with early developing cataracts. In Down syndrome, a cataract usually does not develop until the age of 10. Another reason is Fabry disease. A persistent hyperplastic primary vitreous (PHPV), i.e. persistence of the primary vitreous, can also lead to a cataract. Lens opacification in congenital cataracts can vary in severity. Peripheral opacities are common and hardly noticeable. A cataracta zonularis or cataracta coronaria and coerulea may also be present. However, amblyopia can develop, especially if it is unilateral. There is a risk of secondary glaucoma after surgery at an early age (< 9 months). Surgery for congenital cataracts requires modified vitrectomy techniques and is performed at specialized centers.

Keywords Congenital cataract · Oil-droplet cataracts · Lamellar cataract · Blue-dot cataract · Wedge cataract · Posterior polar cataract · Anterior polar cataract · Cataract surgery

4.1 Introduction

A meta-analysis calculated the prevalence of congenital cataract, based on 8,302,708 children from 17 population studies from different continents between 1959 and 2010. The overall pooled prevalence was 4.24 cases per 10,000 children [1].

Pediatric cataract is a significant cause of preventable childhood blindness, impacting around 200,000 children globally, with a prevalence of three to six per 10,000 live births. Early diagnosis and treatment are crucial to prevent irreversible stimulus-deprivation amblyopia. Congenital of infantile cataracts maybe isolated or associated with systemic conditions. Evaluating the whole child is extremely

I. Broekaert et al., *Infantile Anterior Segment Disorders*,
https://doi.org/10.1007/978-3-031-68558-3_4

important and family members to ensure that there is no underlying molecular cause that maybe overlooked. Recent advances in surgical techniques, intraocular lens (IOL) designs, and early postoperative use of contact lenses have improved outcomes after pediatric cataract surgery. However, issues specific to pediatric eyes, such as increased postoperative inflammation, implant-power calculation, and amblyopia management, remain challenges in achieving good visual outcomes. Management of pediatric cataract should be customized based on various factors, including the age of onset, laterality, and associated ocular and systemic comorbidities. Visual rehabilitation is of paramount importance, and this includes treating any amblyopia that is likely to exist. Without these last two the best surgery in the world will be a failure with respect to visual outcome.

4.2 Embryology

The development of the human lens is a fascinating and complex process that begins early in embryonic life. This process is intricately linked with the overall development of the eye and is influenced by a series of cellular and molecular events.

Early Stages of Eye Development

The journey of lens development starts with the formation of the optic vesicles, which are outgrowths from the forebrain, a part of the early developing brain. Around the third week of gestation, as the neural tube (which eventually forms the central nervous system) closes, these optic vesicles start to form on either side of the forebrain [2]. The optic vesicles play a crucial role in the early stages of eye development, including the formation of the lens.

Formation of the Lens Placode

As the optic vesicles extend outward, they come into contact with the surface ectoderm, the outermost layer of the embryo. This contact induces changes in the ectoderm, leading to the thickening of a specific region known as the lens placode at 27 days [2, 3]. This induction process is a prime example of how tissues interact during development to influence each other's fate.

Development of the Lens Vesicle

Following the formation of the lens placode, it begins to invaginate, or fold inward, at 6 weeks towards the optic vesicle. This invagination process results in the formation of the lens pit. As the invagination deepens, the lens pit eventually detaches from the surface ectoderm, forming a structure known as the lens vesicle [3, 4]. This detachment marks a critical step in the lens's development, as the lens vesicle will give rise to the mature lens.

Differentiation into the Mature Lens

After the formation of the lens vesicle, the cells within start to differentiate into the mature structures of the lens.

At week 7 anterior cells migrate toward equator and form secondary lens fibers that surround embryonal nucleus and form Y sutures. The cells at the back (posterior) of the lens vesicle elongate to form the primary lens fibers, which eventually fill the interior of the vesicle, forming the embryonic nucleus of the lens. Meanwhile, the anterior (front) part of the lens vesicle develops into the lens epithelium, a layer of cells that will continue to produce new lens fibers throughout life, contributing to the growth of the lens [4, 5].

Nutritional Support and Further Development

Initially, the developing lens obtains nutrition via derivatives of the hyaloid artery. However, after the regression of the hyaloid artery, the lens's nourishment is supplied by the aqueous humor [6]. This transition is part of the broader changes occurring in the eye, preparing the lens and other ocular structures for their roles in vision.

Genetic and Molecular Regulation

The development of the lens, like other aspects of eye formation, is tightly regulated by a network of genetic and molecular signals. The Pax6 gene plays a pivotal role in initiating eye development, including the formation of the lens [2]. Other molecular pathways, involving signaling molecules such as Sonic hedgehog, Wnt, and fibroblast growth factors (FGFs), also contribute to the regulation of lens development [2].

Conclusion

The embryology of the human lens is a testament to the complexity of developmental biology [7]. From the initial contact between the optic vesicles and the surface ectoderm to the formation of the lens placode and vesicle, and finally to the differentiation into the mature lens, each step is precisely coordinated.

Understanding these processes not only sheds light on normal eye development but also helps in diagnosing and treating congenital eye disorders.

4.3 Clinical History and Examination of Child

Evaluation of a child with cataract has two aims: the first is to assess how visually significant the lens opacity and the second is to assess why the lens opacity is there.

In order to evaluate a child with a cataract a detailed history including family history; a prenatal history including maternal drug use and febrile illnesses with rash; and birth history, especially birth weight, since low birth weight may be associated with idiopathic bilateral congenital cataracts are needed. Family history should include any details of other family members with any ocular disease but especially childhood cataracts. If such a history is discovered then a family pedigree should be constructed to try and elucidate whether the inheritance is dominant, recessive, or X-linked [8].

A developmental history should be taken and metabolic or systemic related etiologies assessed for. A history of the onset of the lenticular opacities, laterality, and progression is also important. Sometimes asking parents to show old photos of the child can be helpful to ascertain the onset of the cataract, though with smartphone pictures on the rise a red reflex is often not discernible even in normal eyes.

Asking about the visual interaction of the child at home with the family members, also helps in determining the severity of visual dysfunction (Fig. 4.1).

Cataracts present at birth are considered congenital and those developing after birth in the first year of life, infantile. Unilateral cataracts are usually isolated, but they are most commonly found to be associated with persistent fetal vasculature (PFV) (see Fig. 4.2); also, other ocular abnormalities, such as lenticonus/lentiglobus may be associated [9]. The eye affected by PFV is usually smaller than the unaffected eye. Schematic 1 shows a flow for initial evaluation of an infant with cataracts.

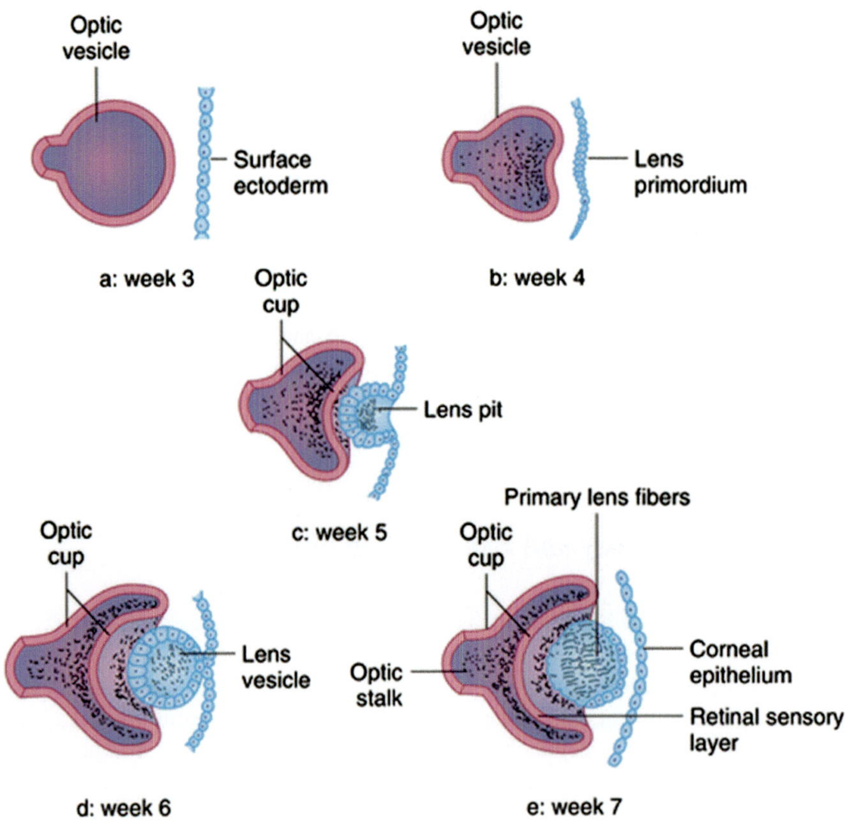

Fig. 4.1 Schematic view of the formation of the optic cup and lens vesicle through the interaction of the optic vesicle and the overlying surface ectoderm

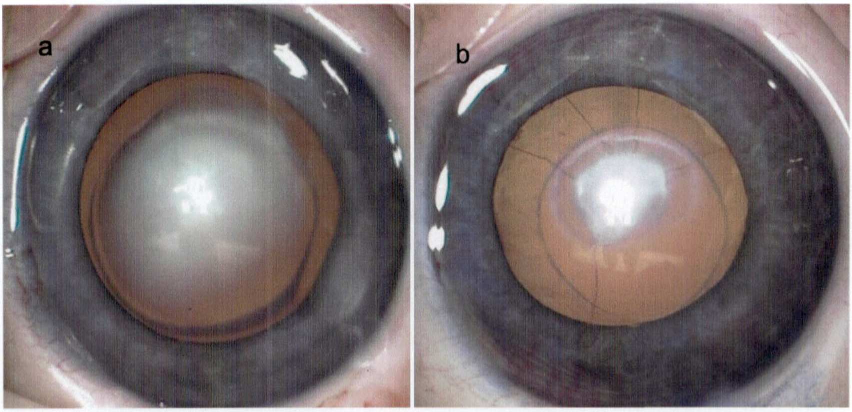

Fig. 4.2 (a) Central opacity in an infant; (b) After removal of the nuclear cataract, a posterior plaque with radiating vessels due to PFV

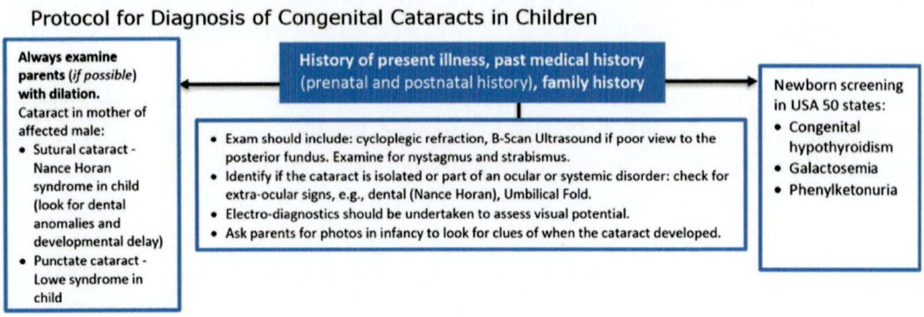

Schematic 1 Evaluation of a child with Cataract(s): taken from UPMC Children's Hospital of Pittsburgh, Eye Center, Clinical Effectiveness Guideline

A detailed ocular examination is carried out either in the office or in the operating room. In infants, if possible, the parents are asked to have the child fast for 4 h and then have the parent feed the child, usually with milk. The child will often fall into a deep sleep and a thorough examination can be done with the child asleep. In infants a handheld slit lamp should be used, while older children may be able to cooperate at a regular slit lamp. In either cases assessment should be made of the size, location, density of lenticular opacity, capsular changes, such as preexistent posterior capsular defects, and other associated anterior-segment developmental anomalies. Additionally, intraocular pressures and corneal diameters are measured. Rebound tonometry has become the method of choice but the possibility of artefactually high or low readings should be borne in min and digital palpation used to corroborate the rebound tonometry values.

Fundus examination in partial cataracts and ultrasound examination in total cataracts may reveal posterior-segment abnormalities that may affect the visual outcome. Linear ultrasound is much more helpful in assessing the cataract itself and the state of the posterior segment. The state of the vitreous and state of the retina can also be assessed and with the use of linear ultrasound a Doppler ultrasound evaluation can also be done to rule out the possibility of persistent fetal vasculature by looking for a persistent hyaloid artery.

Most ophthalmic ultrasound machines use a vector ultrasound probe and therefore in order to get an evaluation of the lens a water bath or some kind of coupling medium that stands the probe away from the lid would be needed. With linear ultrasound this is not the case. Similarly with vector ultrasound a Doppler evaluation cannot be made [10, 11] (Fig. 4.3).

Ultrasound biomicroscopy can be informative in children with anterior-segment developmental anomalies and PFV [9], and also in the assessment of posterior capsular support while considering secondary IOL implantation.

In preverbal children who are uncooperative for standard visual acuity testing, fixation behavior, fixation preference, and objection to occlusion should be checked. In younger infants with poorly developed fixation, a red reflex test can be performed in a darkened room with a direct ophthalmoscope along with undilated retinoscopy to assess the visual significance of the lens opacity. A central cataract larger than 3 mm in diameter, unilateral cataract associated with strabismus, and bilateral cataract with nystagmus are considered visually significant [12].

It is important to check the visual acuity in older cooperative children, if possible, with preferential looking cards (Teller acuity card, Keeler, etc.), or other vision tests such as "E" charts or Snellen chart appropriate to the age of the child. In cases of lamellar or posterior subcapsular cataracts, the visual acuity in an examination lane with dim light may appear normal or reasonable, but glare testing where visual acuity drops by two or more lines, will reveal potential difficulty in daylight. The glare test is performed by shining a bright light to the side of each eye as the child attempts to read the vision chart [8].

Members of the family must be examined [1, 8]; a dilated slit-lamp examination of the parents and any sibling should be performed, which may reveal previously undiagnosed lenticular changes indicative of an inherited cause for the child's cataract. Female carriers of X-linked conditions associated with males presenting with congenital cataracts may show lenticular changes.

Important examples include are punctate lens opacities in a mother of a male child with Lowe syndrome, and Y-sutural opacities in a mother of a male child with Nance–Horan syndrome [13, 14] (see Schematic 1).

For preverbal, less cooperative, children, pattern visual evoked potential (VEP) can be used to assess the effect of the opacity on the visual pathway (Fig. 4.4). Flash VEPs may be useful in complete cataracts to establish the gross integrity of the visual pathways [15].

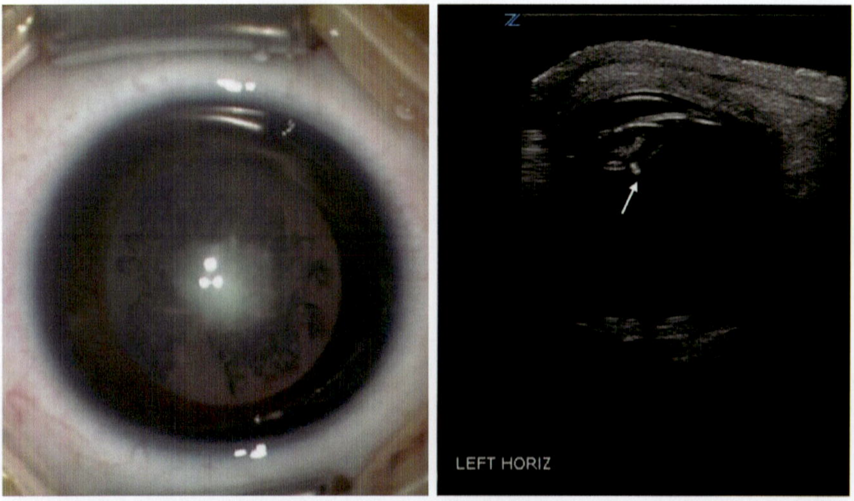

Fig. 4.3 Infant with congenital cataract. The linear ultrasound show a possible posterior defect (white arrow). The linear ultrasound shows the anterior chamber very well, as well as the posterior segment

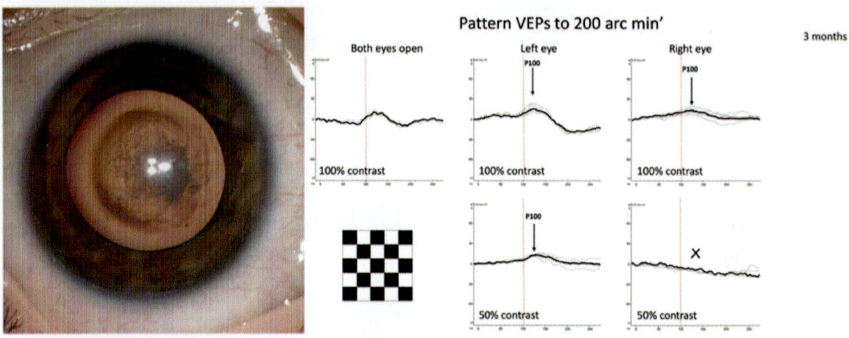

Fig. 4.4 3-month-old child with a right partial cataract. The pattern reversal VEP shows that the P100 disappears when the contrast is reduced to 50%. This suggests that in low light (late afternoon, evenings) the child is likely not getting enough visual stimulation. The option here is to keep the eye dilated and repeat the VEP or consider surgical intervention

➢ ***Note: Clinical History Examination should include:***

- Family history
- Prenatal history including maternal drug use and febrile illnesses
- Birth history of the child: especially birth weight
- Presence of metabolic or systemic related etiologies/disorders
- Visual interaction of the child at home

> ***Note: Ocular Examination Should Include:***
>
> - Detection of size, location, density of the lenticular opacity
> - Presence of capsular changes
> - Presence of anterior-segment developmental anomalies
> - Measurement of intraocular pressures and corneal diameters
> - Fundus examination, e.g. by additional use of linear ultrasound
> - Visual acuity (in older cooperative children)

It is important for the clinician to have a clear algorithm for investigation of a child with cataract (see Schematic 2). If a child has multiple congenital anomalies and dysmorphic features, then a genetic consult should be sought. Chromosomal anomalies where cataracts maybe seen include Trisomy 18,13,21 and Turner syndrome. If the chromosomal analysis is normal then depending on whether the child has a cardiac abnormality, microcephaly, hydrocephaly certain conditions need to be excluded (see Schematic 2).

In a child with bilateral cataracts, it is best to assess whether the child is systemically well or unwell. In a well child TORCH infections, galactosemia and homocystinuria should be excluded; in many parts of the developed world galactosemia screening at or soon after birth is usually performed. Genetic evaluation using a panel may reveal mutations in crystallin or connexin genes. If the child is unwell then depending on whether the child has jaundice, hypotonia or seizures certain conditions need to be excluded (see Schematic 2).

4.4 Clinical Features and Molecular Diagnosis of Congenital Cataracts

It is very important to ensure that the morphology of the cataract(s) is accurately documented. In order to so it is important to understand the various locations of the opacity. Figures 4.5 and 4.6, help with terminology of lens opacity location.

It is important to appreciate that the nucleus of the lens is bound anteriorly and posteriorly by the Y sutures [16]. Any opacity within the sutures is a nuclear opacity; if there is a large space between the nuclear opacity and the Y sutures then this is likely an embryonal nuclear cataract; if there is little or no space from the nuclear cataract to the Y sutures then is called a fetal nuclear cataract. A lamellar cataract (see Fig. 4.7) is one layer of the cataract that has become opaque. The lens fibers are produced much like the layers of an onion. If one layer is opaque, the visual effect may not be severe. Figure 4.8 shows a blue-dot cataract, but the position of the opacities is supranuclear cortical (see Figs. 4.5 and 4.6). There are some clinical features of opacities that can point to a systemic diagnosis. If a lamellar cataract opacifies in

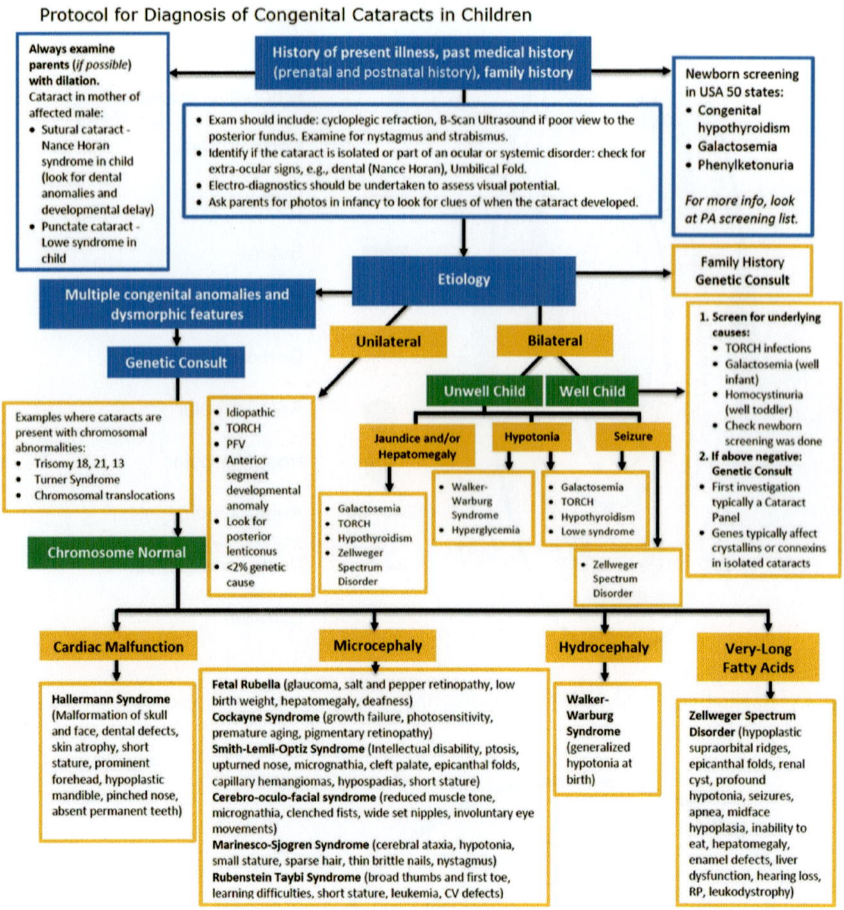

Schematic 2 Algorithm for evaluating a child with cataracts – the most important or relevant systemic conditions are discussed. Taken from UPMC Children's Hospital of Pittsburgh, Eye Center, Clinical Effectiveness Guideline

only one region, this can look like a 'wedge'. The wedge cataract (Fig. 4.11) is most commonly seen Stickler syndrome [16].

In female carriers of Nance Horan syndrome prominent Y sutural cataracts are seen, while female carriers of Lowe syndrome exhibit punctate opacities or vacuoles.

Nuclear cataracts seen in an infant should alert the clinician to the possibility of TORCH in utero infections especially if there are systemic features e.g. an infant with microcephaly, congenital cardiac abnormalities and bilateral nuclear or total cataracts should raise the possibility of congenital rubella. Congenital zika infection should also be considered if the mother was in an area where Zika infection was endemic during pregnancy [8].

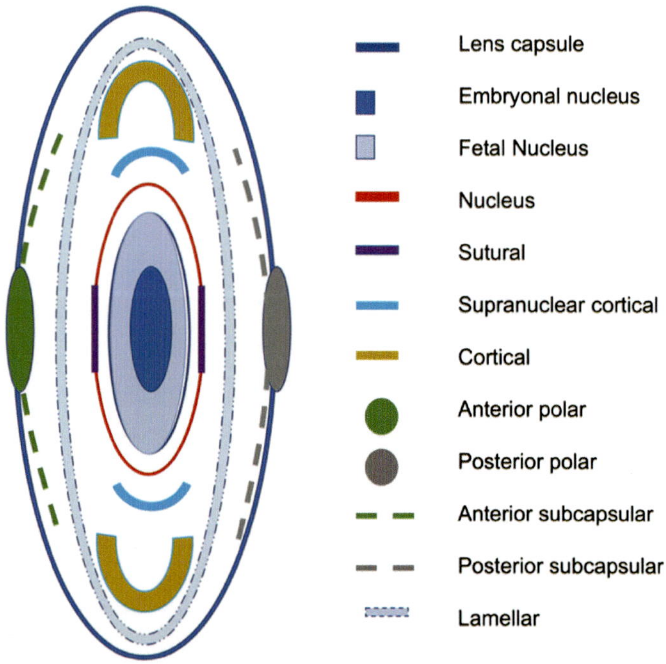

Fig. 4.5 Sagittal view schematic showing location of opacities. the color codes are the same for Figs. 4.4 and 4.5

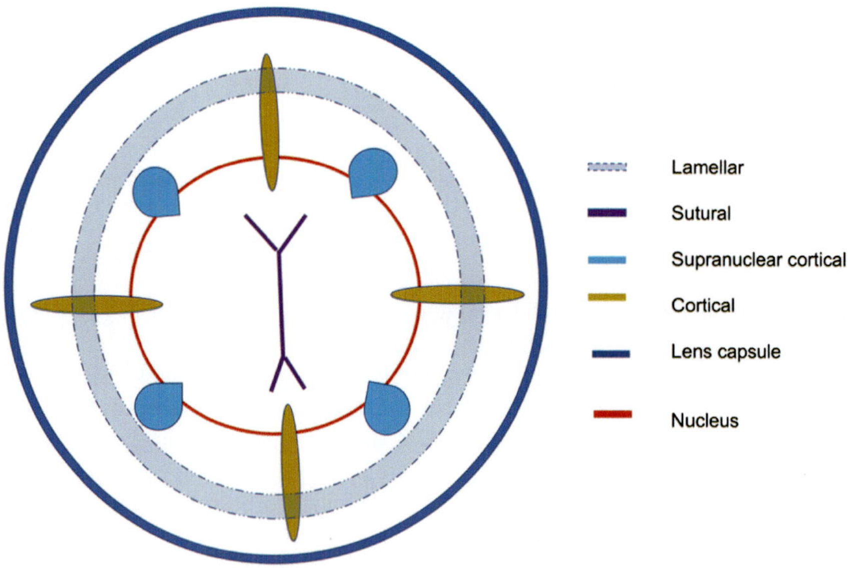

Fig. 4.6 Coronal view schematic showing location of opacities: the color codes are the same for Figs. 4.4 and 4.5

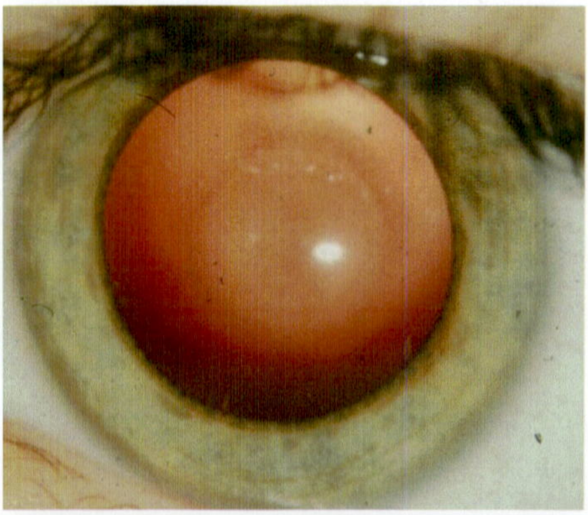

Fig. 4.7 Lamellar cataract giving the appearance of an 'oil droplet'

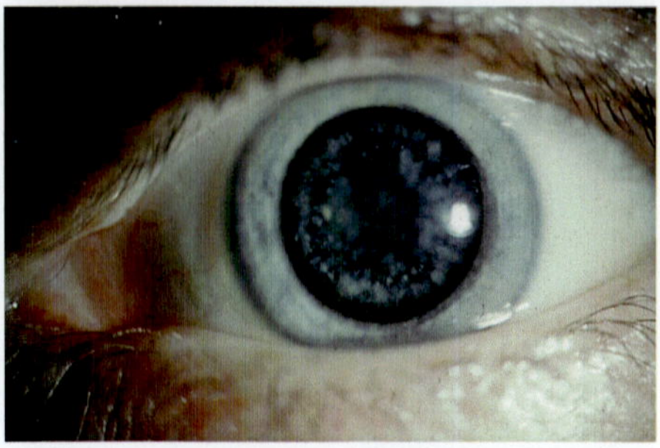

Fig. 4.8 Blue dot cataract showing supranuclear cortical opacities

The morphology of a pediatric cataract may not only help in the diagnosis of a specific condition but also in planning either non-surgical or surgical management.

Morphologically, pediatric cataracts can be broadly classified into the cataracts involving the entire lens, central cataracts, anterior cataracts, posterior cataracts, punctate lens opacities, cortical cataracts, sutural cataracts, wedge-shaped cataract, and cataracts associated with PFV [8].

Total cataracts can be sporadic or hereditary in nature but they can also be seen in Down's syndrome and congenital rubella syndrome [19]. Early surgical intervention is necessary to prevent amblyopia development.

Anterior polar cataracts are commonly seen in patients with aniridia (Fig. 4.9). They may appear dot-like, plaque-like, or in the form of a pyramid. Pyramidal cataracts are seen protruding into the anterior chamber, and have also been described in children with retinoblastoma and Ehlers–Danlos syndrome.They are associated with corneal astigmatism (Fig. 4.10).

Congenital anterior subcapsular cataracts are also seen in aniridia (Fig. 4.9). Anterior lenticonus is a bilateral condition seen in Alport syndrome [8]. The renal function must be evaluated.

Oil-droplet cataracts were thought to be pathognomonic for galactosemia but they are not (see Fig. 4.7).

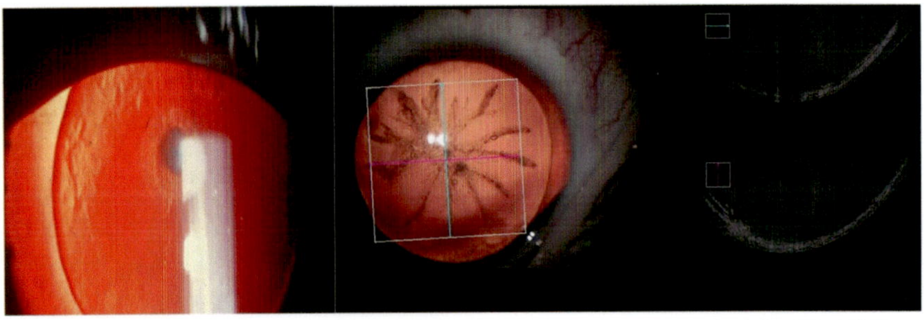

Fig. 4.9 Anterior polar cataract with a component of anterior subcapsular cataract in a child with aniridia left. In another child with aniridia a posterior subcapsular cataract is seen, as confirmed on the AS-OCT

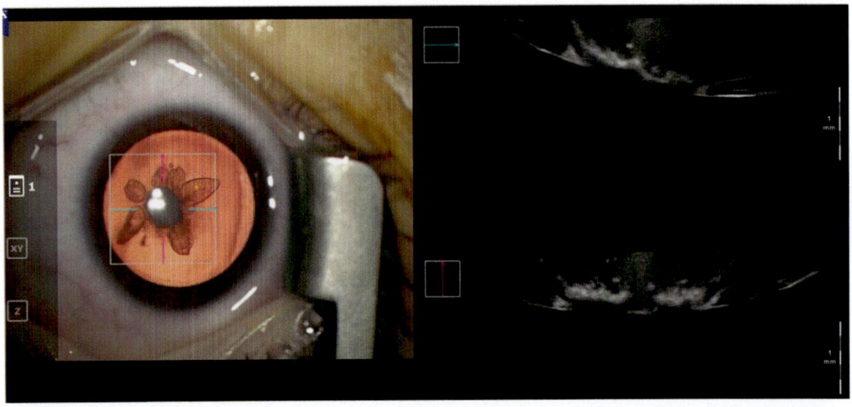

Fig. 4.10 Posterior polar cataract with posterior subcapsular opacities: the OCT shows the location of the opacities

Congenital posterior subcapsular cataract can be seen in aniridia (see Fig. 4.9) and in systemic conditions, such as Turner's syndrome, Fabry's disease, Bardet–Biedl syndrome, and neurofibromatosis type 2 [20].

Membranous cataracts are the disk-like opacities formed after spontaneous resorption of lens material typically seen in Hallermann–Streiff syndrome but also described in congenital rubella syndrome, Lowe syndrome, and PFV.

Radiating spoke-like cortical punctate opacities are also consistent with Fabry's disease.

Before embarking on molecular evaluation, as shown in Schematic 2, chromosome analysis should be considered in children with dysmorphic features and multiple congenital anomalies.

Over 200 syndromes have been associated with pediatric cataract including metabolic disorders such as lysosomal storage diseases, mitochondrial conditions, and congenital disorders of glycosylation.

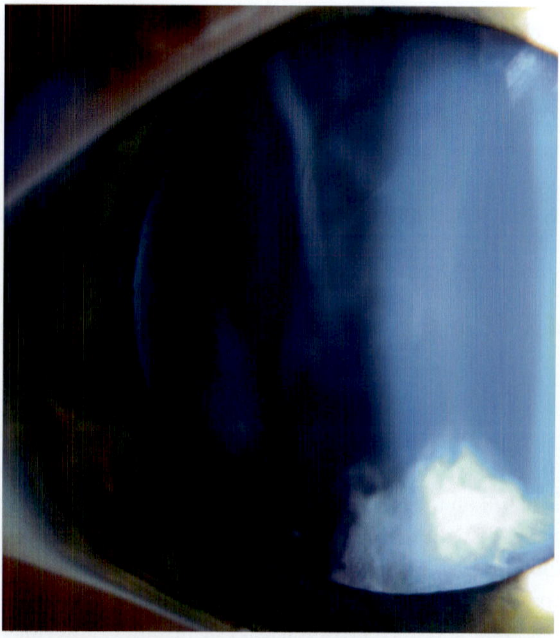

Fig. 4.11 Wedge cataract seen in a child with Stickler Syndrome

While congenital cataracts maybe the major ocular finding for some conditions e.g. Oculofaciocardiodental (*BCOR*), Marinesco-Sjogren (*SIL1*), and Lowe (*OCRL*) syndromes,in other conditions e.g. Branchiooculofacial syndrome (*TFAP2A*), Norrie disease (*NDP)* and Warburg Micro syndrome (*RAB3GAP1, RAB3GAP2, RAB18*, or *TBC1D20*) they are part of generalized ocular maldevelopment along with other anomalies such as microphthalmia, coloboma and anterior segment developmental anomalies [17].

Isolated pediatric cataracts maybe caused by mutations in over 52 genes, most frequently in crystallin genes. Crystallins are proteins in the human lens and provide transparency and refraction of light. They are classed as α-, β-, γ- crystallins and each further divided into individual proteins eg αA or αB each encoded for by separate genes *CRYAA* and *CRYAB*. Other genes that are known to cause isolated cataracts include transcription factors (*HSF4, PITX3, MAF, PAX6, FOXE3*), membrane proteins (GJA8, GJA3, MIP, LIM2, CHMP4B, EPHA2, SLC16A12), cytoskeletal proteins (VIM, BFSP2, BFSP2), and numerous additional genes with other/unknown functions. Some genes have been reported in causing isolated cataracts in some pedigrees but in others are syndromic e.g. CRYAB (can cause a myopathy), MAF (can cause Ayme-Gripp syndrome) [17]. Some conditions that are syndromic may only present initially with what appear to be isolated cataracts; two such that are noteworthy include CTX (cerebrotendinous xanthomatosis) caused by mutations in CYP27A1- this disrupts cholesterol and bile acid metabolism. The clinical features are cataracts, diarrhea and neurological impairment and xanthomas. The child may present with bilateral congenital cataracts. Galactokinase deficiency due to recessive mutations in *GALK1* results in cataracts that can be arrested by diet restriction [18].

Evaluation of a child with congenital cataracts depends on a deep phenotype of the ocular features and a deep phenotype of the systemic features. If the cataracts are truly isolated on exam either a panel can be performed for the gens known to cause isolated cataracts. Whole exome sequence can also be considered if there are systemic features which do not readily fall into a clear diagnosis e.g. Lowe syndrome.

4.5 Conservative and Surgical Procedures for Congenital Cataract

The approach to managing congenital cataracts is influenced by whether the cataracts are unilateral or bilateral and their impact on vision. The decision to perform surgery is based on the extent to which visual function is compromised. Not all lens opacities necessitate surgical intervention. Peripheral lens opacities, punctate opacities with clear areas in between, and opacities smaller than 3 mm in diameter can be monitored closely. Management strategies include treating any associated amblyopia with patching and corrective lenses. For instance, anterior polar and pyramidal cataracts, while not inherently affecting vision, can lead to significant corneal astigmatism and, consequently, reduced visual acuity and amblyopia.

Additionally, pharmacological pupil dilation can enlarge the clear visual axis in cases of small central opacities. A study by Birch et al. [21]. highlighted that young children with partial cataracts exhibiting abnormal visual acuity and contrast sensitivity faced poor long-term visual outcomes. This underscores the importance of cautious conservative treatment, incorporating tests like glare testing to confirm that the lens opacity does not significantly impair vision. Serial visual evoked potentials can also be used to assess central visual function [22].

The initial weeks of life, particularly the first six, are a crucial phase for visual development. During this time, vision is primarily processed below the cortex, and infants show a relative immunity to amblyopia. Removing unilateral congenital cataracts by 4–6 weeks and bilateral ones within 6–8 weeks can avert the onset of stimulus-deprivation amblyopia, as well as strabismus and nystagmus.

Early and appropriate optical rehabilitation combined with occlusion therapy can lead to satisfactory visual acuity, along with the ability to fuse images and perceive depth.

Pediatric eyes are distinct from those of adults, not only in size but also in their developmental trajectory. At birth, the average axial length of an infant's eye is 16.5 mm, which grows significantly in the first 18 months, reaching 23 mm by the age of 13 [23].

The corneal curvature also evolves, shifting from 51.2 diopters in newborns to 43.5 diopters in adults. Children's eyes have a thinner and more flexible sclera, a more pliable lens capsule, and are more susceptible to intense inflammatory responses post-surgery. Additionally, after cataract removal, children have a longer remaining lifespan, which increases the risk of irreversible vision loss from amblyopia. Therefore, assessing a child's eye before surgery is somewhat complex, and the process of emmetropization can be disrupted by these interventions.

> ➢*Note*
>
> - Average axial length of an infant's eye is at birth 16.5 mm, which grows within the first 18 months significantly, reaching 23 mm by the age of 13.
> - The corneal curvature also evolves: Shifting from 51.2 diopters in newborns to 43.5 diopters in adult.

4.5.1 Pre-operative Evaluation

Following pediatric cataract surgery, visual correction can be achieved through the use of aphakic glasses, contact lenses, or the direct implantation of an intraocular lens (IOL). Although the direct implantation of IOLs is becoming more common, especially for younger infants, accurately predicting the growth of the eye over time and selecting the correct IOL power to avoid unexpected changes in refractive error remains challenging. A survey revealed that around 70% of members of the American Association of Pediatric Ophthalmology and Strabismus globally prefer to implant IOLs in children [24].

Given the likelihood of a myopic shift as the eye grows, it's crucial to accurately predict eye growth and perform precise biometry to select the most suitable IOL power for each child at the time of surgery and for the future. Obtaining accurate measurements of axial length and keratometry can be difficult due to challenges with patient cooperation and fixation, often requiring biometry to be conducted under sedation or general anesthesia in the operating room.

Immersion biometry has proven to be more reliable than contact methods for calculating IOL power in children.

The prevailing view among pediatric cataract surgeons globally is to slightly undercorrect during surgery to account for the myopic shift that occurs postoperatively. However, research findings on how this surgery affects axial elongation in young children are mixed, with some studies noting a decrease and others an increase in axial length. It has been observed that axial elongation tends to be greater following the removal of a unilateral cataract compared to bilateral cataract surgery. Recent studies have shown axial growth in children who underwent surgery at the age of 10, recommending aiming for a slight hyperopia at the time of surgery in older children. Given these considerations, selecting the IOL power should be tailored to the individual needs of the child and, in cases of unilateral cataract, the refractive status of the unaffected eye.

Choosing the right IOL power requires an accurate calculation formula. Various formulas such as SRK II, Holladay 1, Holladay 2, Hoffer Q, SRK/T, and the Pediatric IOL Calculator have been employed with mixed outcomes [8]. Factors contributing to prediction errors include inaccuracies in measuring axial length, especially in the supine position, biometry techniques, keratometry readings, the phenomenon of pseudo-accommodation, variability in IOL positioning due to capsular fibrosis, and the increased elasticity of the corneoscleral complex in children. Moreover, children under two years old, with their smaller axial lengths, shallower anterior chambers, and changes in corneal curvature and thickness, are more prone to higher prediction errors. The Infant Aphakia Treatment Study (IATS) found that less than half of the children achieved within 1.00 D of the target refraction, with the largest errors in eyes with axial lengths of 18 mm or less.

The IATS later recommended the Holladay 1 and SRK/T formulas for infant eyes, despite observing a wide range of refractive errors (+5.00 to -19.00 D) at 5 years, attributing it to the challenge of predicting axial elongation in infant Eyes [25].

It's important to note that the Hoffer Q formula uses an anterior-chamber depth (ACD) value, which is predicted postoperatively and typically larger in adults than in children. To achieve a more accurate ACD value for children, the author suggests measuring the ACD of both eyes and then predicting the ACD, adjusting the preoperative ACD by 1 mm, though adjustments may be made in unilateral cases based on the ACD of the unaffected eye. An empirical rule is applied for prescribing postoperative refraction, adjusting the values based on the child's age and, in unilateral cases, the refraction of the other eye.

Hydrophobic acrylic intraocular lenses (IOLs) have become more favored than polymethyl methacrylate (PMMA) IOLs due to their higher biocompatibility, the ability to use a smaller incision owing to their foldable nature, and a reduced incidence and delayed onset of posterior capsule opacification (PCO). A significant majority, 93%, of pediatric cataract surgeons opt for hydrophobic acrylic IOLs.

The preference leans towards one-piece lenses for in-the-bag placement and three-piece lenses (MA series) for sulcus placement [24]. Silicone IOLs are less commonly used due to a higher risk of capsule contraction.

The capsular bag diameter can be measured using linear ultrasound to check to see if an IOL can be placed [8, 23] (see Fig. 4.12). The capsular bag diameter is the equator to equator distance with the addition of 1 mm [23]; for a 12.5 mm diameter IOL to be placed safely into the bag the capsular bag diameter should be 8 mm at least [23].

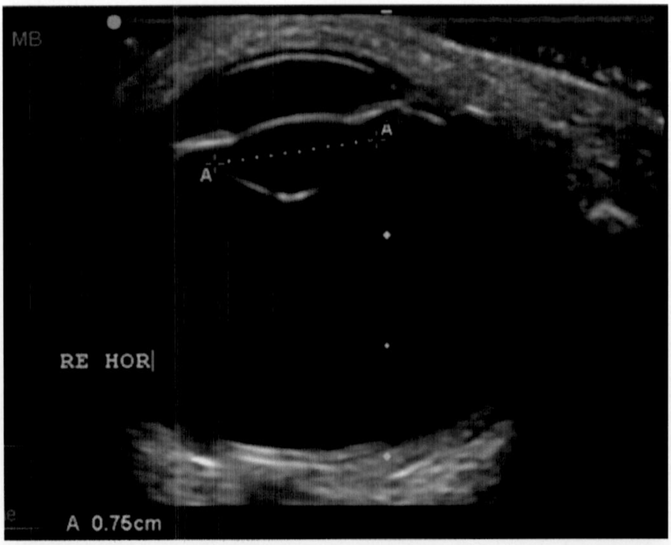

Fig. 4.12 Linear USS showing a crystalline lens. The capsular bag diameter is the equator to equator distance with the addition of 1 mm. In this example the equator to equator distance is 7.5 mm;the capsular bag diameter is 7.5 mm + 1 mm + 8.5 mm. The capsular bag diameter must be at least 8 mm for a 12.5 mm diameter lens to be placed safely in the bag

4.5.2 Wound Healing

Performing cataract surgery on children presents unique challenges due to factors such as the increased elasticity of the sclera, thicker corneas, a higher likelihood of trauma from eye rubbing, difficulties in adhering to activity restrictions, and the critical impact of postoperative astigmatism on the development of amblyopia. Although scleral tunnel incisions were once the preferred method among pediatric cataract surgeons for their supposed reduction in postoperative astigmatism, recent studies have indicated that the difference in astigmatism between scleral tunnel and other incision types is clinically negligible, with astigmatism often resolving naturally over time. Superior incisions are more commonly used than temporal ones, likely due to a perceived lower risk of injury and postoperative endophthalmitis. Temporal incisions tend to induce with-the-rule astigmatism in young children due to corneal flattening along the incision meridian. The temporal approach is favored for eyes that are deep-set or in children who have had or are planning to have superior filtration surgery. However, there is a lack of studies directly comparing astigmatic outcomes between superior and temporal incisions in pediatric cataract surgery. If immediate IOL insertion is not planned, lensectomy via the pars plana approach is also an option [8].

To prevent wound leakage for the reasons mentioned, it is recommended to suture all wounds, including paracentesis, with either 10–0 or 9–0 Vicryl or nylon sutures. Absorbable sutures are generally preferred to avoid the need for a follow-up visit for suture removal. Studies have shown that the use of 10–0 Vicryl can induce astigmatism, but this effect typically resolves within six weeks.

> ***Note: Challenging factors in cataract surgery in children:***
>
> - ***Intraoperative***
>   - Increased elasticity of the sclera
>   - Thicker corneas
>   - Tight chamber conditions
> - ***Postoperative***
>   - Difficulties in adhering the child to activity restrictions
>   - Critical impact of postoperative astigmatism
>   - Development of amblyopia

4.5.3 Capsolutomy

Achieving a continuous, smooth, and well-centered anterior capsulotomy is essential for the safe placement of a lens implant. Current methods for creating anterior capsulotomies in pediatric patients include vitrectorhexis, manual continuous curvilinear capsulorhexis (CCC), can-opener technique, and radio-frequency diathermy. Other tools, such as the plasma blade, diacapsulotomy, and pulsed-electron avalanche knife, have been proposed to reduce zonular stress and avert the unintended extension of the CCC, yet they have not gained widespread acceptance. The elasticity and thickness of the anterior capsule in young children make manual CCC particularly challenging, with a significant learning curve. This technique can be executed using either a cystotome or forceps. Manual CCC is known to create the most flexible capsulotomy with the smoothest edges, as observed under scanning electron microscopy in animal models.

While manual CCC is considered the benchmark, some surgeons opt for the vitrector in very young patients and manual CCC for older children due to the vitrectorhexis technique's lack of robustness compared to manual CCC. The two-incision push–pull technique [26], has been shown to yield consistently sized capsulorhexis openings with minimal risk of extension or tearing. Dick and Schultz [27] have reported encouraging outcomes with femtosecond laser-assisted anterior and posterior capsulotomies in a small group of children. Titiyal et al. [28] have suggested using multiple small anterior capsulorhexisotomies to prevent anterior capsule phimosis. For optimal IOL centration, the anterior capsulotomy should be smaller than the optic of the IOL. An ideal capsulotomy for an IOL with an optic diameter of 5.5–6 mm should measure 4–5 mm. Smaller capsulotomies may lead to severe capsular phimosis, considering that the capsular bag diameter typically shrinks by 15% over six months (Fig. 4.13 and 4.14).

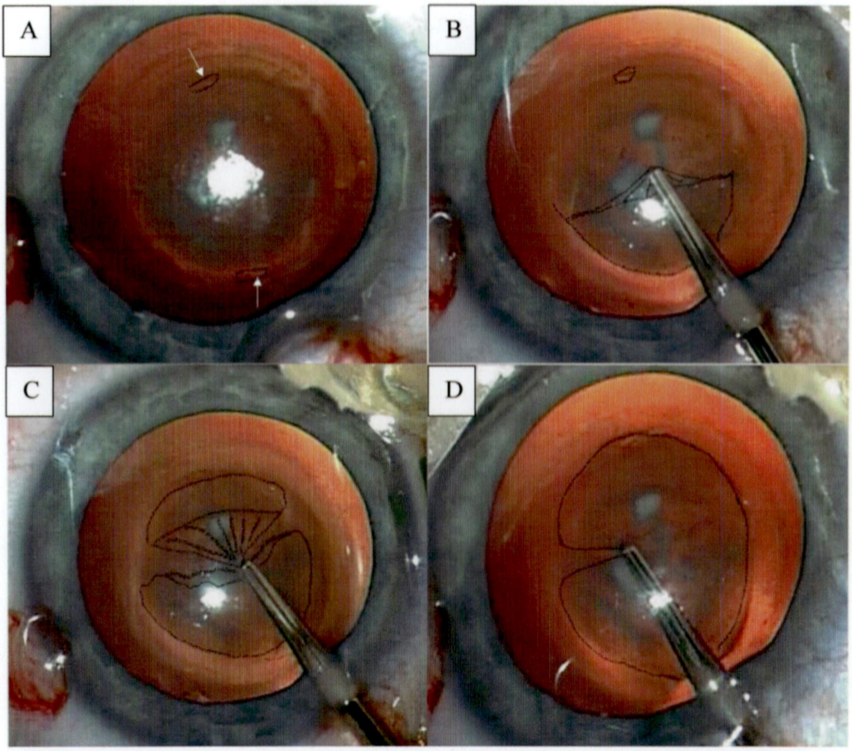

Fig. 4.13 The two incision push pull rhexis. Two stab incisions are made with an MVR blade for the desired diameter of the anterior capsular opening (A)- two white arrows pointing to stab incisions. The proximal stab is pushed to create a flap (B) -black outline shows the tear and the hatched black lines show the flap being held and pushed by the intraocular forceps. The distal flap is now grasped and pulled to create a second tear (C). The two tears are joined (D)

Fig. 4.14 The TIPP rhexis performed in Fig. 4.12 is seen more clearly after aspiration of the lens

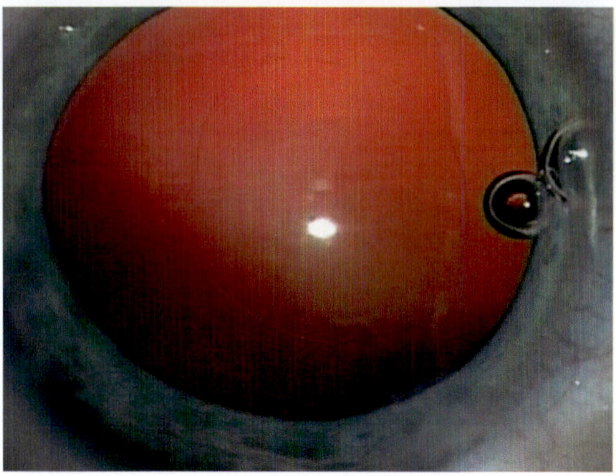

4.5.4 Technique for Cataract Extraction

Pediatric cataract surgery techniques continue to advance to reduce complications. The soft nature of pediatric cataracts eliminates the need for phacoemulsification. Lens removal can be performed through an anterior approach using manual irrigation and aspiration, or through the pars plana with a vitrector. In cases of membranous cataracts or retro-lenticular membranes associated with persistent fetal vasculature (PFV), intraocular scissors may be necessary. An anterior-chamber maintainer is used during surgery for continuous irrigation to prevent the anterior chamber from collapsing when instruments are removed.

It also helps dilate the pupil when epinephrine is added to the balanced salt solution.

The addition of heparin to the balanced salt solution and the use of intracameral recombinant tissue-plasminogen activator have been shown to reduce fibrin formation and pigment deposits on the IOL, although the effectiveness of heparin in reducing early postoperative inflammation has been recently questioned. The transconjunctival 25-gauge vitrectomy system is becoming more popular for lens removal in pediatric patients [8].

4.5.5 Posterior-Capsule Management

Ensuring a clear visual axis is crucial for achieving favorable visual outcomes after pediatric cataract removal. If the posterior capsule remains intact, all children under the age of 4 are at risk of developing significant posterior capsule opacification (PCO). The anterior vitreous surface serves as a foundation for lens epithelial cells (LECs) to proliferate, making it vital to perform a primary posterior capsulotomy (PPC) alongside anterior vitrectomy in infants and young children. This approach may also be beneficial for older children who are not suitable candidates for neodymium-doped yttrium aluminum garnet (Nd:YAG) laser capsulotomy. PPC can be executed via a limbal or pars plana route, and the PPC opening should be smaller than the anterior capsulotomy. Utilizing trypan blue 0.1% to stain the posterior capsule can ease the PPC process. The two-incision push–pull technique for PPC has been recognized for delivering consistent outcomes without the risk of vitreous loss [26]. Triamcinolone-assisted vitrectomy has been highlighted by Praveen et al. for better visualization of the anterior vitreous during surgery in children.

Optic capture of the intraocular lens (IOL) has been considered a method to avoid anterior vitrectomy and prevent PCO development. However, Vasavada et al. [29] have argued that anterior vitrectomy remains necessary with optic capture, even in older children, and performing this technique with single-piece IOLs without haptic angulation is challenging.

A technique involving posterior vertical capsulectomy with optic entrapment, as demonstrated by Grieshaber et al. [30], showed promising long-term visual axis clarity in 68 children aged 2 months to 8 years, observed over 5–12 years postoperatively. Despite its technical demands, anterior vitrectomy is rarely needed with this method.

Post-surgery, the use of subconjunctival or intracameral steroids is advised to mitigate inflammation shortly after the operation. Intracameral recombinant tissue-plasminogen activator has been effective in reducing fibrinous reactions and pigment deposits on the IOL following pediatric cataract surgery, though it carries a risk of hyphema. While the intracameral application of antibiotics has been reported to lower postoperative endophthalmitis rates in adults, its efficacy in the pediatric population has yet to be demonstrated through studies.

Despite the Infant Aphakia Treatment Study suggesting that visual axis opacification is very common in infants operated below the age of 7 months this is not a consistent finding in studies based outside the USA [32, 33].

4.6 Complications

Children undergoing cataract surgery may experience an increased inflammatory response, leading to complications such as fibrinous reactions, pigment deposits on the intraocular lens (IOL), IOL decentration, and posterior synechiae. Toxic anterior-segment syndrome, a recognized complication in adults post-cataract surgery, has also been linked to the development of secondary glaucoma.

Research by Mataftsi et al. [34] suggests that the risk of glaucoma following infantile cataract surgery is higher when surgery is performed within the first month of life or when additional intraocular surgeries are required, rather than being directly related to primary IOL implantation. The exact factors contributing to postoperative glaucoma risk remain unclear.

Measuring central corneal thickness in both aphakic and pseudophakic eyes is crucial for accurately diagnosing glaucoma, making glaucoma monitoring essential for any child who has undergone cataract surgery early in life. Retinal detachment is a less common but serious late complication, and it is uncertain if the pars plana approach increases this risk.

Visual axis opacification (VAO) is the most frequent complication after pediatric cataract surgery. Techniques such as primary posterior capsulotomy (PPC), anterior vitrectomy, using hydrophobic acrylic IOLs, or placing the IOL in the bag have been effective in preventing or delaying VAO, yet it remains a significant concern, especially in young eyes.

Severe capsular phimosis can also block the visual axis, which can be addressed with Nd: YAG laser capsulotomy or surgical membranectomy. Techniques like sealed-capsule irrigation with distilled water or 5-fluorouracil have shown success in adult eyes by eliminating lens epithelial cells (LECs) and could help pediatric surgeons manage PCO, though the risk to endothelial cells is a consideration. The bag-in-the-lens technique developed by Tassignon et al. [35] offers a promising approach by trapping LECs between the anterior and posterior capsules, significantly reducing the rate of PCO.

➢ ***Note : Challenging factors in cataract surgery in children*:**

- Increased inflammatory response
- Fibrinous reactions
- Posterior synechiae
- Pigment deposits on the intraocular lens (IOL)
- IOL decentration
- Toxic anterior-segment syndrome
- Secondary glaucoma.

4.6.1 Vision Rehabilitation

Options for visual rehabilitation following pediatric cataract removal encompass IOL implantation, aphakic glasses, and contact lenses. Aphakic glasses serve as an effective rehabilitation method for children up to 4 years old, with the addition of a bifocal segment necessary for those aged 4 and above. Contact lenses are generally well-received, allowing for adjustments in power until the child is prepared for IOL implantation with a stable postoperative refraction. The majority of clinicians prefer rigid gas-permeable contact lenses. Achieving good visual acuity with contact lens use within three weeks post-surgery is possible for unilateral aphakic patients.

A study by the Infant Aphakia Treatment Study (IATS) comparing contact lens and IOL correction outcomes indicated no significant difference in median visual acuity at 5 years between the two groups, though the IOL group experienced more complications. Regardless of the rehabilitation method chosen, ongoing monitoring is crucial.

For children, the success of cataract surgery in terms of visual outcomes heavily relies on prompt and effective amblyopia management, particularly after unilateral cataract removal. Patching post-surgery is typically continued until the risk of developing amblyopia is deemed no longer present. However, there's no widely agreed-upon standard for the extent and duration of patching needed to secure optimal visual results. Excessive occlusion therapy in early infancy could interfere with binocular vision development.

Adherence to patching is linked to better postoperative visual outcomes in both unilateral and bilateral cataract cases, especially in cases of monocular cataract. Thus, educating parents on the significance of post-surgery amblyopia therapy is essential.

Acknowledgements of Sarah Barbara Zwingelberg: With eternal love for my loving mother and my wonderful brother. My special thanks also go to Prof. Dr. Claus Cursiefen, PD Dr. Alexandra Lappa, and Prof. Dr. Thomas Dietlein, for allowing me to learn so much about children with congenital cataracts at the University Hospital Cologne.

References

1. Bremond-Gignac D, Daruich A, Robert MP, Valleix S. Recent developments in the management of congenital cataract. Ann Transl Med. 2020;8(22):1545.
2. Ludwig PE, Lopez MJ, Czyz CN. Embryology, Eye Malformations. [Updated 2023 Apr 3]. In: StatPearls [Internet]. Treasure Island (FL): StatPearls Publishing; 2024 Jan-. Available from: https://www.ncbi.nlm.nih.gov/books/NBK482496/
3. https://en.wikipedia.org/wiki/Eye_development
4. Bales TR, Lopez MJ, Clark J. Embryology, Eye. [Updated 2023 Mar 27]. In: StatPearls [Internet]. Treasure Island (FL): StatPearls Publishing; 2024 Jan-. Available from: https://www.ncbi.nlm.nih.gov/books/NBK538480/
5. Rosen D, Mahabadi N. Embryology, Optic Cup. [Updated 2023 May 1]. In: StatPearls [Internet]. Treasure Island (FL): StatPearls Publishing; 2024 Jan-. Available from: https://www.ncbi.nlm.nih.gov/books/NBK545150/
6. https://eyewiki.aao.org/Embryology_of_the_Eye_and_Ocular_Adnexa
7. George K. SMELSER; Embryology and Morphology of the Lens. Invest Ophthalmol Vis Sci. 1965;4(4):398–410.
8. Medsinge A, Nischal KK. Pediatric cataract: challenges and future directions. Clin Ophthalmol. 2015;7(9):77–90.
9. Mackeen LD, Nischal KK, Lam WC, Levin AV. High-frequency ultrasonography findings in persistent hyperplastic primary vitreous. J AAPOS. 2000;4(4):217–24.
10. Shazlee MK, Ali M, SaadAhmed M, Hussain A, Hameed K, Lutfi IA, Khan MT. Diagnostic Accuracy of Ultrasound B scan using 10 MHz linear probe in ocular trauma;results from a high burden country. Pak J Med Sci. 2016;32(2):385–8.
11. Silverman RH. Focused ultrasound in ophthalmology. Clin Ophthalmol. 2016Sep;27(10):1865–75.
12. Taylor D, Wright KW, Amaya L, et al. Should we aggressively treat unilateral congenital cataracts? Br J Ophthalmol. 2001;85(9):1120–6.
13. Ding X, Patel M, Herzlich AA, Sieving PC, Chan CC. Ophthalmic pathology of Nance-Horan syndrome: case report and review of the literature. Ophthalmic Genet. 2009;30(3):127–35.
14. Lavin CW, McKeown CA. The oculocerebrorenal syndrome of Lowe. Int Ophthalmol Clin. 1993;33(2):179–91.
15. Lin D, Chen J, Liu Z, Lin Z, Li X, Wu X, Cao Q, Lin H, Chen W, Liu Y. Impairments of visual function and ocular structure in patients with unilateral posterior lens opacity. Transl Vis Sci Technol. 2018;7(4):9.
16. Amaya L, Taylor D, Russell-Eggitt I, Nischal KK, Lengyel D. The morphology and natural history of childhood cataracts. Surv Ophthalmol. 2003 Mar-Apr;48(2):125–44.
17. Reis LM, Semina EV. Genetic landscape of isolated pediatric cataracts: extreme heterogeneity and variable inheritance patterns within genes. Hum Genet. 2019;138(8–9):847–63.
18. Gillespie RL, Urquhart J, Anderson B, Williams S, Waller S, Ashworth J, Biswas S, Jones S, Stewart F, Lloyd IC, Clayton-Smith J, Black GC. Next-generation Sequencing in the Diagnosis of Metabolic Disease Marked by Pediatric Cataract. Ophthalmology. 2016 Jan;123(1):217–20.
19. Stewart F, Lloyd IC, Clayton-Smith J, Black GC. Next-generation sequencing in the diagnosis of metabolic disease marked by pediatric cataract. Ophthalmology. 2016;123(1):217–20.

20. Trumler AA. Evaluation of pediatric cataracts and systemic disorders. Curr Opin Ophthalmol. 2011;22(5):365–79.
21. Birch EE, Subramanian V, Patel CC, Stager D Jr. Preoperative visual acuity and contrast sensitivity in children with small, partial, or non-central cataracts. J AAPOS. 2013;17(4):357–62.
22. McCulloch DL, Skarf B. Pattern reversal visual evoked potentials following early treatment of unilateral, congenital cataract. Arch Ophthalmol. 1994;112(4):510–8.
23. Wilson ME, Apple DJ, Bluestein EC, Wang XH. Intraocular lenses for pediatric implantation: biomaterials, designs, and sizing. J Cataract Refract Surg. 1994;20(6):584–91.
24. Wilson ME, Trivedi RH. Choice of intraocular lens for pediatric cataract surgery: survey of AAPOS members. J Cataract Refract Surg. 2007;33(9):1666–8.
25. VanderVeen DK, Nizam A, Lynn MJ, et al. Predictability of intraocular lens calculation and early refractive status: the Infant Aphakia Treatment Study. Arch Ophthalmol. 2012;130(3):293–9.
26. Nischal KK. Two-incision push-pull capsulorhexis for pediatric cataract surgery. J Cataract Refract Surg. 2002;28(4):593–5.
27. Dick HB, Schultz T. Femtosecond laser-assisted cataract surgery in infants. J Cataract Refract Surg. 2013;39(5):665–8.
28. Titiyal JS, Sinha R, Sharma N, Vajpayee RB. Postage stamp multiple anterior capsulorhexisotomies in pediatric cataract surgery. BMC Ophthalmol. 2005;5:3.
29. Vasavada AR, Trivedi RH, Singh R. Necessity of vitrectomy when optic capture is performed in children older than 5 years. J Cataract Refract Surg. 2001;27(8):1185–93.
30. Grieshaber MC, Pienaar A, Stegmann R. Posterior vertical capsulotomy with optic entrapment of the intraocular lens in congenital cataracts—prevention of capsule opacification. J Cataract Refract Surg. 2005;31(5):886–94.
31. Plager DA, Lynn MJ, Buckley EG, Wilson ME, Lambert SR; Infant Aphakia Treatment Study Group. Complications in the first 5 years following cataract surgery in infants with and without intraocular lens implantation in the Infant Aphakia Treatment Study. Am J Ophthalmol. 2014;158(5):892–8.
32. Magnusson G, Gyllén J, Haargaard B, Nyström A, Rosensvärd A, Scurei C, Kjellström U, Tornqvist K. The prevalence of visual axis opacification in the Swedish Pediatric Cataract Register. Acta Ophthalmol. 2024 Jan 22.
33. Trivedi RH, Wilson ME, Vasavada AR, Shah SK, Vasavada V, Vasavada VA. Visual axis opacification after cataract surgery and hydrophobic acrylic intraocular lens implantation in the first year of life. J Cataract Refract Surg. 2011;37(1):83–7.
34. Mataftsi A, Haidich AB, Kokkali S, Rabiah PK, Birch E, Stager DR Jr, Cheong-Leen R, Singh V, Egbert JE, Astle WF, Lambert SR, Amitabh P, Khan AO, Grigg J, Arvanitidou M, Dimitrakos SA, Nischal KK. Postoperative glaucoma following infantile cataract surgery: an individual patient data meta-analysis. JAMA Ophthalmol. 2014;132(9):1059–67.
35. Tassignon MJ, De Veuster I, Godts D, Kosec D, Van den Dooren K, Gobin L. Bag-in-the-lens intraocular lens implantation in the pediatric eye. J Cataract Refract Surg. 2007;33(4):611–7.

Chapter 5
Pediatric Diseases in the Context of Infantile Anterior Segment Disorders

Ilse Broekaert and Sarah Zwingelberg

Abstract Disorders of the anterior segment of the eye encompass a variety of diseases affecting the cornea, the iris, and the lens. Developmental disorders of the anterior segment of the eye are often associated with systemic manifestations, such as posterior embryotoxon in Alagille syndrome, aniridia in WAGR syndrome, congenital iris ectropion syndrome in Prader-Willi syndrome or neurofibromatosis. Further affections of the anterior segment of the eye are e.g. congenital glaucoma and the corneal dystrophies (which can also be found in Alport syndrome) There are several risk factors (systemic disease and environmental factors) predisposing to keratoconus. Inherited metabolic disorders can initially present with symptoms affecting the eye (e.g., neonatal cataract in disorders of galactose metabolism), but eye disorders can also evolve later in the natural history of an already diagnosed metabolic disorder (e.g., cornea verticillata in Fabry disease). There are also infectious causes for diseases of the anterior segment, such as herpes keratitis, Chlamydia keratoconjunctivitis and gonococcal conjunctivitis which play an important role on a global scale. Other conditions associated with anomalies of the anterior segment are Goldenhar Gorlin syndrome where patients may show a dermoid and X-chromosomal ichthyosis.

Keywords Anterior segment of the eye · Developmental disorders of the anterior segment · Syndrome · Inherited metabolic disorders · Infectious disease of the anterior segment of the eye

5.1 Developmental Disorders of the Anterior Segment of the Eye

Developmental disorders of the anterior segment of the eye, also known as anterior segment developmental anomalies (ASDA) or anterior segment dysgenesis (ASD), exhibit significant phenotypic and genetic heterogeneity, leading to a spectrum of ocular and systemic manifestations. In ASD, there is a disruption in late gestational

I. Broekaert et al., *Infantile Anterior Segment Disorders*,
https://doi.org/10.1007/978-3-031-68558-3_5

development, resulting in retained primitive endothelium, failure of the peripheral iris to migrate posteriorly, and/or incomplete differentiation of the corneal endothelium.

Approximately 60% of patients with ASD are prone to developing increased intraocular pressure during infancy or later life. The ciliary body of the iris produces aqueous humor, which is drained via the trabecular meshwork into the Schlemm's canal and the uveoscleral outflow pathway. Disruptions in this process are frequent in ASD, often leading to secondary glaucoma [1]. Consequently, regular monitoring for the development of glaucoma is crucial for patients with ASD. ASD is frequently associated with syndromes, as described below.

When fetal ultrasound abnormalities during pregnancy (e.g., polyhydramnios, cardiac, genitourinary or gastrointestinal anomalies) are present, genetic counseling including prenatal diagnostics can be performed even before birth. Nowadays, trio exome sequencing is a useful addition to prenatal diagnostics due to its high diagnostic yield and short processing time as it covers a wide spectrum of genetic changes [2]. Comprehensive interdisciplinary counseling before and after diagnostics is indispensable.

5.1.1 *Posterior Embryotoxon*

A posterior embryotoxon is an anteriorly displaced and thickened Schwalbe's line (Fig. 5.1).

Posterior embryotoxon most often occurs in Axenfeld-Rieger syndrome (see below) and Alagille syndrome [3]. Alagille syndrome is an autosomal dominant disorder usually caused by pathogenic variants in the *JAG1* on chromosome 20p12 (95%) or NOTCH2 (2.5%) [4]. Alagille syndrome affects multiple organ system and has a wide range of clinical severity even within families. The most clinically important manifestations are cholestatic liver disease due to a paucity of bile ducts, congenital heart disease (most often stenosis or hypoplasia of the pulmonary arteries) and cerebrovascular anomalies. Other features include a characteristic facies (Fig. 5.2), renal disease, posterior embryotoxon, skeletal abnormalities (e.g., butterfly vertebrae), and growth failure.

5.1.2 *Axenfeld-Rieger Spectrum*

Axenfeld-Rieger spectrum (ARS) is a rare autosomal dominant continuum of phenotypes with an estimated prevalence of 1:200,000. It has been associated with loci on chromosomes 4, 6, 13, and 16 [1, 5–7]. Mutations in transcription factors *PITX2* (chromosome 4) and *FOXC1* (chromosome 6) have been associated with the ocular and hearing symptoms found in ARS [4]. In ARS, patients present with ocular and systemic symptoms (see Table 5.1). Penetration of symptoms varies ranging from iris hypoplasia and polycoria to microdontia (compare Fig. 5.3) [1].

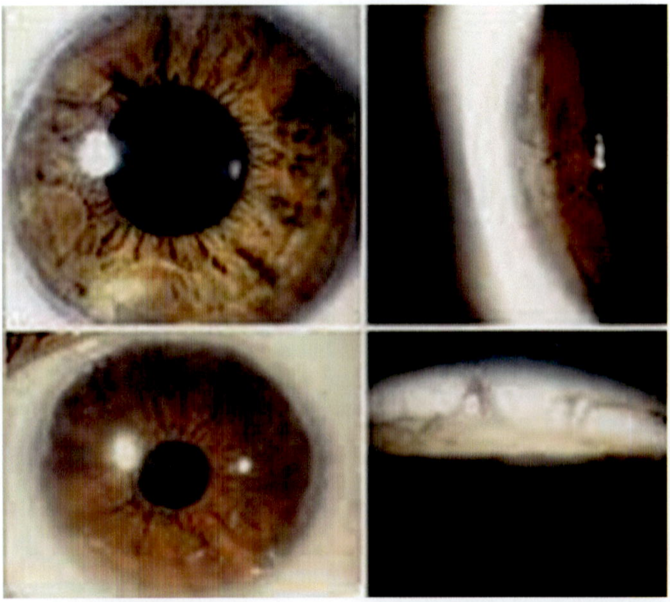

Fig. 5.1 Posterior embryotoxon

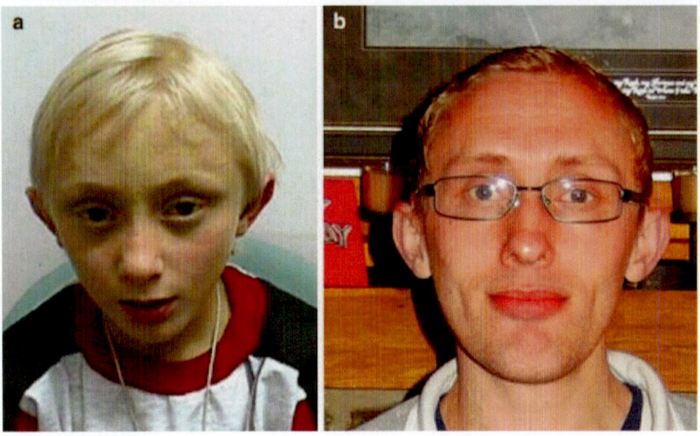

Fig. 5.2 Characteristic facies evolve from childhood to adulthood in a patient with Alagille syndrome: (a) Characteristic facial features in children with ALGS include a triangular face, deeply set eyes, and a straight nose with a bulbous tip. (b) Facial features in adults with ALGS are distinct, with a square jaw and prominent chin

Table 5.1 Manifestations of Axenfeld-Rieger spectrum [8–10]

Anterior segment dysgenesis	Posterior embryotoxon	
	Abnormalities of the iris	Iris hypoplasia
		Corectopia
		Polycoria
		Anirdia
	Glaucoma	
Dysmorphic facial features	Prominent forehead	
	Broad and flat nasal bridge	
	Mid-facial abnormalities	
	Maxillary hypoplasia	
	Hypertelorism	
	Telecanthus	
	Prognathism	
	Prominent eyes	
	Saddle nose	
Systemic developmental abnormalities	Dental	Hypodontia
		Microdontia
		Delayed eruption
		Cone shaped teeth
		Increased spacing between teeth
	Redundant periumbilical skin	Failure of involution of the periumbilical skin in the abdominal region leads to the typical "elephant trunk" umbilicus
		Increased incidence of umbilical hernia
	Others	Hypospadias in males
		Pituitary abnormalities
		Growth retardation
		Anal stenosis
		Cardiac anomalies (atrial septal defect, valvular defects, patent ductus arteriosus)
		Abnormal ears, hearing loss
		Intellectual disability
		Cerebellar vermis hypoplasia

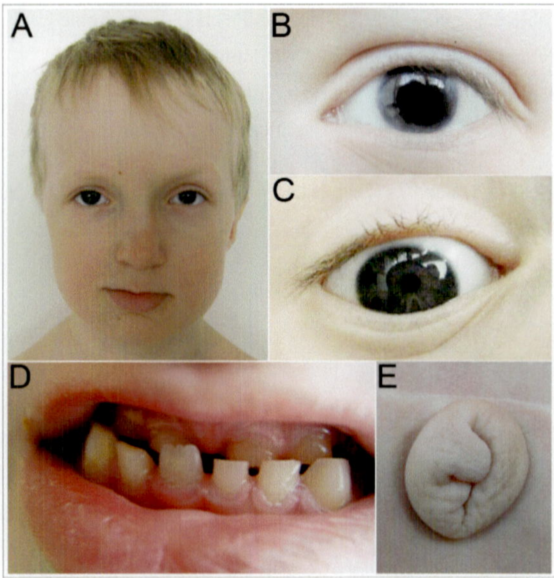

Fig. 5.3 Systemic symptoms in Axenfeld-Rieger spectrum: Patient with PITX2 regulatory region deletion and AXS. (A) Facial photograph showing maxillary hypoplasia, thin upper lip, and broad nasal bridge. (B) Left eye corectopia. (C) Right eye posterior embryotoxon. (D) Dental anomalies, including maxillary hypodontia. (E) Redundant periumbilical skin

5.1.3 Peters Anomaly and Peters Plus Syndrome

Peters anomaly is associated with mutations in *PAX6, PITX2*, and *CYP1B1* [1]. Inheritance can be sporadic, autosomal dominant, or autoxomal recessive. Peters plus syndrome is an autosomal recessive disease and is associated with defects in glycosylation due to mutation in the *B3GLCT* gene [11].

In Peters anomaly, the anterior segment is affected heterogeneously, presenting with a central corneal opacity and a defect in the endothelium and the Descemet's membrane of the cornea. The whitish plaque on the cornea (leukoma) is due to a central defect in the corneal endothelium with various degrees of adhesion of the iris and lens capsule to the central cornea. The presence of a central corneal opacity is required for diagnosis, but the extent of the opacity varies among patients [1, 12].

Peters plus syndrome is characterized by defects in the anterior chamber as well as systemic anomalies (compare Table 5.2).

5.1.4 Primary Congenital Glaucoma

Primary congenital glaucoma (PCG) is an autosomal recessive disorder and is defined as having elevated intraocular pressure with onset in the first year of life. Primary congenital glaucoma is present at birth, whereas primary infantile glaucoma has an onset in the first two to three years of life [14]. Onset after four to five years of life is referred to as juvenile glaucoma. The later the onset, the less severe the structural

Table 5.2 Symptoms described in Peters plus syndrome [1, 9, 13]

Prenatal manifestations	Polyhydramnios	
Growth	Low birth weight	
	Intrauterine and postnatal growth restriction	
Head and neck	Face	Long face
		Prominent forehead
		Maxillary hypoplasia
		Long philtrum
		Micrognathia
	Ears	Low-set ears
		Small posteriorly rotated ears
		Preauricular pit
		Hearing loss
	Eyes	Hypertelorism
		Upslanting palpebral fissures
		Reduced vision
		Anterior chamber anomaly (Peters anomaly, cataract, glaucoma)
	Mouth	Thin vermilion border
		Cupid-bow shaped upper lip
		Cleft lip, cleft palate
	Teeth	Widely spaced teeth
	Neck	Short neck
Cardiovascular	Heart	Atrial septal defect
		Ventricular septal defect
		Pulmonary stenosis
		Patent ductus arteriosus
	Chest	Widely spaced nipples
Abdomen	Gastrointestinal	Anteriorly placed anus
		Gastrointestinal malrotation
		Feeding problems
	Genitourinary	Small kidneys
		Hyperechoic kidneys
Skeletal	Limbs	Rhizomelic shortening
	Hands	Brachydactyly
		Fifth finger clinodactyly
	Feet	Short toes
		Short feet

(continued)

Table 5.2 (continued)

Prenatal manifestations	Polyhydramnios	
Neurologic		Developmental delay
		Corpus callosum hypoplasia or agenesis
		Enlarged ventricles

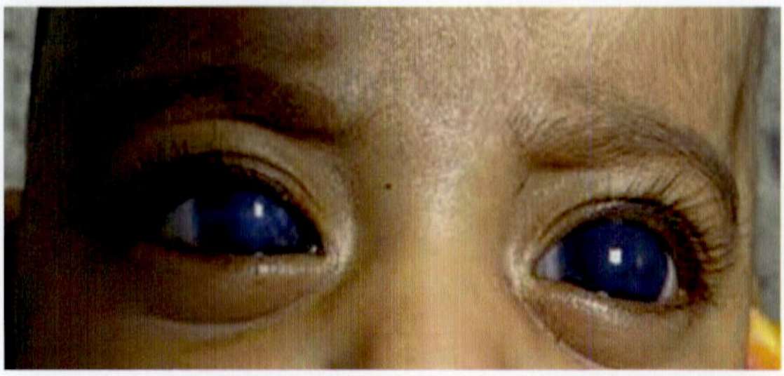

Fig. 5.4 Primary congenital glaucoma with buthalmos

anomaly and the more likely the glaucoma will respond to treatment. PCG has been linked to mutations in the *GLC3A* locus (2p21) involving the gene *CYP1B1*, which produces a member of the cytochrome P450 family of enzymes [15]. Other genetic loci include *GLC3B (1p36)*, *GLC3C (14q24.3)*, and more recently *GLC3D (14q24)*, involving the gene *LTBP2*. The gene myocilin (*MYOC*) has also been implicated PCG [16, 17]. PCG is considered a part of ASD as it frequently involves malformations of the structures involved in aqueous humor outflow, such as Schlemm's canal and the trabecular meshwork. Although the pathogenesis of infantile and juvenile glaucoma is similar, the presenting signs and symptoms differ.

Juvenile glaucoma presents insidiously and vision loss due to optic nerve damage may be the first presenting symptoms. Peripheral vision is affected first, and if left untreated, central vision loss and blindness may occur. In congenital/ infantile glaucoma, the cornea and sclera are more elastic, and patients may present with enlarged and edematous cornea, buphthalmos (compare Fig. 5.4), tearing, photophobia, headache, and eye pain.

5.1.5 *Aniridia*

Aniridia, or iris hypoplasia, is a rare congenital abnormality caused by mutations in the *PAX6* gene, which is involved in the early development of the eyes, brain, and central nervous system. Mutations in the genes *FOXC1* and *CYP1B1* (chromosomes 6 and 2, respectively) have also been linked to aniridia [4]. The majority of cases are sporadic, with occasional familial cases. The familial cases are autosomal dominant and involve deletion of chromosome 11p13, a deletion that increases the risk of Wilms

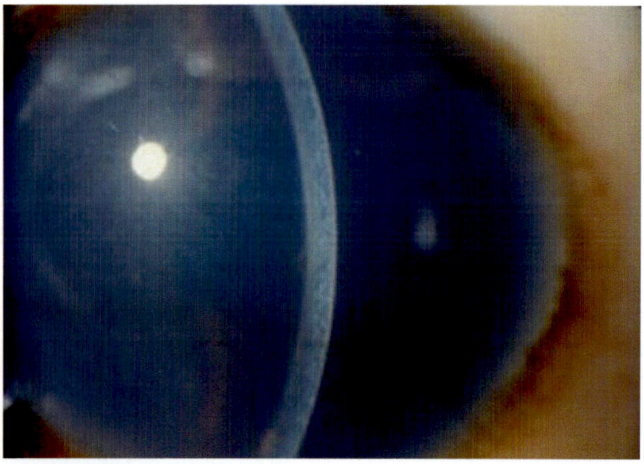

Fig. 5.5 Congenital hereditary endothelial dystrophy (CHED)

tumor (also known as the WAGR syndrome [Wilms tumor, aniridia, genitourinary anomalies, and mental retardation]) [18]. Other ocular manifestations include foveal hypoplasia, nystagmus, optic nerve hypoplasia, glaucoma, and progressive corneal degenerative changes. Glaucoma often presents in infancy but can present at any time, therefore, patients should be regularly monitored for the development of glaucoma.

5.1.6 Corneal Dystrophies

5.1.6.1 Congenital Hereditary Endothelial Dystrophy

Congenital hereditary endothelial dystrophy presents with corneal edema and opacifications at birth (compare Fig. 5.5). Associated epiphora and photophobia are uncommon. Nystagmus is very common. The cornea is of normal size horizontally and very thickened (up to two to three times), the intraocular pressure is usually normal, and the optic nerve and angle are normal (albeit difficult to visualize). Congenital hereditary endothelial dystrophy is inherited in an autosomal recessive pattern and may be due to mutations in the *ZEB1* gene in PPCD3 and *SLC4A11* on chromosome 20p13 [19, 20].

5.1.6.2 Posterior Polymorphous Corneal Dystrophy

Posterior polymorphous corneal dystrophy is an autosomal dominant disease of the corneal endothelium with thickening of Descemet's membrane, which can present with bilateral corneal opacities and corneal edema in severe cases (compare Fig. 5.6). Several loci on chromosomes 1, 8, 10 and 20 have been identified that may affect embryological development of the cornea, such as mutations in the PPCD1 locus

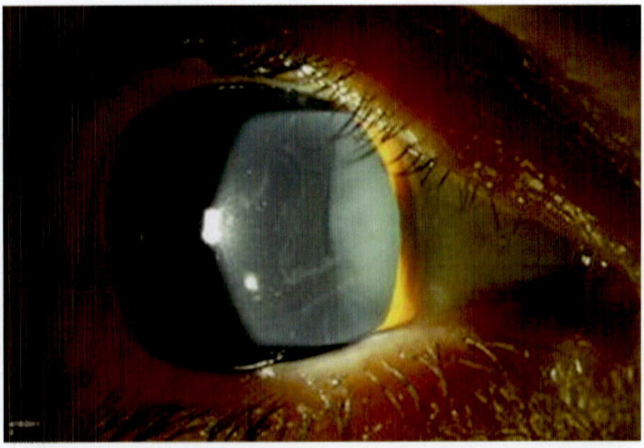

Fig. 5.6 Posterior polymorphous corneal dystrophy

on chromosome 20q11, PPCD2 locus on chromosome 1p34.3 and PPCD3 on chromosome 10p [19, 21].

Posterior polymorphous corneal dystrophy may be associated with Alport syndrome, an inherited progressive form of glomerular disease that is often associated with sensorineural hearing loss and ocular abnormalities.

5.1.7 Sclerocornea

Sclerocornea is a congenital malformation of the cornea in which the limits of the cornea and sclera are indistinct. The cornea is hazy because collagen fibrils are irregularly arranged by ingrowth of vascularized, opaque scleral tissue extending into the peripheral cornea (compare Fig. 5.7). Additional ocular anomalies (e.g., aniridia, cataracts, coloboma) usually are present.

Sclerocornea may be part of PHACE (posterior fossa anomalies, hemangioma, arterial anomalies, cardiac anomalies, and eye anomalies) syndrome, a rare disorder

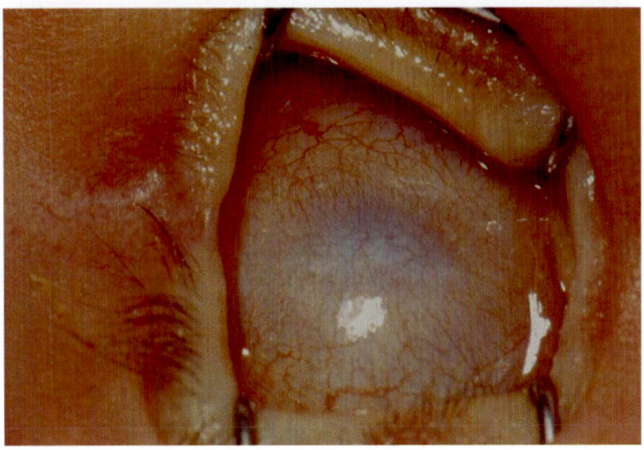

Fig. 5.7 Sclerocornea in a newborn

of unknown etiology characterized by large segmental hemangiomas of the face and various developmental defects. Genes implicated in sclerocornea have significant overlap with other forms of anterior segment disorders, such as congenital cataracts, and include *FOXE3, RAX, SOX2, PITX3, PAX6*, and *PXDN* [22].

5.1.8 Megalocornea

Primary megalocornea is an inherited eye disorder that may be confused with infantile glaucoma. Megalocornea usually is inherited as an X-linked recessive trait and occurs almost exclusively in males. In patients with primary megalocornea, the intraocular pressure is normal; corneal edema, epiphora, and photophobia are absent; and the optic nerve is normal. Unilateral high myopia, proptosis, lid retraction, microphthalmos, enophthalmos, or ptosis can give the appearance of an enlarged cornea because one eye is larger, more prominent, or more visible than the other (compare Fig. 5.8) [23]. *CHRDL1* mutations have been shown to cause X-linked megalocornea. The gene has been linked to development of the corneal stroma and endothelium [23]. X-linked megalocornea caused by mutations in CHRDL1 identifies an essential role for ventroptin in anterior segment development [23].

5.1.9 Iridogoniodysgenesis Syndrome

Iridogoniodysgenesis is a rare autosomal dominant disease associated with malformations of the iris stroma and trabecular meshwork, leading to iris hypoplasia and glaucoma [24–26]. The iridogoniodysgenesis locus is mapped to 6p25, and is thought to be associated with a malfunction in the migration or induction of neural crest cells involved in the formation of the anterior segment [26]. Mutations in the *RIEG* gene at locus 4q25 have also been found to be associated with Iridogoniodysgenesis syndrome [26].

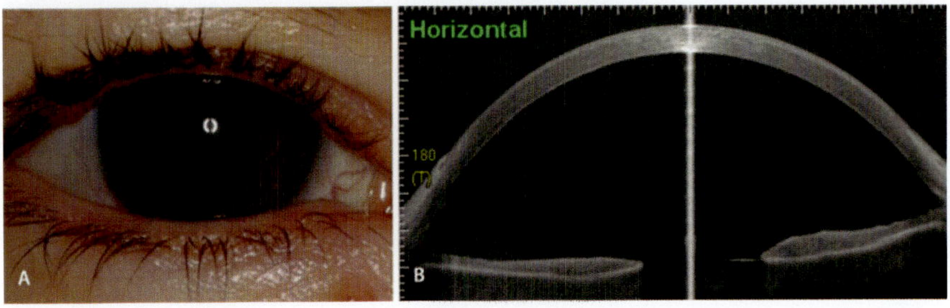

Fig. 5.8 Megalocornea in a child

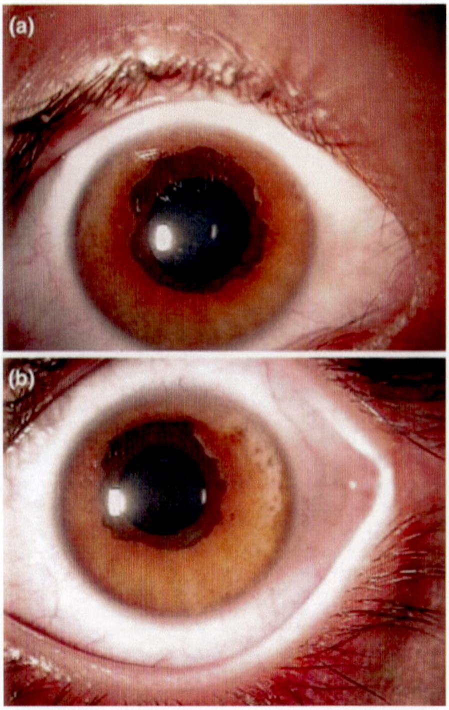

Fig. 5.9 Congenital iris ectropion syndrome

5.1.9.1 Congenital Iris Ectropion Syndrome

Congenital iris ectropion is a rare neural crest disorder that commonly presents with developmental glaucoma. It is characterized by posterior iris epithelium presenting on the anterior side of the stroma (compare Fig. 5.9) [27]. Congenital iris ectropion is inherited in an autosomal recessive pattern and has been linked to mutation of the *PAX-6* gene on chromosome 1 [28]. It most commonly presents in males [29].

Congenital iris ectropion has been associated with neurofibromatosis, primary facial hemihypertrophy, Rieger anomaly and Prader-Willi syndrome [27].

5.1.9.2 Keratoconus and Keratoglobus

Keratoconus is a noninflammatory disorder of the cornea of unknown etiology. It is characterized by progressive thinning and cone-shaped protrusion of the cornea leading to visual impairment (see Fig. 5.10).

In keratoglobus, there is a generalized thinning and globular protrusion of the cornea [30]. In keratoconus, patients may present with blurry vision or a sudden decrease in visual acuity. Corrective lenses may be difficult to fit and require frequent changes due to progressive myopia and irregular astigmatism. Visual impairment can be managed initially with corrective lenses but may require corneal cross-linking to

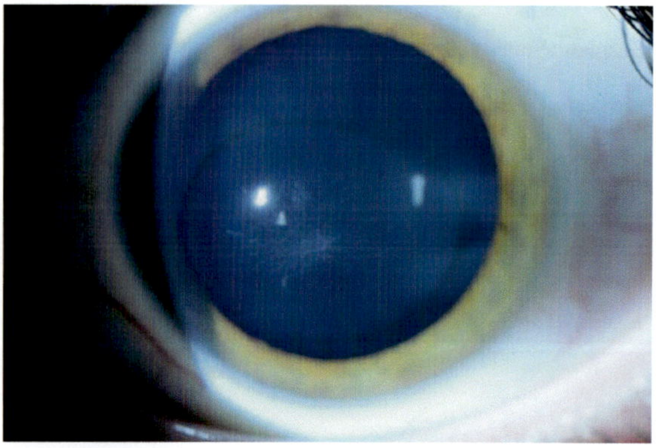

Fig. 5.10 Keratoconus with typical circular corneal hemosiderin deposits (Fleischer rings), corneal opacities as well as Vogt striae

prevent disease progression or penetrating keratoplasty in more advanced disease. Risk factors for the development of keratoconus are described in Table 5.3.

Table 5.3 Risk factors for the development of keratoconus (uptodate)

Risk factor	Associated symptoms	Diagnosis	Reference
Systemic disorders			
Down syndrome	Dysmorphic features, cognitive impairment, congenital heart disease (e.g. septal defects), duodenal atresia/ stenosis, imperforate anus, esophageal atresia, celiac disease, Hirschsprung disease, small stature, low birth weight, ophthalmologic disorders (refractive errors, strabismus, nystagmus, cataracts), hearing problems, otitis media, thyroid dysfunction, type 1 diabetes, atlantoaxial instability, hematologic abnormalities, immunological impairments	Characteristic phenotype, genetic testing	[31]
Ehlers-Danlos syndrome	Skin hyperextensibility, joint hypermobility, tissue fragility, fatigue, hernias, vascular complications	Characteristic phenotype, genetic testing	[32]

(continued)

Table 5.3 (continued)

Risk factor	Associated symptoms	Diagnosis	Reference
Osteogenesis imperfecta	Bone fragility, blue or greyish sclerae, hearing loss, skin hyperlaxity, joint hyperextensibility, dentinogenesis imperfecta, facial dysmorphism, cardiovascular, neurologic and respiratory manifestations	Bone imaging, genetic testing	[33]
Turner syndrome	Short stature, dysmorphic features, primary amenorrhea due to ovarian failure, cardiovascular malformations (e.g. aortic valve abnormalities, coarctation of the aorta), congenital lymphedema, liver function abnormalities, neurocognitive deficits, autoimmune diseases (thyroiditis), ocular abnormalities (refractive errors, strabismus, amblyopia, ptosis), otitis media, hearing loss	Characteristic phenotype, genetic testing	[34]
Marfan syndrome	Aortic root disease (aortic aneurysm, aortic regurgitation, aortic dissection), mitral valve prolapse, excess linear growth, arachnodactyly, pectus carinatum, joint hypermobility, ectopia lentis, myopia, dural ectasia	Characteristic phenotype, echocardiography, family history, genetic testing	[35]
Alport syndrome	Glomerular disease (initially microscopic haematuria) progressing to kidney failure, sensorineural hearing loss	Family history, kidney or skin biopsy, genetic testing	[36]

(continued)

Table 5.3 (continued)

Risk factor	Associated symptoms	Diagnosis	Reference
Silver-Russell syndrome	Intrauterine growth restriction, short stature, dysmorphic features (e.g. clinodactily 5th finger, triangular face), feeding difficulties, mild developmental delay	Genetic testing	[37, 38]
Noonan syndrome	Short stature, dysmorphic features, congenital heart disease (e.g. pulmonary valve stenosis, hypertrophic cardiomyopathy), feeding difficulties, macrocephaly, pectus carinatum/ excavatum, mild developmental delay, cryptorchidism, lymphedema	Family history, genetic testing	[39]
Mulvihill-Smith syndrome	Premature aging, short stature, microcephaly, premature aging, lack of facial subcutaneous fat, hearing loss, cognitive impairment, multiple pigmented nevi, immunodeficiency	Genetic testing	[40]
Environment			
Atopic disease	Perennial or saisonal; allergic rhinoconjunctivitis: sneezing, rhinorrhoea, nasal obstruction, postnasal drainage, itchy eyes/ nose, fatigue, irritability Asthma: (chronic) cough, wheezing,	History, allergen-specific testing (skin, specific IgE), allergen challenge, lung function testing, exhaled nitric oxide, bronchoprovocation testing, chest radiograph	[41]
Sleep apnea	Risk factors: snoring, enlarged adenoids/ tonsils, obesity, craniofacial abnormalities, neuromuscular disorders, mucopolysaccharidosis, Down syndrome, sickle cell disease	Polysomnography	[42]
Eye-rubbing	Ocular irritation/ dryness leading to itching; atopic disease; emotional stress	History	[43]

5.2 Inherited Metabolic Disorders Associated with Anomalies of the Anterior Segment

Inherited metabolic disorders are a large group of rare disorders affecting biochemical pathways. Many metabolic disorders can initially present with symptoms affecting the eye (e.g., neonatal cataract in disorders of galactose metabolism), but eye disorders can also evolve later in the natural history of an already diagnosed metabolic disorder (e.g., cornea verticillata in Fabry disease).[32] Awareness of an inherited metabolic disorder is important to facilitate early diagnosis and, in some cases, initiate early treatment if a child presents with eye involvement suggestive of a metabolic disorder. Ophthalmological interventions are an important component of the multidisciplinary approach to treating children with inherited metabolic disorders.

Diagnostical Approach

Identification of an inherited metabolic disorder requires a low threshold of clinical suspicion. Further extra-ocular features should be sought to determine of the presenting eye signs or symptoms are within the context of a multisystem disease. The family history, presence of consanguinity, achievement of developmental milestones, presence of hepato/splenomegaly or dysmorphic feature may allude to an inherited metabolic disorder. Specific biochemical and metabolic tests including enzyme assays and ultimately genetic testing may lead to the diagnosis. A multidisciplinary team approach including at least the geneticist, and the specialists involved with treatment of the child's symptoms including the ophthalmologist is indispensable [44]. A list of relevant inherited metabolic disorders associated with anterior segment disorders of the eye is found in Table 5.4 [45].

5.3 Infectious Causes for Diseases of the Anterior Segment

5.3.1 Herpes Keratitis

Keratitis (corneal infection and inflammation) caused by herpes simplex virus (HSV) is a major cause of blindness worldwide, due to corneal scarring and opacity [72]. Keratitis is the most prevalent form of ocular HSV-1 disease besides eyelid lesions (herpetic blepharitis), conjunctivitis, uveitis, retinitis, and, rarely, scleritis [73]. The diagnosis of herpes simplex keratitis is mainly clinical. Patients often present with an acute onset of symptoms including pain, visual blurring, photophobia, watery ocular discharge, and a red eye.

Physical examination is notable for conjunctivitis, decreased corneal sensation, and characteristic dendritic lesions of the cornea. Serologic testing is not helpful. The treatment of herpes simplex keratitis is dependent upon whether the episode of disease is caused by active viral replication (epithelial herpes simplex keratitis) or immune response to past infection (stromal keratitis or endotheliitis).

Table 5.4 Overview of metabolic disorders associated with anterior segment disorders of the eye

Ophthalmic finding	Metabolic disease	Extraocular findings	Diagnostic tests	Treatment	References
Cornea					
Dendritic keratitis, corneal ulcers	Hereditary tyrosinaemia type II	Hyperkeratotic plaques in pressure areas, intellectual disability	Plasma amino acids, urine organic acids, genetic testing	Diet low in tyrosine and phenylalanine	[46]
Cornea verticillata	Fabry disease	Acroparaesthesia, hypertrophic cardiomyopathy, progressive renal impairment, stroke	Lyso-Gb3, enzymology, genetic testing	ERT, migalastat, symptomatic therapy	[47]
Corneal crystal deposits	Cystinosis	nephropathy, end stage renal failure, hypothyroidism, growth retardatation	Cystine in leucocytes, genetic testing	Symptomatic therapy; eyes: topical cysteamine	[48]
Corneal clouding/ opacities	Mucopolysaccharidosis (type I, IV, VI)	Dysmorphic features, HSM, dysostosis multiplex, developmental delay, short stature	Urine glycosaminoglycans, enzymology, genetic testing	ERT	[49]
	I-cell disease (mucolipidosis type II)	Early onset dysmorphic features	I-cell screen enzymology, genetic testing	symptomatic	[50]
	Galactosialidosis	Dysmorphic features, cherry red spot	Urine sialic acid, glycosaminoglycans, genetic testing	symptomatic	[51]
	Alpha mannosidosis	Dysmorphic features, frequent infections, hepatosplenomegaly	Urine oligosaccharides, enzymology, genetic testing	BMT, ERT	[52, 53]
	Tangier disease	Orange coloured tonsils, hepatosplenomegaly, peripheral neuropathy	Cholesterol, lipoproteins, genetic testing	Low fat diet	[54]

(continued)

Table 5.4 (continued)

Ophthalmic finding	Metabolic disease	Extraocular findings	Diagnostic tests	Treatment	References
	Infantile free sialic acid storage disease	Hepatosplenomegaly, dysmorphic features, cardiomegaly	Urine sialic acid, genetic testing	Symptomatic	[55]
	Lecithin cholesterol acyltransferase (LCAT) deficiency	Corneal lipid deposits, renal failure, anaemia	Genetic testing	Symptomatic	[56]
Lens					
Ectopia lentis	Homocystinuria	Marfanoid habitus, thromboembolic events	Plasma amino acids, genetic testing	Diet, medication	[35]
	Sulfite oxidase deficiency	Severe neonatal seizure disorder, microcephaly, psychomotor retardation	Urine sulphocysteine, genetic testing	Symptomatic	[57]
Cataract					
Congenital (at birth)	Cockayne syndrome	Cachectic dwarfism, microcephaly, cognitive impairment, pigmentary retinopathy, sensorineural deafness	DNA repair studies, genetic testing	Symptomatic	[54]
	Lowe syndrome	Renal Fanconi syndrome, arthropathy, growth impairment	Genetic testing	Symptomatic	[58]
	Peroxisomal biogenesis disorder	Hepatopathy, hypotonia, developmental delay, ataxia, peripheral neuropathy	VLCFA, plasmalogens, genetic testing	Symptomatic	[59]
	Sorbitol dehydrogenase deficiency	Isolated lens SDH deficiency	Genetic testing	Symptomatic	[60]
Neonatal	Galactosaemia	Hepatopathy, renal tubular dysfunction, premature ovarian failure, neurodevelopmental impairment	Neonatal screening, enzymology, genetic testing	Dietary	[61]

(continued)

Table 5.4 (continued)

Ophthalmic finding	Metabolic disease	Extraocular findings	Diagnostic tests	Treatment	References
Infancy	Alpha mannosidosis	Dysmorphic features, frequent infections, hepatosplenomegaly	Urine oligosaccharides, enzymology, genetic testing	BMT, ERT	[52, 53]
	Mitochondrial disease (e.g., FBXL4-mutation)	Multisystem disease	Genetic testing	Symptomatic	[62]
	Sialidosis	Cherry red spot; myoclonus, dysmorphism	Urine sialic acid, enzymology, genetic testing	Symptomatic	[63]
Childhood	Mevalonic aciduria (hyper IgD syndrome)	Periodic fever, inflammatory disorder	Urine mevalonic acid, IgD, genetic testing	Symptomatic	[64]
Later	Cerebrotendinous xanthomatosis (sterol 27-hydroxylase deficiency)	neonatal cholestasis, intellectual dysability, later tendon xanthomata, progressive spasticity, tremor, ataxia	Plasma sterol profile, (cholestanol), genetic testing	Chenodeoxycholic acid	[65]
	Fabry disease	Cornea verticillata, later corneal opacity,acroparaesthesia, hypertrophic cardiomyopathy, progressive renal impairment, stroke	Lyso-Gb3, enzymology, genetic testing	ERT, migalastat, symptomatic therapy	[47]
	Homocystinuria	Marfanoid habitus, thromboembolic events, ectopia lentis, myopia	Homocystine levels, genetic studies	Diet, medication	[47]
	Ornithine aminotransferase deficiency (gyrate atrophy of choroid and retina)	Posterior subcapsular cataract, visual field defect, retinopathy	Plasma amino acids, urine amino acids, genetic testing	Diet, medication (pyridoxine)	[66]
	Tangier disease	Orange coloured tonsils, hepatosplenomegaly, peripheral neuropathy; corneal infiltration in adulthood	Cholesterol, lipoproteins, genetic testing	Low fat diet	[54]

(continued)

Table 5.4 (continued)

Ophthalmic finding	Metabolic disease	Extraocular findings	Diagnostic tests	Treatment	References
	Peroxisomal biogenesis disorder PEX7	Late onset ataxia, cognitive impairment	VLCFA, phytanic acid, genetic testing	Symptomatic, diet	[59, 67]
	Glycogen storage disease type 1 and 3	Hypoglycaemia, cardiomyopathy, hepatomegaly	Enzymology, genetic testing	Diet	[68]
	Vici (defect in autophagy)	Multisystem disorder	Genetic testing	Symptomatic	[69]
Glaucoma	Congenital disorders of glycosylation	Multisystem disease, dysmorphic features, protein losing enteropathy	Transferrin isoelectric focussing, enzymology, genetic testing	Symptomatic (monosaccharides for specific disorders)	[70]
	Leber hereditary optic neuropathy	Multisystem disease	Biochemistry, genetic testing	Symptomatic	[71]
	Mucopolysaccharidoses	Dysmorphic features, hepatosplenomegaly, dysostosis multiplex, developmental delay, short stature	Urine glycosaminoglycans, enzymology, genetic testing	ERT	[49]

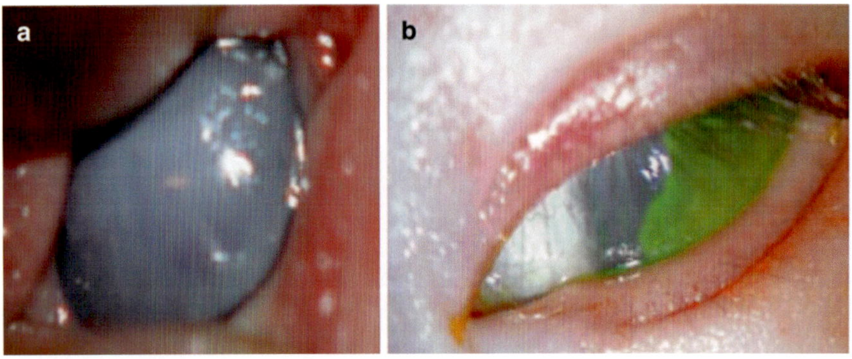

Fig. 5.11 Severe Herpes keratitis in a newborn

Topical glucocorticoids should not be used when active HSV epithelial disease is present. For patients with epithelial herpes simplex keratitis, antiviral therapy with oral or topical acyclovir or valacyclovir can be used. For patients with stromal keratitis, a combination therapy with a topical glucocorticoid and antiviral treatment should be used (Fig. 5.11).

5.3.2 Chlamydia Keratoconjunctivitis

Chronic keratoconjunctivitis caused by recurrent infection with Chlamydia trachomatis, also called trachoma, is the leading infectious cause of blindness worldwide [74]. Trachoma is endemic in remote, resource-limited areas across Africa, Asia, Latin America, the Middle East, and the Pacific Rim [75]. The clinical manifestations of trachoma include two phases: active trachoma (conjunctivitis) occurring largely in young children and cicatricial disease (conjunctival scarring) in adults.

In the initial phase, most patients are asymptomatic, but some may present with chronic conjunctivitis showing redness, discomfort, light sensitivity, and mucopurulent discharge. Repeated episodes of infection cause marked conjunctival inflammation, leading to eyelid scarring and ultimately entropion (inward rolling of the eyelid) and trichiasis (eyelashes rubbing against the eyeball).

The diagnosis of trachoma is clinical and should be suspected in patients with follicular conjunctivitis and/or conjunctival scarring in areas where trachoma is endemic or in areas with risk for trachoma. Treatment of trachoma consists of antibiotic therapy, e.g. azithromycin or tetracycline. In addition, patients with trichiasis need surgery tailored to individual physical findings.

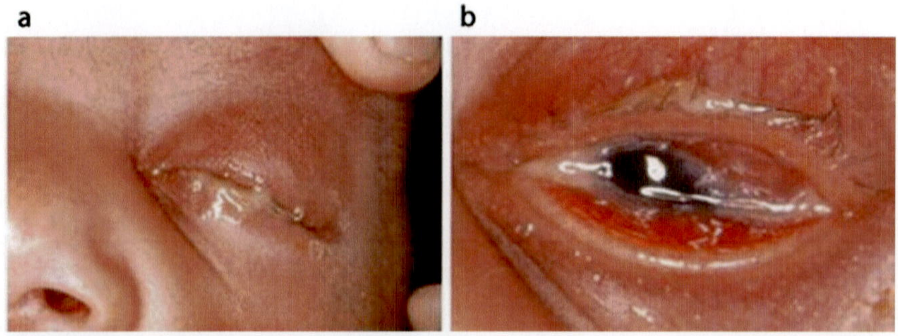

Fig. 5.12 Gonoccocal ophthalmia neonatorum

5.3.3 Gonococcal Conjunctivitis

The eye is the most frequent site of gonococcal infection in the newborn.

The incidence of gonococcal ophthalmia neonatorum has decreased with the use of routine antibiotic prophylaxis and maternal screening for sexually transmitted infections. Also children and adolescents can present with gonococcal conjunctivitis. There is purulent conjunctivitis with profuse exudate and swelling of the eyelids (Fig. 5.12).

Without treatment, the infection can extend from the superficial epithelial layers into the subconjunctival connective tissue and the cornea, leading to ulceration, scarring, and visual impairment. The diagnosis is confirmed by PCR and/or culture of the exudate.

Treatment consists of a single dose of ceftriaxone intravenously or intramuscularly. Alternative antibiotics include cefotaxime, or ceftazidime. Infants with confirmed gonococcal disease should also be evaluated for coinfection with Chlamydia trachomatis.

5.4 Other Diseases Associated with Anomalies of the Anterior Segment

5.4.1 X-chromosomal Ichthyosis

X-linked ichthyosis, also known as steroid sulfatase deficiency, is a recessive, nonsyndromic genetic skin disorder predominantly affects males. Affected patients can produce skin cells but cannot shed them correctly, leading to dry skin that accumulates in the form of polygonal scales. Extracutaneous manifeststions include asymptomatic punctate corneal opacities, cryptorchidism, and cognitive or behavioural symptoms, such as attention-deficit hyperactivity disorder. Diagnosis is based on

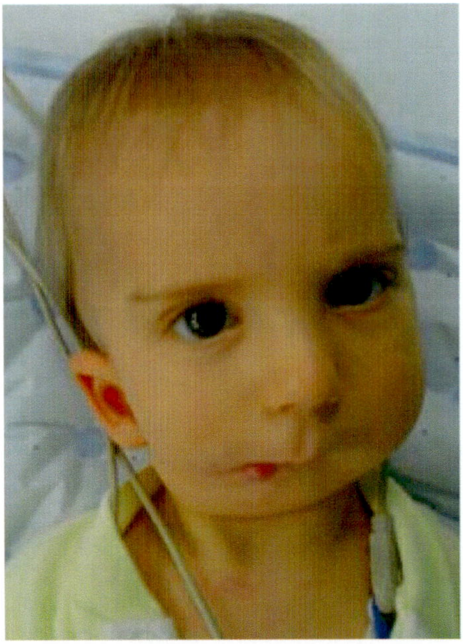

Fig. 5.13 Typical craniofacial findings in Goldenhar-Gorlin syndrome

clinical findings, family history, and genetic testing. Treatment is symptomatic with lubricating bath oils and emollients; systemic retinoids are an option, e.g. during winter, when ichthyosis is more severe [75].

5.4.2 Goldenhar Gorlin Syndrome

Goldenhar-Gorlin syndrome, also called craniofacial macrosomia, hemifacial microsomia, oculo-auriculo-vertebral spectrum, or first and second branchial arch syndrome is an association of anomalies that results from a defect in development of the first and second branchial arches. It is typically sporadic, but autosomal-dominant inheritance has been reported [76, 77]. The defects in craniofacial microsomia involve the orbit, mandible, ear, facial nerve, and soft tissue and are typically unilateral (Fig. 5.13). Patients may also show epibulbar of limbal dermoids (Fig. 5.14). Further ocular manifestations are microphthalmia, lipodermoids, and coloboma [78]. Diagnosis is based on the clinical picture. Surgical corrections of the facial deformity are reserved for severe cases.

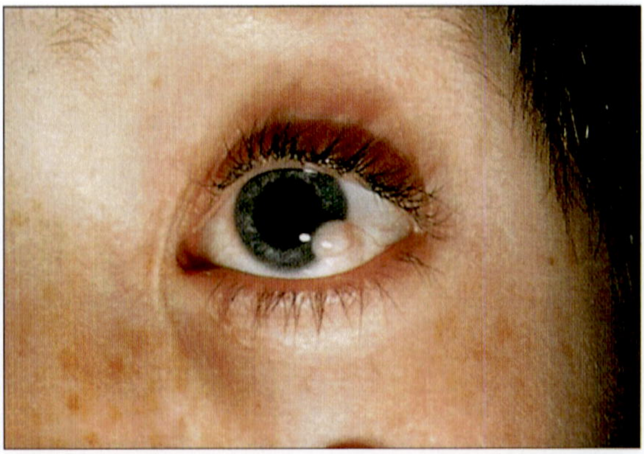

Fig. 5.14 Epibulbar limbal dermoid in a child

References

1. Ito YA, Walter MA. Genomics and anterior segment dysgenesis: a review. Clin Experiment Ophthalmol. 2014;42(1):13–24. https://doi.org/10.1111/ceo.12152.
2. Gabriel H. Trio exome sequencing is highly relevant in prenatal diagnostics. Prenat Diagn. 2022;42(7):845–51. https://doi.org/10.1002/pd.6081. Epub 2021 Dec 27. PMID: 34958143; PMCID: PMC9305182.
3. Rennie CA, Chowdhury S, Khan J, et al. The prevalence and associated features of posterior embryotoxon in the general ophthalmic clinic. Eye. 2005;19(4):396–9. https://doi.org/10.1038/sj.eye.6701508.
4. Reis LM, Semina EV. Genetics of anterior segment dysgenesis disorders. Curr Opin Ophthalmol. 2011;22(5):314–24. https://doi.org/10.1097/ICU.0b013e328349412b.
5. Phillips JC, del Bono EA, Haines JL, et al. A second locus for Rieger syndrome maps to chromosome 13q14. Am J Hum Genet. 1996;59(3):613–9.
6. Idrees F, Vaideanu D, Fraser SG, Sowden JC, Khaw PT. A review of anterior segment dysgeneses. Surv Ophthalmol. 2006;51(3):213–31. https://doi.org/10.1016/j.survophthal.2006.02.006.
7. Levin AV, Enzenauer RE. The eye in pediatric systemic disease. https://doi.org/10.1007/978-3-319-18389-3.
8. Levin AV, Enzenauer RW. The eye in pediatric systemic disease. https://doi.org/10.1007/978-3-319-18389-3.
9. Papanagnu E. Iridocorneal anomalies in infants. https://www.aao.org/education/disease-review/iridocorneal-anomalies-in-infants-2.
10. https://www.omim.org/clinicalSynopsis/602482?highlight=axenfeld%20rieger.
11. Lesnik Oberstein SA, Ruivenkamp CAL, Hennekam RC. Peters plus syndrome. Seattle: University of Washington; 1993.
12. Hanson IM, Fletcher JM, Jordan T, et al. Mutations at the PAX6 locus are found in heterogeneous anterior segment malformations including Peters' anomaly. Nat Genet. 1994;6(2):168–73. https://doi.org/10.1038/ng0294-168).
13. https://www.omim.org/clinicalSynopsis/261540.
14. Sinha G, Patil B, Sihota R, Gupta V, Nayak B, Sharma R, Sharma A, Gupta N. Visual field loss in primary congenital glaucoma. J AAPOS. 2015;19(2):124–9.
15. Chouiter L, Nadifi S. Analysis of CYP1B1 gene mutations in patients with primary congenital glaucoma. J Pediatr Genet. 2017;06(04):205–14. https://doi.org/10.1055/s-0037-1602695.
16. Lim S-H, Tran-Viet K-N, Yanovitch TL, et al. CYP1B1, MYOC, and LTBP2 mutations in primary congenital glaucoma patients in the United States. Am J Ophthalmol. 2013;155(3):508-517.e5. https://doi.org/10.1016/j.ajo.2012.09.012.

17. Faiq M, Sharma R, Dada R, Mohanty K, Saluja D, Dada T. Genetic, biochemical and clinical insights into primary congenital glaucoma. J Curr Glaucoma Pract. 2013;7(2):66–84. https://doi.org/10.5005/jp-journals-10008-1140.
18. Beck AD. Diagnosis and management of pediatric glaucoma. Ophthalmol Clin North Am. 2001;14(3):501.
19. Weiss JS, Rapuano CJ, Seitz B, Busin M, Kivelä TT, Bouheraoua N, Bredrup C, Nischal KK, Chawla H, Borderie V, Kenyon KR, Kim EK, Møller HU, Munier FL, Berger T, Lisch W. IC3D classification of corneal dystrophies-edition 3. Cornea. 2024. https://doi.org/10.1097/ICO.0000000000003420.
20. Aldave AJ, Han J, Frausto RF. Genetics of the corneal endothelial dystrophies: an evidence-based review. Clin Genet. 2013;84(2):109.
21. Cibis G, Gulani AC. Posterior polymorphous corneal dystrophy. StatPearls Publishing; 2019.
22. Ma AS, Grigg JR, Prokudin I, Flaherty M, Bennetts B, Jamieson RV. New mutations in GJA8 expand the phenotype to include total sclerocornea. Clin Genet. 2018;93(1):155–9. https://doi.org/10.1111/cge.13045.
23. Webb TR, Matarin M, Gardner JC, Kelberman D, Hassan H, Ang W, Michaelides M, Ruddle JB, Pennell CE, Yazar S, Khor CC, Aung T, Yogarajah M, Robson AG, Holder GE, Cheetham ME, Traboulsi EI, Moore AT, Sowden JC, Sisodiya SM, Mackey DA, Tuft SJ, Hardcastle AJ. X-linked megalocornea caused by mutations in CHRDL1 identifies an essential role for ventroptin in anterior segment development. Am J Hum Genet. 2012;90(2):247–59. https://doi.org/10.1016/j.ajhg.2011.12.019.
24. Knezević T, Novak-Laus K, Skunca J, Mandić Z. Iridogoniodysgenesis syndrome: a case report. Acta Clin Croat. 2008;47(3):161–4.
25. Mears AJ, Mirzayans F, Gould DB, Pearce WG, Walter MA. Autosomal dominant iridogoniodysgenesis anomaly maps to 6p25. Am J Hum Genet. 1996;59(6):1321.
26. Pearce WG, Mielke BC, Kulak SC, Walter MA. Histopathology and molecular basis of iridogoniodysgenesis syndrome. Ophthalmic Genet. 1999;20(2):83–8.
27. Grieshaber MC, Orgul S, Bruder E, Hadziselimovic F, Flammer J. Congenital iris ectropion and glaucoma associated with intestinal neuronal dysplasia: a manifestation of a neural crest syndrome. Arch Ophthalmol. 2006;124(10):1495. https://doi.org/10.1001/archopht.124.10.1495.
28. Kim WJ, Kim JH, Cho NC. Newly identified paired box 6 mutation of variant familial aniridia: congenital iris ectropion with foveal hypoplasia. Indian J Ophthalmol. 2017;65(1):55–6. https://doi.org/10.4103/0301-4738.202305.
29. Nischal KK. Developmental anomalies of the anterior segment and globe. In: Pediatric ophthalmology and strabismus. New York, NY: Springer New York; 2003. p. 369–90. https://doi.org/10.1007/978-0-387-21753-6_24.
30. Wallang BS et al. Eye (Lond). 2013;27(9):1004–12. https://doi.org/10.1038/eye.2013.130. Epub 2013 Jun 28.
31. Ostermaier K. Down syndrome: clinical features and diagnosis. 2024. Available from: https://www.uptodate.com/contents/down-syndrome-clinical-features-and-diagnosis?search=down%20syndrom&source=search_result&selectedTitle=1%7E150&usage_type=default&display_rank=1.
32. Pauker SP. Clinical manifestations and diagnosis of Ehlers-Danlos syndrome. 2024. Available from: https://www.uptodate.com/contents/clinical-manifestations-and-diagnosis-of-ehlers-danlos-syndromes?search=Ehlers-Danlos%20syndrome&source=search_result&selectedTitle=2%7E141&usage_type=default&display_rank=2.
33. Balasubramanian M. Osteogenesis imperfecta: an overview. 2024. Available from: https://www.uptodate.com/contents/osteogenesis-imperfecta-an-overview?search=Osteogenesis%20imperfecta&source=search_result&selectedTitle=1%7E78&usage_type=default&display_rank=1.
34. Backeljauw P. Clinical manifestations and diagnosis of Turner syndrome. 2024. Available from: https://www.uptodate.com/contents/clinical-manifestations-and-diagnosis-of-turner-syndrome?search=Turner%20syndrome&source=search_result&selectedTitle=1%7E150&usage_type=default&display_rank=1.

35. Wright MJ. Genetics, clinical features, and diagnosis of Marfan syndrome and related disorders. 2024. Available from: https://www.uptodate.com/contents/genetics-clinical-features-and-diagnosis-of-marfan-syndrome-and-related-disorders?search=Marfan%20syndrome&source=search_result&selectedTitle=1%7E150&usage_type=default&display_rank=1.
36. Kashtan CE. Clinical manifestations, diagnosis, and treatment of Alport syndrome (hereditary nephritis). 2024. Available from: https://www.uptodate.com/contents/clinical-manifestations-diagnosis-and-treatment-of-alport-syndrome-hereditary-nephritis?search=Alport%20syndrome&source=search_result&selectedTitle=1%7E46&usage_type=default&display_rank=1.
37. Richmond EJ. Causes of short stature. 2024. Available from: https://www.uptodate.com/contents/causes-of-short-stature?search=Silver-Russell%20syndrome&source=search_result&selectedTitle=1%7E10&usage_type=default&display_rank=1.
38. Silver-Russell Syndrome 1; SRS1. 2024. Available from: https://www.omim.org/entry/180860.
39. Burkitt-Wright EM. Noonan syndrome. 2024. Available from: https://www.uptodate.com/contents/noonan-syndrome?search=Noonan%20syndrome&source=search_result&selectedTitle=1%7E73&usage_type=default&display_rank=1.
40. Progeroid Short Stature with Pigmented Nevi. 2024. Available from: https://www.omim.org/entry/176690?search=Mulvihill-Smith%20syndrome&highlight=%22mulvihill%20smith%22%2C%28syndrome%7Csyndromic%29%2Cmulvihillsmith.
41. Hamrah P. Atopic keratoconjunctivitis. 2024. Available from: https://www.uptodate.com/contents/atopic-keratoconjunctivitis?search=keratoconus%20allergy&source=search_result&selectedTitle=6%7E22&usage_type=default&display_rank=6.
42. Pellegrini M, Bernabei F, Friehmann A, Giannaccare G. Obstructive sleep apnea and keratoconus: a systematic review and meta-analysis. Optom Vis Sci. 2020;97(1):9–14.
43. Najmi H, Mobarki Y, Mania K, Altowairqi B, Basehi M, Mahfouz MS, et al. The correlation between keratoconus and eye rubbing: a review. Int J Ophthalmol. 2019;12(11):1775–81.
44. Davison JE. Eye involvement in inherited metabolic disorders. Ther Adv Ophthalmol. 2020;29(12):2515841420979109. https://doi.org/10.1177/2515841420979109.
45. Search—UpToDate; Home—OMIM; List of Rare Diseases | A-Z Database | NORD.
46. Grompe M. Disorders of tyrosine metabolism. 2024. Available from: https://www.uptodate.com/contents/disorders-of-tyrosine-metabolism?search=Hereditary%20tyrosinaemia%20type%20II&sectionRank=2&usage_type=default&anchor=H12&source=machineLearning&selectedTitle=1%7E150&display_rank=1#H12.
47. Giugliani R. Fabry disease: neurologic manifestations. 2024. Available from: https://www.uptodate.com/contents/fabry-disease-neurologic-manifestations?search=Fabry%20disease%20cornea&source=search_result&selectedTitle=2%7E150&usage_type=default&display_rank=2.
48. Niaudet P. Cystinosis. 2024. Available from: https://www.uptodate.com/contents/cystinosis?search=Cystinosis&source=search_result&selectedTitle=1%7E34&usage_type=default&display_rank=1.
49. Hahn S. Mucopolysaccharidoses: clinical features and diagnosis. 2024. Available from: https://www.uptodate.com/contents/mucopolysaccharidoses-clinical-features-and-diagnosis?search=Mucopolysaccharidosis&source=search_result&selectedTitle=1%7E69&usage_type=default&display_rank=1.
50. I Cell Disease. 2024. Available from: https://rarediseases.org/rare-diseases/i-cell-disease/.
51. Galactosialidosis; GSL. 2024. Available from: https://omim.org/entry/256540?search=galactosialidosis&highlight=galactosialidosi.
52. Alpha-Mannosidosis. 2023. Available from: https://rarediseases.org/rare-diseases/alpha-mannosidosis/.
53. Mannosidosis, ALPHA B, Lysosomal; MANSA. 2024. Available from: https://omim.org/entry/248500?search=Alpha-Mannosidosis&highlight=%22alpha%20mannosidosi%22%20%22alpha%7Cmannosidosi%22%20%28alphamannosidosi%7C%20%29%20alphamannosidosi.

54. Kang PB. Neuropathies associated with hereditary disorders. 2024. Available from: https://www.uptodate.com/contents/neuropathies-associated-with-hereditary-disorders?search=Cockayne%20syndrome&sectionRank=1&usage_type=default&anchor=H26&source=machineLearning&selectedTitle=1%7E31&display_rank=1#H26.
55. Infantile Sialic Acid Storage Disease; ISSD. 2024. Available from: https://omim.org/entry/269920?search=Infantile%20free%20sialic%20acid%20storage%20disease&highlight=acid%20disease%20free%20infantile%20sialic%20storage.
56. Ledithin: Cholesterol Acyltransferase Deficiency. 2024. Available from: https://www.omim.org/entry/245900?search=Lecithin%20cholesterol%20acyltransferase&highlight=acyltransferase%2Ccholesterol%2Clecithin.
57. Sulfite Oxodase Deficiency, Isolated; ISOD. 2024. Available from: https://omim.org/entry/272300.
58. Lowe Oculocerebral Syndrome; OCRL. 2024. Available from: https://www.omim.org/entry/309000.
59. Wanders RJA. Peroxisomal disorders. 2024. Available from: https://www.uptodate.com/contents/peroxisomal-disorders?search=Peroxisomal%20biogenesis%20disorder&source=search_result&selectedTitle=1%7E146&usage_type=default&display_rank=1.
60. Sorbitol Dehydrogenase; SORD. 2024. Available from: https://omim.org/entry/182500?search=%22sorbitol%20dehydrogenase%20deficiency%22&highlight=%22sorbitol%20dehydrogenase%20deficiency%22.
61. Sutton VR. Galactosemia: Clinical features and diagnosis. 2024. Available from: https://www.uptodate.com/contents/galactosemia-clinical-features-and-diagnosis?search=Galactosaemia&source=search_result&selectedTitle=1%7E50&usage_type=default&display_rank=1.
62. F-Box and Leucine-Rich Repeat Protein 4; FBXL4. 2024. Available from: https://omim.org/entry/605654?search=%22fbxl4%20gene%22&highlight=%22fbxl4%20gene%22.
63. Sialidosis. 2016. Available from: https://rarediseases.org/rare-diseases/sialidosis/.
64. Padeh YC. Hyperimmunoglobulin D syndrome: Clinical manifestations and diagnosis. 2024. [Available from: https://www.uptodate.com/contents/hyperimmunoglobulin-d-syndrome-clinical-manifestations-and-diagnosis?search=Mevalonic%20aciduria%20&source=search_result&selectedTitle=1%7E5&usage_type=default&display_rank=1.
65. Waldman AT. Cerebrotendinous xanthomatosis. 2024. Available from: https://www.uptodate.com/contents/cerebrotendinous-xanthomatosis?search=Cerebrotendinous%20xanthomatosis%20&source=search_result&selectedTitle=1%7E13&usage_type=default&display_rank=1.
66. Michaud J, Thompson GN, Brody LC, Steel G, Obie C, Fontaine G, et al. Pyridoxine-responsive gyrate atrophy of the choroid and retina: clinical and biochemical correlates of the mutation A226V. Am J Hum Genet. 1995;56(3):616–22.
67. Peroxisome Biogenesis Factor 7; PEX7. 2024. Available from: https://omim.org/entry/601757?search=Peroxisomal%20biogenesis%20disorder%20PEX7&highlight=biogenesi%2Cdisorder%2Cperoxisomal%2Cpex7.
68. Allegrini D, Autelitano A, Fogagnolo P, De Cilla S, Piozzi E, Mazza M, et al. Lens opacities in glycogenoses type I and III. Can J Ophthalmol. 2015;50(6):480–4.
69. Vici Syndrome; VICIS. 2024. Available from: https://www.omim.org/entry/242840?search=vici%20autophagy&highlight=autophagy%2Cvici.
70. Krasnewich DM. Overview of congenital disorders of glycosylation. 2024. Available from: https://www.uptodate.com/contents/overview-of-congenital-disorders-of-glycosylation?search=Congenital%20disorders%20of%20glycosylation&source=search_result&selectedTitle=1%7E15&usage_type=default&display_rank=1.
71. Lin YH, Wang NK, Yeung L, Lai CC, Chuang LH. Juvenile open-angle Glaucoma associated with Leber's hereditary optic neuropathy: a case report and literature review. BMC Ophthalmol. 2018;18(1):323.
72. Liesegang TJ. Herpes simplex virus epidemiology and ocular importance. Cornea. 2001;20(1):1–13. https://doi.org/10.1097/00003226-200101000-00001.

73. Gonzalez-Gonzalez LA, et al. Clinical features and presentation of infectious scleritis from herpes viruses: a report of 35 cases. Ophthalmology. 2012;119(7):1460–4. https://doi.org/10.1016/j.ophtha.2012.01.033.
74. Taylor HR. Trachoma: a blinding scourge from the bronze age to the twenty-first century. Melbourne: Centre for Eye Research Australia; 2008.
75. https://www.orpha.net/consor/cgi-bin/Disease_Search.php?lng=EN&data_id=42.
76. Ala-Mello S, et al. Further evidence for a relationship between the 5p15 chromosome region and the oculoauriculovertebral anomaly. Am J Med Genet A. 2008;146A(19):2490–4. https://doi.org/10.1002/ajmg.a.32479.
77. Skarzyński H, et al. Treatment of otological features of the oculoauriculovertebral dysplasia (Goldenhar syndrome). Int J Pediatr Otorhinolaryngol. 2009;73(7):915–21. https://doi.org/10.1016/j.ijporl.2009.01.015.
78. https://eyewiki.aao.org/Goldenhar_Syndrome.
79. World Health Organization. WHO alliance for the global elimination of trachoma by 2020: progress report on elimination of trachoma, 2020. https://reliefweb.int/sites/reliefweb.int/files/resources/WER9631-eng-fre.pdf.
80. https://www.uptodate.com/contents/syndromes-with-craniofacial-abnormalities?search=goldenhar&source=search_result&selectedTitle=1~22&usage_type=default&display_rank=1#H3.
81. Kohut TJ. Alagille syndrome. 2024. Available from: https://www.uptodate.com/contents/alagille-syndrome?search=alagille&source=search_result&selectedTitle=1~30&usage_type=default&display_rank=1.
82. Reis LM, Semina EV. Genetics of anterior segment dysgenesis disorders. Curr Opin Ophthalmol. 2011;22(5):314–24.

Index

I. Broekaert et al., *Infantile Anterior Segment Disorders*,
https://doi.org/10.1007/978-3-031-68558-3